PATHOLOGY
OF THE
PROSTATE

CONTEMPORARY ISSUES IN SURGICAL PATHOLOGY VOLUME 15

SERIES EDITOR

Lawrence M. Roth, M.D.

Professor of Pathology
Director, Division of Surgical Pathology
Indiana University School of Medicine
Indianapolis, Indiana

Previously published

PATHOLOGY
OF THE
PROSTATE

Edited by

David G. Bostwick, M.D.

Associate Clinical Professor
Department of Pathology
University of Maryland School of Medicine
Chairman
Department of Pathology
Mercy Medical Center
Baltimore, Maryland

Churchill Livingstone
New York, Edinburgh, London, Melbourne

Library of Congress Cataloging-in-Publication Data

Pathology of the prostate / edited by David G. Bostwick.
      p. cm.—(Contemporary issues in surgical pathology ; v. 15)
   Includes bibliographical references.
   ISBN 0–443–08655–9
    1. Prostate—Biopsy. 2. Prostate—Tumors—Diagnosis.
3. Pathology, Surgical. I. Bostwick, David G. II. Series.
   [DNLM: 1. Pathology, Surgical. 2. Prostate—pathology.
3. Prostatic Neoplasms—diagnosis. 4. Prostatic Neoplasms—
pathology. W1 CO769MS v. 15 / WJ 752 P297]
RC280.P7P37 1990
616.99′26307′58—dc20
DNLM/DLC   89–71192
for Library of Congress   CIP

Distributed in the United Kingdom by Churchill Livingstone, Robert Stevenson
House, 1–3 Baxter's Place, Leith Walk, Edinburgh EH1 3AF, and by associated
companies, branches, and representatives throughout the world.

Accurate indications, adverse reactions, and dosage schedules for drugs are provided
in this book, but it is possible that they may change. The reader is urged to review
the package information data of the manufacturers of the medications mentioned.

The Publishers have made every effort to trace the copyright holders for borrowed
material. If they have inadvertently overlooked any, they will be pleased to make
the necessary arrangements at the first opportunity.

Acquisitions Editor: *Robert A. Hurley*
Copy Editor: *Kathleen P. Lyons*
Production Supervisor: *Christina Hippeli*

Printed in the United States of America

First published in 1990

In memory of James G. Timbers (1918–1988)

Contributors

Alberto G. Ayala, M.D.
Professor, Deputy Chairman, and Director, Surgical Pathology Section, Department of Pathology, The University of Texas Medical School at Houston, M. D. Anderson Cancer Center, Houston, Texas

David G. Bostwick, M.D.
Associate Clinical Professor, Department of Pathology, University of Maryland School of Medicine; Chairman, Department of Pathology, Mercy Medical Center, Baltimore, Maryland

Michael K. Brawer, M.D.
Assistant Professor, Department of Urology, University of Washington School of Medicine; Chief, Section of Urology, Veterans Administration Medical Center, Seattle, Washington

John N. Eble, M.D.
Associate Professor, Departments of Pathology and Experimental Oncology, Indiana University School of Medicine; Chief, Department of Pathology, Richard L. Roudebush Veterans Administration Medical Center, Indianapolis, Indiana

Jonathan I. Epstein, M.D.
Assistant Professor, Departments of Pathology and Urology, Johns Hopkins University School of Medicine, Baltimore, Maryland

Cirilo F. Galang, M.D.
Medical Director, Aspiration Biopsy Laboratory, Inc.; Director, Department of Laboratory Medicine, Saint Vincent Charity Hospital and Health Center, Cleveland, Ohio

Donald F. Gleason, M.D., Ph.D.
Clinical Assistant Professor Emeritus, Department of Laboratory Medicine and Pathology, University of Minnesota Medical School—Minneapolis; Staff Pathologist, Fairview Hospital, Minneapolis, Minnesota (retired)

R. Warren J. Hartwick, M.D., F.R.C.P.(C)
Staff Pathologist, Mount Sinai Hospital; Lecturer, Department of Pathology, University of Toronto Faculty of Medicine, Toronto, Ontario, Canada

Paul W. Johenning, M.D.

Consulting Urologist, Aspiration Biopsy Laboratory, Inc.; Chief of Urology, Department of Surgery, Saint Vincent Charity Hospital and Health Center, Cleveland, Ohio

Ileana Lopez-Plaza, M.D.

Senior Resident, Department of Pathology, University of Maryland School of Medicine, Baltimore, Maryland

John A. Maksem, M.D.

Chief, Department of Pathology, Mercy Hospital Medical Center, Des Moines, Iowa; Former Medical Director, Aspiration Biopsy Laboratory, Inc., Cleveland, Ohio

John E. McNeal, M.D.

Clinical Assistant Professor, Division of Urology, Department of Surgery, Stanford University Medical Center, Stanford University School of Medicine, Stanford, California

Nelson G. Ordóñez, M.D.

Professor, and Director, Immunocytochemistry Section, Department of Pathology, The University of Texas Medical School at Houston, M. D. Anderson Cancer Center, Houston, Texas

Chanho H. Park, M.D.

Associate Medical Director, Aspiration Biopsy Laboratory, Inc.; Associate Pathologist, Department of Laboratory Medicine, Saint Vincent Charity Hospital and Health Center, Cleveland, Ohio

Jae Y. Ro, M.D., Ph.D.

Associate Professor, Department of Pathology, The University of Texas Medical School at Houston, M. D. Anderson Cancer Center, Houston, Texas

John R. Srigley, M.D.

Assistant Professor, Department of Pathology, University of Toronto Faculty of Medicine; Director of Surgical Pathology, Department of Pathology, Sunnybrook Medical Centre, Toronto, Ontario, Canada

Myron Tannenbaum, M.D., Ph.D.

Professor, Departments of Pathology and Urology, Mount Sinai School of Medicine of the City University of New York, New York, New York; Chief, Department of Surgical Pathology and Cytopathology, Bronx Veterans Administration Hospital and Research Center, Bronx, New York

Bernard Têtu, M.D.

Assistant Professor, Department of Pathology, Laval University Faculty of Medicine; Staff Pathologist, Department of Pathology, L'Hôtel-Dieu de Québec; Québec City, Québec, Canada

Preface

This volume of the *Contemporary Issues in Surgical Pathology* series is concerned with diagnostic problems encountered in prostatic pathology and is directed primarily at the practicing surgical pathologist. The book also serves to acquaint urologists and oncologists with the morphologic decision-making process and diagnostic tools used in interpreting prostatic specimens.

Each chapter is designed to give comprehensive coverage to its topic, with emphasis on recent developments, controversial issues, new diagnostic techniques, and differential diagnosis. Many of the topics presented have not yet received sufficient consideration in available textbooks. The book is organized so that it may be read in continuity or used as a reference for solving diagnostic dilemmas. There are some differences of opinion and terminology between authors, an unavoidable although frequently enlightening characteristic of a multiauthored text; also, various aspects of specific lesions may be discussed in several chapters. Cited references are as current as possible, and most have been deliberately selected from the last ten years.

I am greatly indebted to Dr. Lawrence Roth for inviting me to contribute a monograph to his series; to Linda Panzarella of Churchill Livingstone for her attention to detail; to my colleagues, Drs. Victor Fazekas and Glenn Jockle, for their support and encouragement; to Margaret Huesman, for editorial assistance; to Dr. Donald Gleason for emerging from retirement to contribute additional thoughts on grading of prostatic carcinoma; and to all the authors, whose cooperation has been outstanding.

David G. Bostwick, M.D.

Contents

1

Anatomy of the Prostate:
Implications for Disease

John E. McNeal and David G. Bostwick

The human prostate is a composite organ made up of several glandular and nonglandular elements tightly fused together within a common capsule. Each of these elements has a characteristic and unique predisposition to disease. In this chapter, the current understanding of the anatomy of the adult prostate is presented. Also discussed are anatomic considerations in tissue sampling and imaging, and implications for disease processes, including atrophy, nodular hyperplasia, prostatitis, and carcinoma.

ANATOMIC LANDMARKS

PROSTATIC URETHRA

The urethra is a key anatomic reference point for the study of the prostate.[1] A single sharp 35-degree bend in the middle of the prostatic urethra creates proximal and distal segments of approximately equal length,[2] and each segment has significantly different anatomic relationships (Fig. 1-1).

The verumontanum is part of the distal urethral segment. It bulges from the posterior wall of the urethra at the point of angulation, and tapers distally to form the crista urethralis. The utricle is a müllerian (paramesonephric) remnant that appears as a small 0.5 cm-long epithelium-lined cul-de-sac extending proximally from the verumontanum. The ducts of more than 90 percent of the glandular prostate empty into the distal prostatic urethra together with the ejaculatory ducts. Periurethral glands are scattered

along the length of the proximal urethral segment, consisting of tiny ducts and abortive acinar systems lined by simple cuboidal to columnar epithelium.

Transitional epithelium lines the prostatic urethra and extends for a variable distance into the large prostatic ducts. This epithelium does not mature toward luminal umbrella cells, distinguishing it histologically from bladder epithelium and female urethral epithelium; instead, the surface is lined by a single layer of columnar secretory cells (Fig. 1-2) that produces prostatic acid phosphatase and prostate specific antigen.[3]

The entire length of the prostatic urethra is surrounded by sphincteric muscle. The preprostatic sphincter (Figs. 1-1 and 1-3) is a sleeve of smooth muscle fibers surrounding the proximal urethral segment. It is thought to function during ejaculation to prevent retrograde flow of seminal fluid, and to maintain closure of the proximal prostatic urethra.[2, 4] Posterior to the urethra, the preprostatic sphincter is compact, but laterally, its fibers split and mingle with the small ducts and acini of the medial transition zone.[5] This sphincter is incomplete anteriorly, with some fibers terminating within the anterior fibromuscular stroma. Distal to the base of the verumontanum, there is a striated sphincter of small compactly arranged striated muscle fibers. This sphincter is incomplete posteriorly where its fibers anchor into the anterior margin of the peripheral zone, and it is continuous with the external urethral sphincter distal to the apex of the prostate.

The anterior fibromuscular stroma (Figs.

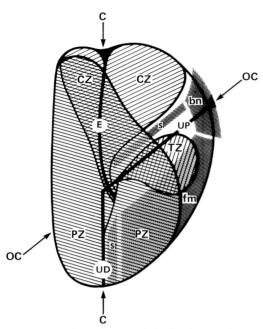

Fig. 1-1. Sagittal diagram of the distal prostatic urethral segment (*UD*), proximal urethral segment (*UP*), and ejaculatory ducts (*E*) showing their relationships to a sagittal section of the anteromedial nonglandular tissues [bladder neck (*bn*), anterior fibromuscular stroma (*fm*), preprostatic sphincter (*s*), distal striated sphincter (*s*)]. These structures are shown in relation to a three-dimensional representation of the glandular prostate [central zone (*CZ*), peripheral zone (*PZ*), transitional zone (*TZ*)]. The coronal plane (*C*) of Figure 1-4 and the oblique coronal plane (*OC*) of Figure 1-3 are indicated by arrows.

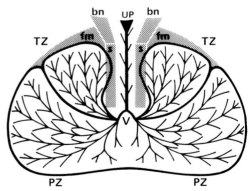

Fig. 1-2. Epithelial lining of the main peripheral zone duct near the urethra is identical to the lining of the prostatic urethra. Multilayered transitional epithelium is surmounted by a single layer of luminal secretory cells.

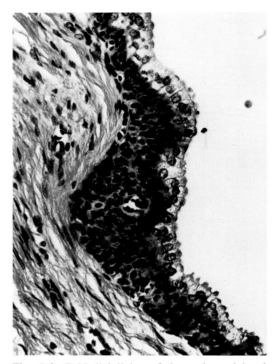

Fig. 1-3. Oblique coronal section diagram of the prostate showing location of the peripheral zone (*PZ*) and transition zone (*TZ*) in relation to the proximal urethral segment (*UP*), verumontanum (*V*), preprostatic sphincter (*s*), bladder neck (*bn*), and periurethral region with periurethral glands. The branching pattern of the prostatic ducts is indicated; medial transition zone ducts penetrate into the sphincter.

1-1 and 1-3) is an apron of tissue that extends downward from the bladder neck over the anteromedial surface of the prostate, narrowing to join the urethra at the prostatic apex.[6] Its lateral margins blend with the capsule, where it covers the border of the peripheral zone. The deep surface is in contact with the preprostatic sphincter and transition zone proximally and with the striated sphincter distally. This stroma is composed of large compact bundles of smooth muscle cells, which are similar to those of the bladder neck, and blend with them proximally. These smooth muscle fibers are more randomly oriented than those in the bladder neck, and are separated in some areas by bands of fibrous connective tissue.

PROSTATIC ZONES

The prostate contains three major glandular regions that differ histologically and biologically: the peripheral zone, the central zone, and the transition zone (Table 1-1).[6]

The central zone (Figs. 1-1 and 1-4) comprises approximately 25 percent of the volume of the glandular prostate. Its ducts exit from the convexity of the verumontanum adjacent to the ejaculatory duct orifices. The ducts branch directly toward the base of the prostate along the course of the ejaculatory ducts, fanning out mainly in the coronal plane to form a somewhat flattened conical structure. The base of the cone comprises almost the entire base of the prostate. The most lateral central zone ducts run parallel to the proximal peripheral zone ducts, separated by a narrow band of stroma.

The transition zone (Figs. 1-1 and 1-3) contains approximately 5 to 10 percent of the volume of glandular prostate. It consists of two independent small lobes whose ducts exit from the posterolateral wall of the urethra just proximal to the point of urethral angulation.

The peripheral zone (Figs. 1-1, 1-3 and 1-

Table 1-1. Glandular Zones of the Human Prostate: Histologic Features

	Central Zone	Transition Zone	Peripheral Zone
Volume of normal prostates	25%	5%	70%
Anatomic landmarks			
Intraprostatic relationships	Ejaculatory ducts	Surrounds proximal prostatic urethra	Distal prostatic urethra
Adjacent structures	Seminal vesicles	Bladder neck	Rectum
Urethral orifices of ducts	Verumontanum, adjacent to ejaculatory ducts	Posterolateral wall of proximal prostatic urethra at its distal end	Posterolateral wall of distal prostatic urethra
Distinctive histologic features			
Epithelium	Complex, large polygonal glands with intraluminal ridges	Simple, small rounded glands	Simple, small rounded glands
Stroma	Compact	Compact	Loose
Biochemical differences			
Production of pepsinogen II	Yes	No	No
Production of tissue plasminogen activator	Yes	No	No
Lectin binding patterns[a]			
LCA,Con-A,WGA, PNS-N,RCA-I UEA-1,S-WGA,	Yes	—	Yes
PNA,	Yes	—	No
DBA,SBA,BS-I	No	—	No
Proposed embryonic origin	Wolffian duct	Urogenital sinus	Urogenital sinus

[a] LCA, lens culinaris; Con A, concanavalia ensiformis; WGA, triticum vulgaris (wheat germ); PNA-N, arachis hypogoa (peanut) with neuraminidase predigestion; RCA-I, ricinus communis; UEA-I, ulex europaeus; S-WGA, succinyl-WGA; PNA, arachis hypogea (peanut); DBA, dolichus biflorus; SBA, glycine max (soybean); BS-I, bandeirea simplicifolia; —, not evaluated.

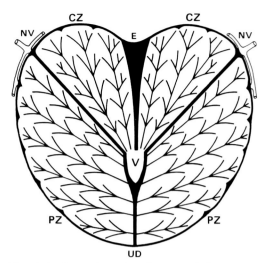

Fig. 1-4. Coronal section diagram of the prostate showing the location of the central zone (*CZ*) and peripheral zone (*PZ*) in relation to the distal urethral segment (*UD*), verumontanum (*V*), and ejaculatory ducts (*E*). The branching pattern of the prostatic ducts is indicated; subsidiary ducts provide uniform density of acini along the entire main duct course. The neurovascular bundle (*NV*) is located at the junction between the central zone and the peripheral zone.

4) consists of approximately 70 percent of the volume of the glandular prostate. Its ducts exit from the posterolateral recesses of the urethral wall as a double row, extending from the base of the verumontanum to the prostatic apex. The ducts course mainly laterally in the coronal plane, with major branches that curve anteriorly and minor branches that curve posteriorly.

Within each zone of the prostate, ducts and acini are morphologically similar (Figs. 1-5 and 1-6), apparently functioning as distensible secretory reservoirs.[1] Both ducts and acini are lined by columnar secretory cells (Figs. 1-7 to 1-9) that show uniform immunohistochemical staining for prostatic acid phosphatase and prostate-specific antigen.

The main ducts of the prostate originate at the urethra and terminate near the capsule, except for the transition zone ducts, which terminate at the anterior fibromuscular stroma[5, 7] (Figs. 1-1 and 1-3). In each zone, acini are

distributed uniformly along the course of the main ducts, except for the few millimeters nearest the urethra.[1] Because ducts and acini within each zone have similar caliber, spacing and histologic appearance, they cannot be reliably distinguished microscopically except in sections cut along the long axis of ducts. Hence, abnormalities of architectural pattern are identified mainly by deviations from normal size and spacing of glandular units. Within the central zone, subsidiary ducts and acini are clustered into lobules around central ducts, and both appear polygonal in contour. Corrugations of the wall form prominent intraluminal ridges, providing for expansion as secretory reservoirs (Fig. 1-5). Transition zone and peripheral zone ducts and acini have simple round contours with undulations of the epithelial borders[7, 8] (Fig. 1-6).

Significant differences are noted in stromal density and pattern between each of the zones. In the central zone, the stroma is composed of compact smooth muscle fibers (Fig. 1-7).

In the peripheral zone, the stroma is loosely woven with randomly arranged muscle bundles (Fig. 1-8). There is an abrupt contrast in stromal morphology marking the boundary between the central zone and peripheral zone. Transition zone stroma is composed of compact interlacing smooth muscle bundles (Fig. 1-9) that blend with the adjacent stroma of the preprostatic sphincter and anterior fibromuscular stroma. The boundary between the transition zone and the peripheral zone is usually marked by an abrupt change in stromal pattern (Fig. 1-10). The ratio of epithelium to stroma is higher in the central zone than in the transition zone and peripheral zone. Stromal distinctions are less evident in older prostates and may be obliterated by disease.

Biochemical differences have been demonstrated in the different zones of the prostate. Pepsinogen II and tissue plasminogen activator, two of the four main proteolytic enzymes of the prostate, are produced only by the central zone.[9, 10] Lectin binding patterns, reflecting selective binding to specific cellular glycoconjugates, are almost identical in the central zone and seminal vesicles, but differ from the periph-

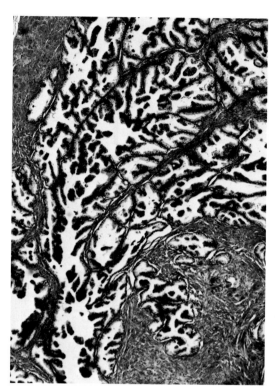

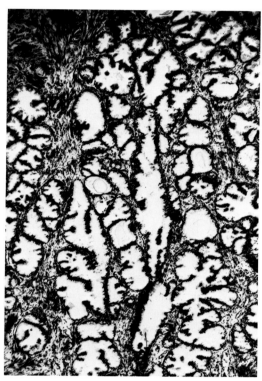

Fig. 1-5. Subsidiary duct and acini in the central zone form a compact lobule with flattened gland borders and prominent intraluminal ridges.

Fig. 1-6. Subsidiary duct and branches in the peripheral zone terminating in small, rounded acini with undulating borders. Ducts and acini have similar caliber and histologic appearance.

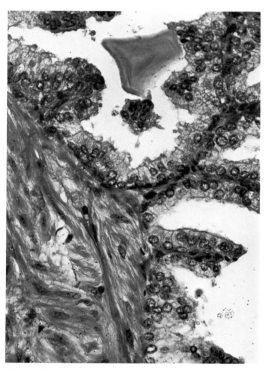

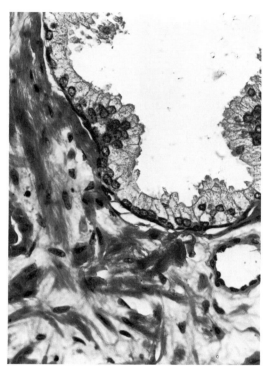

Fig. 1-7. Central zone acinus at the lobule border surrounded by compact muscular stroma. Secretory cells are irregularly arranged with large nuclei at different levels and granular, variably dark cytoplasm. Basal cells are visible.

Fig. 1-8. Peripheral zone acinus set in loosely woven fibromuscular stroma. Secretary cells are more regular than in the central zone, with small basal nuclei and pale cytoplasm. Basal cells are visible.

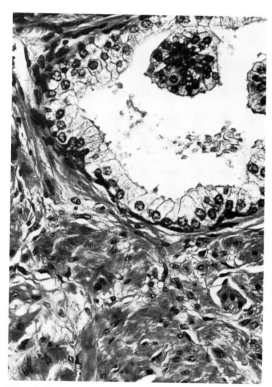

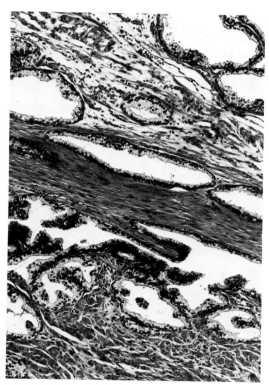

Fig. 1-9. Transition zone acinus set in a compact stroma composed of interlacing, coarse, smooth muscle bundles. Acinar histology is identical to that of the peripheral zone. Basal cells are visible.

Fig. 1-10. The border between the peripheral zone (*above*) and the transition zone shows contrast in stromal texture and a band of smooth muscle at the zone boundary. Glandular histology is similar between zones.

eral zone in binding of 3 of 10 lectins (see Table 1-1).[11]

Morphologic and biologic differences between the zones suggest that the central zone is of wolffian duct origin, similar to the seminal vesicles, and the other zones are of urogenital sinus origin.[6]

CAPSULE

The capsule of the prostate consists of an inner layer of smooth muscle and an outer covering of collagen (Fig. 1-11). There is marked variability in the relative amounts of muscle and fibrous tissue from area to area. As a result, the prostatic capsule cannot be regarded as a well-defined anatomic structure with constant features.[1, 12]

The capsule covers most of the external surface of the prostate. Terminal acini of the central zone and peripheral zone abut on the capsule, and terminal acini of the transition zone abut on the anterior fibromuscular stroma. At the apex of the prostate, there is a defect in the capsule anteriorly and anterolaterally; at this point, there is an admixture of glandular tissue and sphincteric striated muscle. Consequently, in this area the exact boundaries of the prostate are not precisely defined, and, when carcinoma is present at the apex of the prostate, it may be difficult to determine whether it has invaded outside the gland.[13] Also, there is no capsule at the bladder neck and at the site where the ejaculatory ducts enter the prostate, creating similar difficulty in assessing the extent of invasion when carcinoma is present.

NERVE SUPPLY

The prostate is supplied by the prostatic plexus. Paired neurovascular bundles reach the lateral borders of the prostate near the base, only a short distance anterior to the rectal surface.[14] This site overlies the boundary between the central zone and the peripheral zone.[6]

Autonomic ganglia are clustered at the surface of the capsule in the region of the neurovascular bundles (Fig. 1-11). Small nerve trunks originating at this site arborize over the surface of the prostate, giving rise to smaller branches that penetrate through the capsule.[14] Within the prostatic parenchyma, small nerve twigs are in intimate contact with walls of ducts and acini.[15, 16] Infrequently, benign glands lie within the perineural spaces in prostates that contain no foci of carcinoma.[17] Consequently, caution is advised in the interpretation of perineural space invasion as an absolute criterion for the diagnosis of cancer.

BLOOD SUPPLY

The prostate is supplied by one of the branches of the internal iliac artery. Arterial branches ramify within the capsule, and penetrate to extend directly inward toward the distal prostatic urethra between adjacent main ducts of the central and peripheral zones.[18, 19] A major arterial branch enters the prostate at each side of the bladder neck and runs toward the verumontanum parallel to the course of the proximal prostatic urethra. This branch supplies the periurethral region and the medial transition zone. Transurethral resection (TUR) usually obliterates this arterial branch and all of the tissue supplied by it.[19]

Prostatic veins drain directly into the prostatic plexus, and an extensive arborization is present in the capsule. This venous drainage eventually empties into the internal iliac vein.

LYMPHATIC DRAINAGE

Lymphatics from the prostate drain mainly into the internal iliac nodes, although some drain to the external iliac and sacral lymph nodes.

SEMINAL VESICLES

The seminal vesicles consist of two elongated sacs that are superolateral to the central zone of the prostate. They are attached to the posterior wall of the bladder, embedded in a dense sheath of fibrous connective tissue and smooth muscle. The seminal vesicles are separated from the rectum by the rectovesicle pouch and septum.

The coiled glands of the seminal vesicle merge and then join with the corresponding ductus deferens to form the ejaculatory duct. This duct penetrates the base of the prostate, and traverses the long axis of the central zone before entering the prostatic urethra at the verumontanum.

ANATOMY AND IMPLICATIONS FOR DISEASE

TISSUE SAMPLING TECHNIQUES

The regions of the prostate sampled by needle biopsy and by TUR tend to be quite different (Table 1-2). Most needle-biopsy specimens consist of tissue from the peripheral zone, seldom including the central zone or the anterior portion of the transition zone. TUR specimens consist of tissue from the transition zone, urethra, periurethral area, bladder neck, and anterior fibromuscular stroma. We have shown in post-TUR radical prostatectomy specimens that the resection does not usually include tissue from the central or peripheral zones, and that not all of the transition zone is removed.[1] In those cases in which central or peripheral zone fragments are obtained by TUR, there may also be portions of ejaculatory duct, intraprostatic vas deferens, and seminal vesicle.

Well-differentiated carcinoma found incidentally in TUR chips usually represents cancer that has arisen in the transition zone.[20] These tumors are frequently small and may be completely resected by TUR. Poorly differentiated carcinoma in TUR chips usually represents part of a larger tumor that has invaded the transition zone after arising in the peripheral zone. It is important to identify invasion of bladder neck fragments by carcinoma; such a finding usually indicates a large extensive tumor, and, if radical prostatectomy is performed, there may be residual tumor at the bladder neck margin.[1]

ATROPHY

Focal atrophy in the prostate is thought to be the consequence of previous inflammation rather than a normal aging phenomenon[6, 7] (Figs. 1-12 and 1-13). The number and extent of atrophic foci are greater in older men, but their appearance is identical to that of isolated foci found as early as 30 years of age. The histologic features of atrophy are similar to those produced by chronic prostatitis.

Postinflammatory atrophy and cystic atrophy (Fig. 1-14) are common lesions. They are usually present in the peripheral zone, where their distribution is segmental along the ramifications of the duct branches.[4, 6, 7] This segmental distribution is probably due to ductal obstruction, but obstruction is not typically demonstrable. Atrophic and cystically dilated glands may be present in the transition zone, particularly in the stroma adjacent to foci of nodular hyperplasia. Atrophy is infrequent in the central zone.

NODULAR HYPERPLASIA

The transition zone and periurethral region are the exclusive sites of origin of nodular hyperplasia (Table 1-2).[5, 7, 22] These areas are anatomically displaced anteriorly away from the rest of the prostate because of the angulation of the urethra at its midpoint. This anatomic displacement allows foci of nodular hyperplasia to be removed surgically without disturbing the structure and function of the rest of the prostate. Nodular hyperplasia is discussed in Chapter 3.

PROSTATITIS

The peripheral zone is the most susceptible region to inflammation and prostatitis (Table 1-2).[6] The transition zone is less likely to be inflamed, but may exhibit prostatic infarcts with secondary inflammation, usually in the setting of nodular hyperplasia. Postsurgical granulomatous prostatitis may also involve the transition zone. The central zone appears resistant to inflammation.

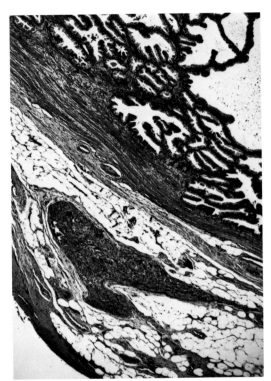

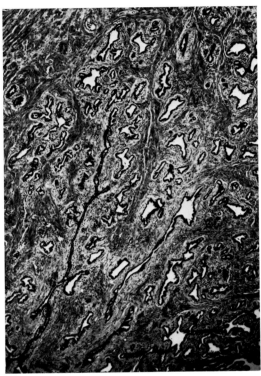

Fig. 1-11. Prostatic capsule, as measured from the glandular border to fat, shows a stepwise twofold increase in thickness from lower right to upper left. The thickest area shows layers of pale collagen between smooth muscle bands in addition to the surface collagen layer. Autonomic ganglion in periprostatic fat is 0.3 mm from the capsule surface.

Fig. 1-12. Focus of postinflammatory atrophy in the peripheral zone. Duct-acinar architecture is apparent but distorted by marked gland shrinkage, with reduced luminal area and perigland fibrosis.

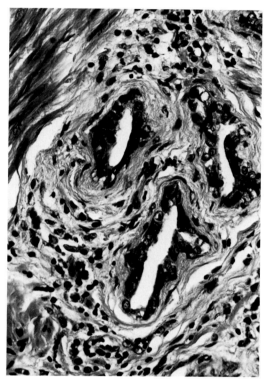

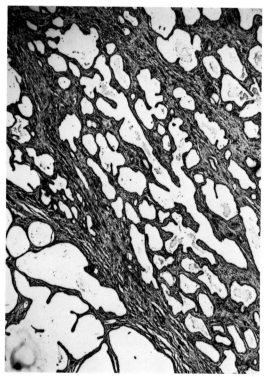

Fig. 1-13. Tiny distorted glands of postinflammatory atrophy. Irregular contour and large nuclei mimic carcinoma, but cytoplasm is scant, and there are periglandular collagenous rings. A few inflammatory cells are present.

Fig. 1-14. Advanced diffuse atrophy of aging in the peripheral zone with ducts and acini of normal caliber and markedly flattened epithelium. A focus of cystic atrophy is seen at the lower left.

Table 1-2. Glandular Zones of the Prostate: Implications for Disease

	Central Zone	Transition Zone	Peripheral Zone
Tissue sampling techniques			
Transurethral resection	Poor	Good	Poor
Needle biopsy	Variable	Poor	Good
Involvement with pathologic processes			
Atrophy	Infrequent	Variable	Frequent
Nodular hyperplasia	Rare	Frequent	Rare
Prostatitis	Infrequent	Variable	Frequent
Carcinoma (% of prostate cancers)	Infrequent (5%)	Frequent (25%)	Frequent (70%)

CARCINOMA

The majority (70 percent) of prostatic carcinomas originate in the peripheral zone (Table 1-2).[21, 23] Although the transition zone accounts for only 25 percent of carcinomas, this frequency is disproportionately high, considering that the transition zone comprises only 5 to 10 percent of the volume of the normal prostate. This increased frequency may be related to the variable expansion of transition zone volume produced by nodular hyperplasia and diffuse enlargement in older men. The susceptibility of the transition zone to cancer is probably comparable to that of the peripheral zone but the marked variability in transition zone size with aging precludes precise estimation. The central zone accounts for about 5 percent of carcinomas, a disproportionately low frequency considering its large volume and increased ratio of epithelium to stroma. Because of this relative resistance to malignant transformation in the central zone, small carcinomas are seldom located at the base of the prostate.[21, 23]

Most carcinomas detected by TUR are transition zone cancers.[20, 21] This zone is the only region sampled by TUR, and the transition zone boundary appears somewhat resistant to invasion by peripheral zone carcinomas.

Transition zone cancers are not usually palpable rectally, except when they are large. Nonpalpable cancers detected in TUR specimens may have a benign prognosis, and these stage A tumors have been considered by some to be a biologically distinctive group. It is now apparent that this clinical presentation (stage A) is simply a reflection of site of origin. Interestingly, TUR appears more sensitive in detecting small transition zone cancers than rectal palpation in detecting small peripheral zone cancers. Since it has been shown that small volume cancers in the prostate have the least aggressive behavior,[3] this probably accounts for the statistically favorable prognosis of stage A carcinoma.

Some transition zone cancers are large, poorly differentiated and clinically aggressive. These tumors usually show more than 5 percent involvement of TUR chips by cancer (stage A2). Also, large peripheral zone cancers may contribute small amounts of typically high-grade cancer to TUR specimens, and these are considered to be stage A2 tumors on the basis of histologic grade.

The histologic classification of stage A2 cancers following TUR is not highly reliable for identifying stage A cancers, which are potentially aggressive.[20] Furthermore, repeat TUR may miss residual cancer, because transition zone carcinomas often grow toward the apex, an area that is not sampled by TUR. The best available technique for evaluation of volume and grade in cancers detected by TUR is probably multiple ultrasound-guided needle biopsies, including biopsies near the apex and biopsies directed anteriorly, lateral to the TUR defect.

IMAGING TECHNIQUES

Imaging techniques should only be applied to the prostate by those understanding the zonal anatomy of the prostate and the predisposition of the different zones to disease. The cystoscopist is unlikely to directly visualize carcinoma within the urethral lumen, except for large infiltrating tumors, transitional cell carcinoma of the urethra, and rare variants such as prostatic adenocarcinoma with endometrioid features.[24]

Ultrasonographers and those employing computed tomography involving the prostate should pay particular attention to the peripheral zone in the search for carcinoma.[25] Comparison of ultrasound-guided biopsy with histologic findings at prostatectomy have revealed numerous hypoechoic lesions mimicking carcinoma, including nodular hyperplasia and infarction.[25] Anatomic structures that appeared hypoechoic by ultrasound included the anterior fibromuscular stroma, ejaculatory ducts, and patulous urethra following TUR. Carcinoma was found most frequently in the peripheral zone, but was not always hypoechoic.

Anatomic studies of the prostate suggest that the central zone is a separate glandular organ within the prostate capsule, with unique morphologic features and relative resistance to inflammation, hyperplasia, and carcinoma.[1]

TREATMENT

New therapeutic techniques should pay heed to anatomic considerations. For instance, nerve-sparing radical prostatectomy allows preservation of erectile function by dissection of the lateral nerve plexus from the neurovascular bundle to the apex away from the capsule.[26, 27] Because the nerve trunks are extremely close to the capsular surface, this operative modification leaves behind a layer of extracapsular fibrofatty tissue that was removed in the traditional radical prostatectomy. This may increase the risk of carcinoma perforating though the capsule laterally at the excision margin. However, the magnitude of this risk has not been determined.[26]

Future studies that evaluate all aspects of tumor morphology, including anatomic considerations, may offer new insights for the diagnosis and treatment of prostatic carcinoma.

REFERENCES

1. McNeal JE: Normal histology of the prostate. Am J Surg Pathol 12:619, 1988
2. McNeal JE: The prostate and prostatic urethra: a morphologic synthesis. J Urol 107:1008, 1972
3. McNeal JE: Developmental and comparative anatomy of the prostate. p.I. In Grayhack J, Wilson J, Scherbenske M (eds): Benign prostatic Hyperplasia. DHEW# (NIH) 76-1113 Washington, D.C., 1976
4. Blacklock NJ: Anatomical factors in prostatitis. Br J Urol 46:47, 1974
5. McNeal JE: Origin and evolution of benign prostatic enlargement. Invest Urol 15:340, 1978
6. McNeal JE: Regional morphology and pathology of the prostate. Am J Clin Pathol 49:347, 1968
7. McNeal JE: The prostate gland: morphology and pathobiology. Monogr Urol 4:3, 1983
8. McNeal JE: Age-related changes in the prostatic epithelium associated with carcinoma. p. 23. In Griffiths K, Pierrepoint CG (eds): Some Aspects of the Aetiology and Biochemistry of Prostatic Cancer. Tenovus Publications, Cardiff, 1970
9. Reese JH, McNeal JE, Redwine EA, et al: Differential distribution of pepsinogen II between the zones of the human prostate and the seminal vesicle. J Urol 136:1148, 1986
10. Reese JH, McNeal JE, Redwine EA, et al: Tissue type plasminogen activator as a marker for functional zones within the human prostate gland. Prostate 12:47, 1988
11. McNeal JE, Leav I, Alroy J, Skutelsky E: Differential lectin staining of central and peripheral zones of the prostate and alterations in dysplasia. Am J Clin Pathol 89:41, 1988
12. Ayala AG, Ro JY, Babaian R, et al: The prostatic capsule: Does it exist? Its importance in the staging and treatment of prostatic carcinoma. Am J Surg Pathol 13:21, 1989
13. McNeal JE, Bostwick DG, Kindrachuk RA, et al: Patterns of progression in prostate cancer. Lancet 1:60, 1986
14. Lepor H, Gregerman M, Crosby R, et al: Precise localization of the autonomic nerves from the pelvic plexus to the corpora cavernosa: a detailed anatomical study of the adult male prostate. J Urol 133:207, 1985
15. Vaalasti A, Hervonen A: Autonomic innervation of the human prostate. Invest Urol 17:293, 1980

16. Freedman SR, Goldman RL: Normal paraganglia in the human prostate. J Urol 113:874, 1975

17. Carstens PHB: Perineural glands in normal and hyperplastic prostates. J Urol 123:686, 1980

18. Clegg EV: The vascular arrangements within the human prostate gland. Br J Urol 28:428, 1956

19. Flocks RH: Arterial distribution within the prostate gland: its role in transurethral prostatic resection. p. 3. In Nesbit RM (ed): Transurethral Prostatectomy. Charles C Thomas, Springfield, IL, 1943

20. McNeal JE, Price H, Redwine EA, et al: Stage A versus stage B adenocarcinoma of the prostate: morphologic comparison and biologic significance. J Urol 139:61, 1988

21. McNeal JE, Redwine EA, Freiha FS, Stamey TA: Zonal distribution of prostatic adenocarcinoma: correlation with histologic pattern and direction of spread. Am J Surg Pathol 12:897, 1988

22. McNeal JE: Anatomy of the prostate and morphogenesis of BPH. Prog Clin Biol Res 145:27, 1984

23. McNeal JE: Origin and development of carcinoma in the prostate. Cancer 23:24, 1969

24. Bostwick DG, Kindrachuk RW, Rouse RV: Prostatic adenocarcinoma with endometrioid features. Am J Surg Pathol 9:595, 1985

25. Hardt N, Kaude J, Wajsman Z, et al: Ultrasound guided prostatic biopsy: explaining ''negative'' results. Lab Invest 60:38A, 1989

26. Catalona WJ, Dresner SM: Nerve-sparing radical prostatectomy: extraprostatic tumor extension and preservation of erectile function. J Urol 134:1149, 1985

27. Eggleston JC, Walsh PC: Radical prostatectomy with preservation of sexual function: pathologic findings in the first 100 cases. J Urol 134:1146, 1985

2

Prostatitis

Ileana Lopez-Plaza and David G. Bostwick

The spectrum of prostatitis encompasses a multitude of inflammatory diseases of the prostate, some of which are rare and poorly understood. Stamey[1] considered prostatitis to be a "wastebasket of clinical ignorance" owing to significant variations in terminology, diagnostic criteria, and treatment. This report reviews the clinical and pathologic features of prostatitis, including acute prostatitis, chronic bacterial and abacterial prostatitis, and granulomatous prostatitis. These varied forms of prostatic inflammation show marked differences in treatment and clinical outcome, and, therefore, require accurate diagnosis.

ACUTE BACTERIAL PROSTATITIS

Acute bacterial prostatitis presents with sudden fever, chills, and pain in the lower back, rectum, and perineum, together with irritative voiding symptoms. There is often a prodromal syndrome of malaise, fever, arthralgia, and myalgia. The prostate is usually swollen, tender, warm, and indurated. Acute cystitis is also frequently present.[2]

Although scattered foci of acute inflammation are commonly seen in prostatic biopsies and resection specimens, the diagnosis of acute prostatitis should be reserved for cases with both clinical and pathologic features.

Microscopically, there are sheets of neutrophils in and around prostatic ducts and acini, with desquamated epithelium and cellular debris. The stroma is edematous and hemorrhagic, and contains variable numbers of lymphocytes, plasma cells, and macrophages. Microabscesses are frequently observed (Fig. 2-1).

Acute (bacterial) prostatitis is most accurately diagnosed by simultaneous culture of expressed prostatic secretions and urine from the urethra and bladder.[3] However, massage of the acutely inflamed prostate carries a high risk for the development of bacteremia; consequently, most clinicians do not undertake prostatic massage when acute prostatitis is suspected, relying instead on urine culture for confirmation of diagnosis.[2, 3]

The bacteria responsible for acute prostatitis are similar to those causing urinary tract infections, and include *Escherichia coli* (80 percent of infections); other Enterobacteriaceae: *Pseudomonas, Serratia,* and *Klebsiella* (10 to 15 percent); and enterococci (5 to 10 percent). Gonococcal prostatitis, due to *Neisseria gonorrhea,* was common in the preantibiotic era, but is infrequently observed today.[2, 3]

Acute bacterial prostatitis is successfully treated by a combination of intravenous and oral antibiotics. These drugs are not able to enter the normal prostate, but the increased blood flow that accompanies acute inflammation allows entry. Therapy for acute prostatitis includes parenteral and oral antibiotics for up to 4 weeks to relieve symptoms and prevent bacteremia and prostatic abscess.[2, 3]

PROSTATIC ABSCESS

Abscess is a rare complication of acute prostatitis, occurring most commonly in immunocompromised patients.[4] Predisposing factors include

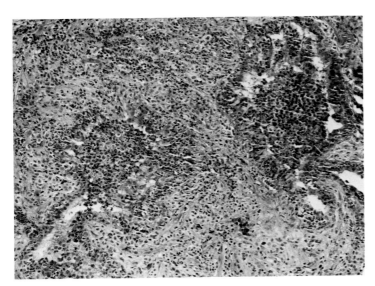

Fig. 2-1. Acute prostatitis. Sheets of neutrophils surround and fill acini, with epithelial destruction and formation of microabscesses.

urethral instrumentation and the use of indwelling catheters. Patients present with prostatic enlargement (75 percent), fever (33 percent), and urinary retention (33 percent).[5] A fluctuant mass is occasionally palpated by rectal examination.

Prostatic abscess is usually caused by aerobic bacteria similar to those of acute prostatitis, including *E. coli* and other gram-negative bacilli. It can also be caused by anaerobic bacteria, including *Actinomyces, Bacteroides, Clostridium, Eubacterium, Peptococcus,* and *Sphaerophorus.*[6] *Candida albicans* is a rare cause of prostatic abscess.

Transrectal ultrasonography is a valuable method for preoperative diagnosis, revealing a hypoechoic mass. Computed tomography is also useful, showing a low-density mass without contrast enhancement. Ultrasound-guided aspiration of pus can facilitate diagnosis, culture, and drainage of prostatic abscesses. The most common therapy is transurethral resection (TUR) and appropriate antibiotics.

Prostatic abscesses have been occasionally observed in adolescent boys requiring intermittent catheterization. These patients present with fever, and voiding cystourethrography shows extravasation of contrast material into the prostate, apparently owing to "chronic" prostatic abscess. When transurethral prostatic drainage was performed in the series of Steinhardt,[7] the prostate appeared to be "destroyed by the suppurative process." Chronic reseeding by bacteria from the bladder was considered the contributing factor. Abscess owing to *Staphylococcus* species has been reported in neonates.[5]

ACQUIRED IMMUNODEFICIENCY SYNDROME-RELATED PROSTATITIS

Patients infected with human immunodeficiency virus (HIV) are susceptible to opportunistic infections, including prostatitis, due in part to abnormalities of T- and B-lymphocyte function.[8] Infectious prostatitis occurs more frequently in patients with the acquired immunodeficiency syndrome (AIDS) (14 percent incidence) than in those with AIDS-related complex (ARC) or asymptomatic HIV infection (3 percent incidence).[9]

A wide variety of pathogens can induce prostatitis in these patients, including *E. coli, Klebsiella, Enterobacter, Serratia, Pseudomonas, Hemophilus parainfluenza, Cryptococcus neoformans,* and *Mycobacterium tuberculosis.*[9-12]

Patients with AIDS-related prostatitis may be asymptomatic, or may present with acute prostatitis, chronic prostatitis, or prostatic abscess. Recurrent infection and relapses are frequently seen despite prolonged antibiotic therapy.[9]

Fig. 2-2. Chronic prostatitis. A dense lymphocytic infiltrate is present within the stroma, extending through the intact glandular epithelium.

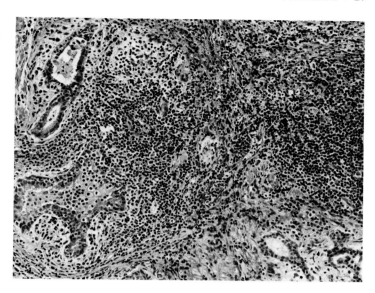

An HIV-related antigen was recently demonstrated in prostatic epithelial cells of AIDS patients at postmortem examination.[13]

CHRONIC PROSTATITIS

The spectrum of chronic prostatitis includes chronic bacterial, chronic abacterial, and granulomatous prostatitis. Granulomatous prostatitis is usually considered as a separate entity (see below).

Clinical features of chronic prostatitis are variable, and include frequency, urgency, dysuria, hematospermia, and pain in the lower back, perineum, and testes.[2, 3] Digital rectal examination of the prostate varies from normal to tender and boggy. Transrectal ultrasonography shows an irregular echo pattern with scattered shadows.[14]

Microscopically, chronic prostatitis is characterized by aggregates of lymphocytes, plasma cells, and macrophages within the prostatic stroma (Fig. 2-2). The epithelium displays reactive atypia, with occasional prominent nucleoli.[15] These histologic findings, in combination with the clinical manifestations, are characteristic of chronic prostatitis, and should not be confused with nonspecific inflammation, which is frequently observed in scattered foci throughout the prostate.[16]

Bacterial and abacterial (idiopathic) chronic prostatitis mimic each other clinically and histologically.[17] In both, expressed prostatic secretions contain increased numbers of white blood cells (more than 10 per high-power field) and lipid-laden macrophages. These two forms of chronic prostatitis are differentiated by the presence or absence of bacteria on culture or gram stain.[2, 3, 17]

Prostatodynia (pain in the prostate) is a clinical syndrome that mimics chronic prostatitis, but examination of expressed prostatic secretions reveals rare or absent white blood cells and macrophages.[2, 3]

Chronic Bacterial Prostatitis

Unlike acute bacterial prostatitis, chronic bacterial prostatitis is difficult to diagnose and treat. It is the most common cause of relapsing urinary tract infections in men with normal intravenous pyelogram studies.[2, 3] Diagnosis is made by bacteriologic localization studies of urine as described by Meares and Stamey[17]; cultures reveal bacteria in expressed prostatic secretions and

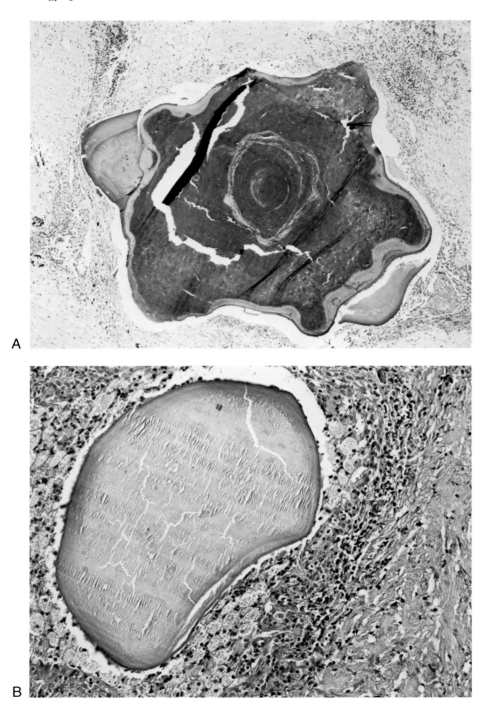

Fig. 2-3. Prostatic concretions. (**A**) Mineralized secretions have caused marked distension of the duct/acinus, with sloughed epithelial lining, circumferential fibrosis, and chronic inflammation. Compare with (**B**), in which the lining has been replaced by a mixture of foamy histiocytes, lymphocytes, and plasma cells.

urine voided after prostatic massage, but not in urethral or bladder specimens.

Most cases of chronic bacterial prostatitis are due to *E. coli*. In patients with prostatic calculi and relapsing urinary tract infections, the stones serve as a nidus of infection, with bacteria embedded in the mineral matrix (Fig. 2-3).[2, 3, 18] The secretory products of the inflamed prostate are alkaline, with decreased levels of zinc, citric acid, spermine, cholesterol, antibacterial factors, and enzyme activity. These patients also have elevated prostatic levels of IgA directed against the offending bacteria.[18]

Most antibiotics are unable to enter the prostate and prostatic fluids in the setting of chronic bacterial prostatitis, hampering treatment.[19] This inability is due in part to poor diffusion into alkaline tissues. Long-term therapy for up to 4 months yields a cure rate of 33 to 70 percent, significantly higher than that following short-term therapy.[18]

Although oral antibiotics are the most common treatment, alternative modalities include direct transperineal antibiotic infiltration of the prostate.[20] This approach circumvents the plasma-prostate barrier. Long-term remissions (6 months or longer) were observed in 71 percent of patients after one or two infiltrations.[20]

CHRONIC ABACTERIAL PROSTATITIS (PROSTATOSIS)

Abacterial or idiopathic chronic prostatitis is more common than bacterial prostatitis, but is rarely preceded by urinary tract infection.[18] Patients frequently complain of painful ejaculation. By definition, cultures and gram stains of expressed prostatic secretions are unrevealing.[2, 3, 18]

Considerable speculation exists concerning the role of *Chlamydia trachomatis, Trichomonas vaginalis,* and *Ureaplasma urealyticum* in chronic abacterial prostatitis. *Chlamydia,* an obligate intracellular parasite closely related to bacteria, is a major cause of other genitourinary tract infections, including nongonococcal urethritis and epididymitis.[21] Since the prostate is in

continuity with the urethra and epididymus, many investigators have proposed that *Chlamydia* is a major cause of chronic abacterial prostatitis. Also, some cases of chronic abacterial prostatitis respond to antibiotics directed against *Chlamydia.*[21] However, the results of published studies are conflicting. Most investigators have shown that *Chlamydia* is not involved in chronic prostatitis.[22-24] Two recent meticulous studies using urethral and prostatic secretions, in combination with transperineal ultrasonography-guided biopsy, failed to identify any pathogens, including *Chlamydia,* as causative.[23, 24] Conversely, Bruce et al.[25] isolated *Chlamydia* in 56 percent of first morning urine specimens in patients with clinical prostatitis. Poletti et al.[26] observed a 33 percent isolation rate in transrectal prostatic biopsies. Shurbaji et al.[27] noted a 31 percent incidence of immunohistochemical staining for *Chlamydia* in paraffin-embedded sections of human prostatic tissues. The precise role of *Chlamydia,* if any, in chronic abacterial prostatitis remains unresolved. *Ureaplasma* has also been proposed as a possible etiologic factor in chronic abacterial prostatitis, present in up to 19 percent of patients with this syndrome.[28] *Trichomonas* is observed in urethral cultures of up to 4 percent of patients.[29]

Chronic abacterial prostatitis has a prolonged indolent course characterized by relapses and remissions. Because the precise etiologic agent has not been identified, treatment is predominantly directed against symptoms.[30, 31]

Immunologic studies have shown an active immune response within the inflammatory infiltrate, with increased numbers of T8-positive lymphocytes and D7-positive macrophages.[32]

GRANULOMATOUS PROSTATITIS

Granulomatous prostatitis is a group of morphologically distinct forms of chronic prostatitis, caused by a wide variety of inciting agents, including infections, tissue disruption after biopsy, and inflammation. It comprises approximately 1 percent of benign inflammatory conditions of the prostate.[33]

Patients range in age from 18 to 86 years, with a mean of 62 years.[33] Presenting symptoms include irritative voiding (59 percent), fever (46 percent), chills (44 percent), acute urinary retention (21 percent), hematuria (11 percent), and flu-like symptoms (2 percent); 11 percent of patients are asymptomatic, with diagnosis made after routine digital examination and biopsy. The majority of patients (71 percent) have a prior history of urinary tract infection 1 to 34 weeks prior to diagnosis, including acute cystitis and prostatitis.[33]

Digital rectal examination reveals diffuse induration (80 percent) or hard, fixed, localized nodules (20 percent), with clinical suspicion of malignancy in up to 77 percent of patients. Urinalysis shows pyuria (82 percent) and hematuria (46 percent). Laboratory studies are usually not helpful in the diagnosis, with normal serum acid phosphatase and alkaline phosphatase levels, erythrocyte sedimentation rate (ESR), and hematology studies. Excretory urography may reveal non-specific prostatic obstruction. Biopsy is required for definitive diagnosis.[33]

The classification of granulomatous prostatitis is controversial. Idiopathic (nonspecific) granulomatous prostatitis ("of unknown cause") comprises the majority of cases (69 percent), and should be differentiated from other causes of granulomatous prostatitis owing to significant differences in treatment and clinical outcome (see Table 2-1).[33]

Towfighi et al.[34] proposed a classification based on histopathologic findings that divided nonspecific granulomatous prostatitis into two categories: eosinophilic and noneosinophilic. Each category was subdivided into those with and without fibrinoid necrosis and vasculitis. The association of eosinophilic granulomatous prostatitis with an allergic and asthmatic history, particularly when fibrinoid necrosis and vasculitis were present, led Towfighi et al. and other investigators to classify such forms of prostatitis as allergic.[34-36] Epstein and Hutchins[37] observed that eosinophilic prostatitis was also frequently seen in patients with no allergic or asthmatic history, regardless of the presence of fibrinoid

necrosis and necrobiotic granulomas. They concluded that eosinophilic granulomatous prostatitis could be attributed to many causes, and should not be considered synonymous with allergic granulomatous prostatitis (see below), a view shared by subsequent investigators. A new classification was proposed, based on clinical and pathologic findings: specific, nonspecific, post-transurethral section, malakoplakia, sarcoid, and allergic.[37] Stillwell et al.[33] emphasized the separation of systemic granulomatous disease-associated cases of granulomatous prostatitis from other cases owing to significant differences in treatment and prognosis. The

Table 2-1. Classification of Granulomatous Prostatitis

Infectious
  Bacterial
    Tuberculosis
    Brucellosis
    Syphilis

  Fungal
    Coccidioidomycosis
    Cryptococcosis
    Blastomycosis
    Histoplasmosis
    Paracoccidioidomycosis

  Parasitic
    Schistosomiasis
    Echinococcus
    Enterobius
    Linguatula

  Viral
    Herpes zoster

Iatrogenic
  Postsurgical
  Postradiation
  BCG-induced

Malakoplakia

Systemic granulomatous disease
  Allergic ("eosinophilic")
  Sarcoidosis
  Rheumatoid
  Autoimmune-vascular
    Wegener's granulomatosis
    Polyarteritis nodosa
    Benign lymphocytic angiitis and granulomatosis
      (BLAG)

Idiopathic ("nonspecific")

classification in Table 2-1 expands on the work of these investigators.

INFECTIOUS GRANULOMATOUS PROSTATITIS

Numerous microorganisms can induce granulomatous prostatitis, including bacteria, fungi, parasites, and viruses (see Table 2-1).

Bacterial

Tuberculosis of the prostate is now rare, and the last case diagnosed at Johns Hopkins Hospital was in 1973.[37] When observed, *Mycobacterium tuberculosis* infection of the prostate is seen only after pulmonary and miliary infection. Microscopically, small 1 to 2-mm caseating granulomas coalesce within the prostatic parenchyma, forming yellow nodules and streaks. Caseation and cavitation can be extensive. Acid-fast stain (Ziehl-Neelsen) and fluorescent stains may be useful in identifying organisms within granulomas. The histologic appearance may be identical to Calmette-Guérin bacillus (BCG)-induced granulomatous prostatitis (see below).

Although rare, involvement of the prostate by brucellosis can mimic tuberculosis clinically and pathologically.[38] *Brucella* is a gram-negative coccobacillus that is not acid fast. It is best identified in tissue by MacCallum-Goodpasture stain[39]; cultures are usually negative.

Syphilitic granulomatous prostatitis, due to *Treponema pallidum,* is rare, although it was occasionally observed in the preantibiotic era.

Fungal

Mycotic infections of the prostate are rare, and virtually always follow fungemia. Most of the deep mycoses induce necrotizing and non-necrotizing granulomas and fibrosis, but candidiasis is usually associated with acute inflammation (see above). Schwarz[40] suggested that prostatic massage is useful for diagnosis owing to the large number of organisms present.

The prostate is involved in up to 4.6 percent of patients with disseminated coccidioidomycosis (Fig. 2-4).[41] Pathologic findings include microabscesses and small granulomas, with large 30 to 60-μm-diameter spherules containing numerous endospores within giant cells, easily identified by periodic acid-Schiff (PAS) and methenamine silver stains.

Cryptococcosis rarely involves the prostate, but should be considered in the differential diagnosis of granulomatous prostatitis, particularly in patients with pulmonary infection.[12, 42] Mucicarmine stain reveals characteristic 4 to 7-μm-diameter budding yeast with thick capsules.

Blastomycosis causes granulomas and acute necrotizing inflammation.[43] The prostate is involved in up to 11.5 percent of cases, with characteristic 8- to 15-μm diameter budding yeast within giant cells.[43]

Histoplasmosis and paracoccidioidomycosis rarely involve the prostate.[40]

Parasitic

Platyhelminths are frequently found in the prostate in patients living in tropical countries. Schistosomiasis (bilharziasis) involves the prostate in 50 percent of males at autopsy in Zambia, and the bladder and seminal vesicles are even more frequently involved (62 and 58 percent, respectively).[44] The organisms lodge in vesicular and pelvic venous plexuses as the final habitat. The adult female migrates into the submucosa of the urinary bladder and prostatic stroma, where she lays eggs that induce granuloma formation and fibrosis. Rare cases have been associated with adenocarcinoma.[45]

Involvement of the prostate by echinococcus is characterized by hydatid cysts with prominent fibrosis.[46]

Other unusual parasites in the prostate have been reported, including *Enterobius* and *Linguatula,* both of which induce granulomatous prostatitis.[47] Interestingly, the prostate is

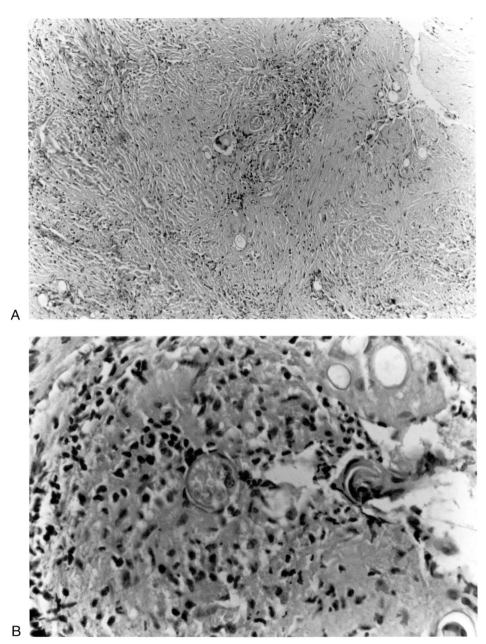

Fig. 2-4. Granulomatous prostatitis owing to coccidioidomycosis. (**A**) There is dense fibrosis and scattered chronic inflammation surrounding multiple intact and disintegrating spherules. (**B**) Higher magnification reveals characteristic thick-walled spherules containing endospores. The patient was a 60-year-old farmer from the San Joaquin Valley of California (an endemic area) who presented with weight loss and decreased mentation. Digital rectal examination revealed stone-hard induration of the prostate, and the clinical impression was prostatic carcinoma with probable metastases to the central nervous system; however, spinal fluid examination revealed coccidioidomycosis, and this was confirmed by prostatic needle biopsy. Despite vigorous antifungal therapy, the patient expired 1 month after presentation.

widely and heavily infiltrated by eosinophils in these infections, with marked peripheral eosinophilia.

Viral

Herpes zoster infection in association with granulomatous prostatitis was first reported by Clason et al.[48] In their two cases, acute urinary retention occurred within days of sacral eruption of herpes zoster. Transurethral resection (TUR) of the prostate demonstrated caseating granulomas typical of herpes, although no inclusion bodies were identified; the bladder was uninvolved. Spontaneous micturition occurred following TUR.[48]

IATROGENIC GRANULOMATOUS PROSTATITIS

Postsurgical

Necrotizing rheumatoid-like granulomas occur up to 5 years after TUR and needle biopsy as a result of cauterization and surgical disruption of tissues.[49-58] The granulomas are characteristically circumscribed, rimmed by palisading histiocytes with central fibrinoid necrosis (Fig. 2-5). Multinucleated giant cells are frequently but not invariably present, and are usually of the foreign-body type, although occasional Touton's and Langhans's types may be present. No polarizable or birefringent foreign material is observed.[57] Mies et al.[50] noted that prostatic glands and ducts were not disrupted in postsurgical granulomatous prostatitis, unlike nonspecific granulomatous prostatitis.

Postsurgical granulomas are usually focal, and should be differentiated from other forms of granulomatous prostatitis that are diffuse and more serious clinically. A similar postsurgical granulomatous lesion occurs in the kidney and other organs.[59]

The striking histologic resemblance of postsurgical granulomatous prostatitis to rheumatoid nodules suggests a hypersensitivity reaction or cell-mediated immune response. Tissue eosinophilia is present in many cases, and this finding has probably been misinterpreted as allergic prostatitis in the past, particularly in patients without a history of allergy or asthma.[36] Epstein and Hutchins[37] noted that eosinophils were most prominent in early lesions of postsurgical granulomatous prostatitis, and decreased in number with time.

No treatment is necessary for postsurgical prostatitis.

Postradiation

Granulomatous inflammation is a rare complication of radiation therapy.[60]

Calmette-Guérin Bacillus-Induced

Since its clinical introduction in the United States in 1976, intravesicular BCG immunotherapy has been shown to decrease the recurrence rate and progression of superficial transitional cell carcinoma of the bladder.[61] Complications of this therapy include granulomatous prostatitis, urethritis (see Ch. 12), hepatitis, cystitis, and pneumonitis. Oates et al. identified granulomatous prostatitis in 100 percent of 13 BCG-treated patients undergoing prostatic biopsy for nodular hyperplasia and carcinoma.

BCG-induced granulomas are characteristically discrete, with and without necrosis. There is no evidence of tissue eosinophilia. Acid-fast bacilli may be identified, particularly within necrotizing granulomas, similar to tuberculous prostatitis. Fine-needle aspiration cytology is useful in establishing the diagnosis.

No therapy is required. Recognition of this entity is necessary to avoid diagnostic and therapeutic confusion.

MALAKOPLAKIA

Malakoplakia is a granulomatous disease attributable to defective intracellular lysosomal digestion of bacteria. It is most commonly found

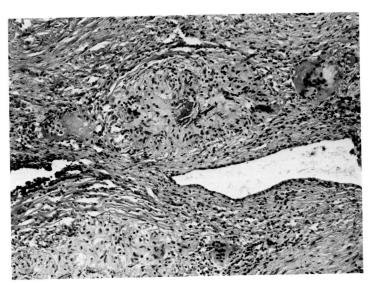

Fig. 2-5. Postsurgical granulomatous prostatitis. Well-circumscribed granulomas are rimmed by palisading histiocytes with central fibrinoid necrosis. Multinucleated foreign-body-type giant cells are present at the periphery.

in the bladder and urinary tract, and occasionally presents in the prostate.[62-66] Patients have obstructive symptoms, including frequency, urgency, dysuria, nocturia, and fever. It occurs in men over 50 years of age with systemic illnesses and other debilitating conditions. Digital rectal examination reveals diffuse induration suggestive of prostatic carcinoma. *E. coli* is commonly isolated from urine cultures.

Prostatic involvement by malakoplakia is characterized by discrete and confluent soft, yellow-brown plaques, with central umbilication or ulceration and peripheral hyperemia. Microscopically, the prostatic architecture is effaced by dense sheet-like aggregates of histiocytes (Van Hansemann cells) admixed with lymphocytes and plasma cells (Fig. 2-6). Intracellular and extracellular Michaelis-Gutmann bodies are identified, appearing as sharply demarcated spherical structures with concentric "owl's eyes," measuring 5 to 10 μm in diameter. Michaelis-Gutmann bodies stain with the following: PAS (polysaccharides), alizarin red (calcium), Prussian blue (iron), and Von Kossa (anionic component of calcium ions). Gram stain, acid-fast stain, and fungal stains are negative.[64]

Electron microscopy shows degenerating bacteria within phagolysomes, with progressive cal-

cification and maturation of these Michaelis-Gutmann bodies.[62]

Biopsy is necessary for diagnosis.[62, 66] Recommended treatment is long-term antibiotic therapy directed against *E. coli*. Surgery is occasionally useful when disease progresses despite antibiotic therapy.[62]

SYSTEMIC GRANULOMATOUS DISEASE

Allergic ("Eosinophilic")

Allergic granulomatous prostatitis is a clinicopathologic entity that requires the following features for diagnosis: clinical history of asthma or allergy with peripheral eosinophilia and systemic lesions (Churg-Strauss syndrome); histologic identification of eosinophilic granulomatous prostatitis with fibrinoid necrosis and vasculitis; prostatic lesions that usually correlate with exacerbation of asthma or allergies. Allergic granulomatous prostatitis can be confused histologically with postsurgical granulomatous prostatitis and parasitic granulomatous prostatitis due to the presence of tissue eosinophilia.[34, 36, 37]

The first reported case of allergic granulomatous prostatitis was in a patient with a history

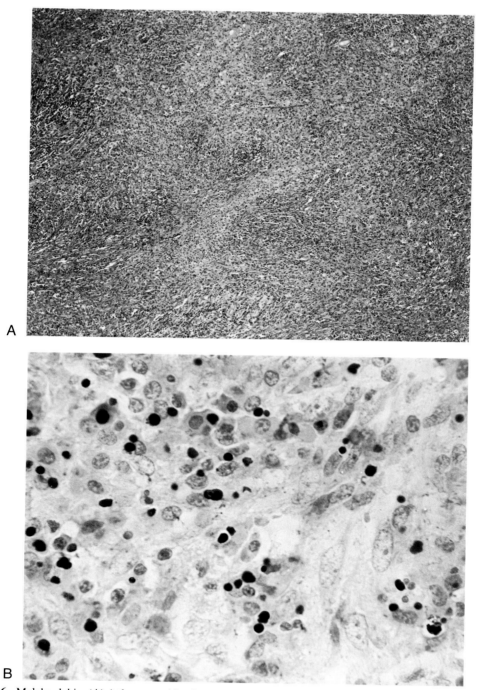

Fig. 2-6. Malakoplakia. (**A**) At low magnification, the prostatic architecture is effaced by sheets of histiocytes, lymphocytes, and plasma cells. (**B**) At high magnification, characteristic extracellular and intracellular Michaelis-Guttman bodies stain black with the von Kossa stain.

of asthma whose symptoms increased in severity in association with acute urinary obstruction.[67] Systemic granulomas were found at autopsy, and involved the seminal vesicles, bladder, rectum, heart, and esophagus. Of 12 documented cases reviewed by Epstein and Hutchins,[37] 9 had active asthma when the prostatic granulomas were first identified; 4 had peripheral eosinophilia; and 3 had extraprostatic granulomas, eosinophilic infiltrates, or systemic allergic reactions.

Allergic granulomatous prostatitis has been successfully treated with steroids.[34] This exceedingly rare condition is reflective of a more generalized allergic reaction, and should be diagnosed with caution, only after complete clinical and pathologic evaluation.

Sarcoidosis

Nonnecrotizing granulomas are occasionally observed in the prostate in patients with sarcoidosis.

Rheumatoid Nodules

The discrete linear necrotizing granulomas of postsurgical granulomatous prostatitis are histologically identical to rheumatoid nodules.[49-50] The recent widespread identification of postsurgical granulomas calls into question the diagnosis of older cases of rheumatoid-like nodules in the prostate, although rheumatoid involvement in the prostate would not be unexpected in such a systemic disease.

Autoimmune-Vascular

The clinical diagnosis of autoimmune and vascular disease is confirmed by histologic identification of necrotizing granulomas and vasculitis in tissue specimens from many organs, including the prostate (see below).

Wegener's Granulomatosis

Wegener's granulomatosis is characterized by systemic necrotizing granulomas with vasculitis. It involves the upper respiratory tract, lungs, kidneys, and other organs in men and women in the fifth decade and older. Prostatic involvement is rare, occurring in 2.3 to 7.4 percent of men with Wegener's granulomatosis.[68] Patients present with urinary obstruction, infection, hematuria, and acute retention, usually after clinical presentation in the upper airways, lungs, or kidneys. Rarely prostatic involvement is the initial clinical manifestation, although most reported cases have been diagnosed postmortem.[68]

Rectal examination reveals diffuse enlargement of the prostate with or without areas of induration. Laboratory tests may reveal microhematuria, red cell casts, or proteinuria, features indicative of renal involvement. The ESR is frequently elevated. At cystoscopy, the prostatic urethra has a ragged, friable mucosa.

Biopsy reveals necrotizing granulomatous prostatitis with vasculitis. Stellate and geographic granulomas are observed, rimmed by palisading histiocytes and scattered multinucleated giant cells. Vasculitis involves small arteries and veins. Special stains and cultures for bacteria, fungi, and parasites are helpful in excluding other causes.

Stillwell et al.[68] considered biopsy diagnosis of prostatic Wegener's granulomatosis to be mandatory. Symptomatic prostatic involvement usually responds to chemotherapy, similar to pulmonary and renal involvement, with treatment consisting of cyclophosphamide and steroids. TUR may also be helpful.

Other vasculitides may involve the prostate, including polyarteritis nodosa, but most are diagnosed at autopsy.

Benign Lymphocytic Angiitis and Granulomatosis

Benign lymphocytic angiitis and granulomatosis (BLAG) is a rare vasculitis usually restricted to the lungs. Microscopically, the lesions of BLAG have a dense lymphocytic infiltrate with an admixture of plasma cells and histiocytes. Fibroblasts and collagen deposition are present, but dense fibrosis does not appear in the lungs. Arteries and veins display inflammation without necrosis.

Prostatic involvement with BLAG was first reported by Weiss et al.[69] in 1984, and is histologically identical to lung involvement.

BLAG has a good prognosis and responds well to chemotherapy.

IDIOPATHIC

Idiopathic (nonspecific) granulomatous prostatitis composes the majority of cases of granulomatous prostatitis (69 percent).[33] As suggested by Stillwell et al.,[33] classification of eosinophilic and noneosinophilic categories is probably not helpful. It is important to recognize the wide variety of inciting agents of granulomatous prostatitis and the occasional histologic clues that allow distinction of these different entities, but most cases will elude definitive classification, and will be considered idiopathic.

Granulomatous prostatitis probably originates in blockage of prostatic ducts and stasis of secretion, regardless of etiology. The epithelium is destroyed, and cellular debris, bacterial toxins, and prostatic secretions escape into the stroma, eliciting an intense localized inflammatory response. Prostatic secretions include corpora amylacea, sperm, and semen products. This process is similar to intraprostatic sperm granuloma formation.[70] Recent evidence indicates that granulomatous prostatitis is not a late stage of chronic prostatitis.[33]

In idiopathic granulomatous prostatitis, the granulomas are usually noncaseating (Fig. 2-7). The inflammation resolves slowly, producing areas of parenchymal loss with marked fibrosis. Fox[71] described a form of nonnecrotizing granulomatous prostatitis composed of histiocytes that he termed *nodular histiocytic prostatitis.*

Treatment has included steroids, antihistamines, antibiotics, and surgery. As described above, specific infections, systemic diseases, and other causes should receive treatment appropriate to the condition. As Stillwell et al.[33] noted, up to 10 percent of patients with idiopathic granulomatous prostatitis will be refractory to conservative management, with severe prostatic obstruction, and such patients may warrant TUR. However, surgery is unsuccessful in up to 50 percent of cases, with some patients requiring multiple procedures. Nonspecific local

Fig. 2-7. Idiopathic granulomatous prostatitis. Patchy diffuse noncaseating granulomatous inflammation is present within and surrounding ducts and acini. The infiltrate is composed of lymphocytes, histiocytes, plasma cells, and scattered eosinophils.

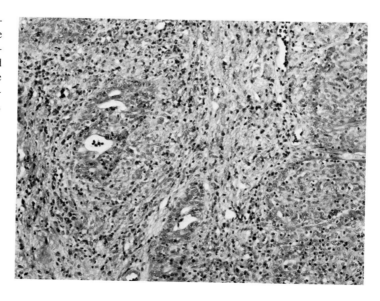

therapy, including sitz baths, fluids, and temporary urinary catheterization as necessary, is probably the treatment of choice. Spontaneous remission occurs in the majority of patients, although induration may persist on physical examination for years. Adenocarcinoma may develop as a late complication, but most investigators do not consider granulomatous prostatitis a cause of malignancy.[33]

REFERENCES

1. Stamey TA: Urinary infections in males. p. 1. In Stamey TA (ed): Pathogenesis and Treatment of Urinary Tract Infections, Williams & Wilkins, Baltimore, 1980

2. Stewart C: Prostatitis. Emerg Med Clin N Am 6:391, 1988

3. Meares EM Jr: Prostatitis syndromes: new perspectives about old woes. J Urol 123:141, 1980

4. Meares EM Jr: Prostatic abscess. J Urol 136:1281, 1986

5. Weinberger M, Cytron S, Servadio C, et al: Prostatic abscess in the antibiotic era. Rev Infect Dis 10:239, 1988

6. Brawer MK, Stamey TA: Prostatic abscess owing to anaerobic bacteria. J Urol 138:1254, 1987

7. Steinhardt GF: Prostatic suppuration and destruction in patients with myelodysplasia: a newly recognized entity. J Urol 140:1002, 1988

8. Witt DJ, Craven DE, McCabe WR: Bacterial infections in adult patients with the acquired immunodeficiency syndrome (AIDS) and AIDS related complex. Am J Med 82:900, 1987

9. Leport C, Rousseau F, Perrone C, et al: Bacterial prostatitis in patients infected with the human immunodeficiency virus. J Urol 141:334, 1989

10. Moreno S, Pacho E, Lopez-Herce JA, et al: *Mycobacterium tuberculosis* visceral abscesses in the acquired immunodeficiency syndrome (AIDS). Ann Intern Med 109:437, 1988

11. Clairmont GJ, Zon LI, Groopman JE: *Hemophilus parainfluenzae* prostatitis in a homosexual man with chronic lymphadenopathy syndrome and HTLV III infection. Am J Med 82:175, 1987

12. Lief M, Sarfarazi F: Prostatic cryptococcosis in acquired immune deficiency syndrome. Urology 28:318, 1986

13. Shevchuk MM, Silva M, Cronin WJ, et al: Detection of HIV-related antigen in testes and prostates of AIDS patients. Lab Invest 58:84A, 1988

14. Gammelgaard J, Holm HH: Transurethral and transrectal ultrasonic scanning in urology. J Urol 124:863, 1980

15. Helpap B: Observations on the number, size and localization of nucleoli in hyperplastic and neoplastic disease. Histopathology 13:203, 1988

16. Nielsen ML, Asnaes S, Hattel T: Inflammatory changes in the non-infected prostate gland: a clinical, microbiological and histological investigation. J Urol 110:423, 1973

17. Meares EM, Stamey TA: Bacteriologic localization patterns in bacterial prostatitis and urethritis. Invest Urol 5:492, 1968

18. Orland SM, Hanno PM, Wein AJ: Prostatitis, prostatosis, and prostatodynia. Urology 25:439, 1985

19. Childs SJ, Goldstein EJC: Ciprofloxacin as treatment for genitourinary tract infection. J Urol 141:1, 1989

20. Baert L, Leonard A: Chronic bacterial prostatitis: 10 years of experience with local antibiotics. J Urol 140:755, 1988

21. Ireton RC, Berger RE: Prostatitis and epididymitis. Urol Clin N Am 11:83, 1984

22. Uehling DT: Abacterial prostatitis: more about what it isn't but what is it? J Urol 141:367, 1989

23. Berger RE, Krieger JN, Kessler D, et al: Case-control study of men with suspected chronic idiopathic prostatitis. J Urol 141:328, 1989

24. Doble A, Thomas BJ, Walker MM, et al: The role of *Chlamydia trachomatis* in chronic abacterial prostatitis: a study using ultrasound guided biopsy. J Urol 141:332, 1989

25. Bruce AW, Chadwick P, Willett WS, O'Shaughnessy M: The role of Chlamydiae in genitourinary disease. J Urol 126:625, 1981

26. Poletti F, Medici MC, Alinovi A, et al: Isolation of *Chlamydia trachomatis* from the prostatic cells in patients affected by nonacute abacterial prostatitis. J Urol 134:691, 1985

27. Shurbaji MS, Gupta PK, Myuers J: Immunohistochemical demonstration of chlamydial antigens in association with prostatitis. Mod Pathol 1:348, 1988

28. Weidner W, Brunner A, Kruase W: Quantitative culture of *Ureaplasma urealyticium* in patients with chronic prostatitis or prostatosis. J Urol 124:622, 1980

29. Krieger JN, Egan KJ: Comprehensive evaluation

and treatment of 75 men with chronic prostatitis. J Urol 141:240A, 1989

30. Thin RN, Simmons PD: Chronic bacterial and nonbacterial prostatitis. Br J Urol 55:513, 1983
31. Greenberg RN, Reilly PM, Luppen KL, Piercy S: Chronic prostatitis: comments on infectious etiologies and antimicrobial treatment. Prostate 6:45, 1985
32. Doble A, Walker MM, Harris JRW, Taylor-Robinson D: Immunological studies in chronic abacterial prostatitis. J Urol 141:530A, 1989
33. Stillwell TJ, Engen DE, Farrow GM: The clinical spectrum of granulomatous prostatitis: a report of 200 cases. J Urol 138:320, 1987
34. Towfighi J, Sadeghee S, Wheeler JE, Enterline HT: Granulomatous prostatitis with emphasis on the eosinophilic variety. Am J Clin Pathol 58:630, 1972
35. Stewart MJ, Wray S, Hall M: Allergic prostatitis in asthmatics. J Pathol Bacteriol 67:423, 1954
36. Yonker RA, Katz P: Necrotizing granulomatous vasculitis with eosinophilic infiltrates limited to the prostate. Am J Med 77:362, 1984
37. Epstein JI, Hutchins GM: Granulomatous prostatitis: distinction among allergic, non-specific, and posttransurethral resection lesions. Hum Pathol 15:818, 1984
38. Kelalis PP, Greene LF, Weed LA: Brucellosis of the urogenital tract: a mimic of tuberculosis. J Urol 38:347, 1962
39. Better LF: Brucellosis. p. 174. In Binford CH, Connor DH (eds): Pathology of Tropical and Extraordinary Diseases. Vol. 1. Armed Forces Institute of Pathology, Washington, DC, 1976
40. Schwarz J: Mycotic prostatitis. Urology 19:1, 1982
41. Kuntze JR, Herman MH, Evans SG: Genitourinary coccidioidomycosis. J Urol 140:370, 1988
42. Braman RT: Cryptococcosis (torulosis) of prostate. Urology 17:284, 1981
43. Inoshita T, Youngberg GA, Boelen LJ, Loangston J: Blastomycosis presenting with prostatic involvement: report of 2 cases and review of the literature. J Urol 130:160, 1983
44. Patil PS, Elem B: Schistosomiasis of the prostate and the seminal vesicles: observations in Zambia. J Trop Med Hyg 91:245, 1988
45. Alexis R, Domingo J: Schistosomiasis and adenocarcinoma of the prostate: a morphologic study. Hum Pathol 17:757, 1986
46. Deklotz RJ: Echinococcal cyst involving the prostate and seminal vesicles: a case report. J Urol 115:116, 1976
47. Symmers W St C: Two cases of eosinophilic prostatitis due to metazoan infestation (with *Oxyuris vermicularis,* and with a larva of *Linguatula serrata*). J Pathol Bacteriol 73:549, 1957
48. Clason AE, McGeorge A, Garland C, Abel BJ: Urinary retention and granulomatous prostatitis following sacral Herpes Zoster infection. A report of 2 cases with a review of the literature. Br J Urol 54:166, 1982
49. Pieterse AS, Aarons I, Jose JS: Focal prostatic granulomas: rheumatoid-like probably iatrogenic in origin. Pathology 16:174, 1984
50. Mies C, Balogh K, Stadecker M: Palisading prostate granulomas following surgery. Am J Surg Pathol 8:217, 1984
51. Castrillon JV, Maurino MLG, Carcavilla CG, et al: Palisading lower urinary tract granuloma. Br J Urol 62:489, 1988
52. Koplovic J, Rivkind A, Sherman Y: Granulomatous prostatitis with vasculitis. A sequel of transurethral prostatic resection. Arch Pathol Lab Med 108:732, 1984
53. Schned AR: Prostatic granuloma (letter). Am J Surg Pathol 8:797, 1984
54. Feiner HD: Reparative granulomas of the prostate (letter). Am J Surg Pathol 8:797, 1984
55. Evans CS, Goldman RL, Klein HZ: More on prostatic granulomas (letter). Am J Surg Pathol 8:798, 1984
56. Eyre RC, Aaronson AG, Weinstein BJ: Palisading granulomas of the prostate associated with prior prostatic surgery. J Urol 136:121, 1986
57. Lee G, Shepherd N: Necrotizing granulomata in prostatic resection specimens: a sequel to previous operation. J Clin Pathol 36:1067, 1983
58. Hedelin H, Johansson S, Nilson S: Focal prostatic granulomas. A sequel to transurethral resection. Scand J Urol Nephrol 15:193, 1981
59. Balogh K: Palisading granuloma in the kidney after open biopsy. Am J Surg Pathol 10:441, 1986
60. Bostwick DG, Egbert BM, Fajardo LF: Radiation injury of the normal and neoplastic prostate. Am J Surg Pathol 6:541, 1982
61. Oates RD, Stilmant MM, Fredlund MC, Siroky MB: Granulomatous prostatitis following bacillus Calmette-Guérin immunotherapy of bladder cancer. J Urol 140:751, 1988
62. Stanton MJ, Maxted W: Malakoplakia: a study of the literature and current concepts of pathogen-

esis, diagnosis and treatment. J Urol 125:139, 1981

63. McClure J: Malakoplakia of the prostate: a report of two cases and a review of the literature. J Clin Pathol 32:629, 1979

64. Altaffer LF, Enghardt M: Malakoplakia of prostate gland. Urology 24:196, 1984

65. Makek M, Lagler U: Malakoplakie der Prostata. Urologe [A] 19:89, 1980

66. Shimizu S, Takimoto Y, Niimura T, et al: A case of prostatic malakoplakia. J Urol 126:277, 1981

67. Melicow MM: Allergic granulomas of the prostate gland. J Urol 65:288, 1951

68. Stillwell TJ, DeRemee RA, McDonald TJ, et al: Prostatic involvement in Wegener's granulomatosis. J Urol 138:1251, 1987

69. Weiss MA, Rolfes DB, Alvir MA, Cohen LJ: Benign lymphocytic angiitis and granulomatosis: a case report with evidence of an autoimmune etiology. Am J Clin Pathol 81:110, 1984

70. Nelson G, Culberson DE, Gardner WA Jr: Intraprostatic spermatozoa. Hum Pathol 19:541, 1988

71. Fox H: Nodular histiocytic prostatitis. J Urol 96:372, 1966

3

The Pathobiology of Nodular Hyperplasia

John E. McNeal

Microscopic changes characteristic of nodular hyperplasia of the prostate, or benign prostate hyperplasia (BPH), take place as early as the fourth decade of life.[1] They comprise a set of specific deviations from normal duct-acinar architecture, and are not simply the result of a generalized increase in cell population. The morphologic features of these architectural deviations, together with the anatomic relationships of the compartments in which they develop, provide important clues to the pathobiology of the hyperplastic process. It has not been established that age-related hormonal changes cause nodular hyperplasia; rather, the normal hormonal milieu may merely provide a growth stimulus to a localized tissue abnormality established years earlier.

ANATOMIC LOCATION OF NODULAR HYPERPLASIA

Nodular hyperplasia arises exclusively within the transition zone and periurethral region (Fig. 3-1).[1, 2] Most clinically significant cases consist of transition zone enlargement, both diffuse and nodular. Diffuse enlargement of this zone is an almost universal accompaniment of aging, and is always present in cases with nodular enlargement, sometimes appearing as the dominant component (Figs. 3-2 and 3-3). Periurethral nodular hyperplasia seldom reaches clinically significant size, except as an occasional midline dorsal mass at the bladder neck protruding into the bladder lumen.

When the precise anatomic distribution of incipient nodules (less than 3 mm in diameter) is plotted, a tight cluster is identified within the medial transition zone near the distal end of the preprostatic sphincter (Figs. 3-2 and 3-3). Many nodules lie within this sphincter, splitting the fiber bundles. This intermingling of sphincteric and glandular tissue occurs only in the transition zone, which is the region of the prostate that experiences the greatest delay in completion of growth and development. The slow development of this zone apparently continues into adult life long after the potential for growth in the rest of the prostate has been suppressed. Morphologic studies indicate that the volume of the transition zone is higher in men over the age of 40 than in younger adults, even in the absence of nodular hyperplasia. These features of delayed prepubertal development, continued growth into adult life, and intermingling of different types of stroma are unique to the transition zone, and may be related to the origin of nodular hyperplasia at this site.

MORPHOLOGY OF NODULAR HYPERPLASIA

Most periurethral nodules are pure stromal nodules. These nodules have a unique histologic appearance, with an abundance of pale ground substance and scant collagen fibers, reminiscent of embryonic mesenchyme.

In the transition zone, however, almost all nodules are glandular from their inception. The smallest foci are represented by a localized increase in the density of glandular structures with-

31

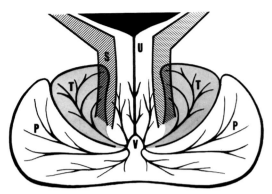

Fig. 3-1. Oblique coronal plane of a section along the proximal segment of the prostatic urethra (*U*) showing the relationships of the transition zone (*T*) to the larger peripheral zone (*P*) and to the preprostatic sphincter (*S*). Periurethral glands arise proximal to the base of the verumontanum (*V*) and remain confined inside the sphincter. (From McNeal,[1] with permission.)

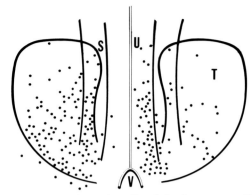

Fig. 3-3. Locations of small nodules from cases with many nodules are graphed as in Figure 3-2. The transition zone is diffusely enlarged. Stromal nodules (right) are more clearly localized to the periurethral region (*U*). Glandular nodules (left) are more widely distributed through the transition zone (*T*). (From McNeal,[1] with permission.)

out an expansile border (Fig. 3-4). The glands differ from the surrounding transition zone tissue only in their architectural arrangement. Incipient nodules arise by budding and branching of new small glands from pre-existing ducts (Fig. 3-

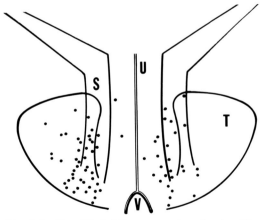

Fig. 3-2. Simplified oblique coronal section (see Fig. 3-1) showing locations of small nodules from cases with few nodules in relation to the transition zone (*T*), preprostatic sphincter (*S*), and urethra (*U*). Locations of nodules with predominant *stromal* composition are all graphed to the right of the urethra. Locations of predominantly *glandular* nodules are graphed on the left. (From McNeal,[1] with permission.)

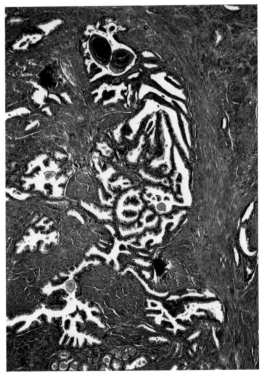

Fig. 3-4. Local increase in gland density without expansile border (center) signals the earliest phase of glandular nodule formation. (H&E, ×70)

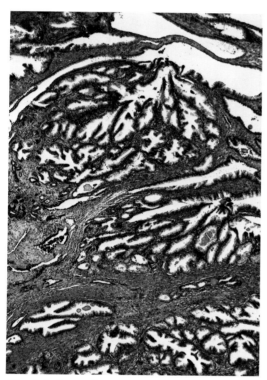

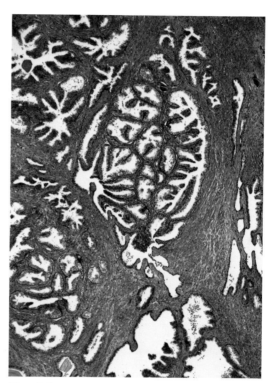

Fig. 3-5. Formation of new small nodules (top and center) results from formation of new duct branches sprouting from two separate foci. (H&E, ×70)

Fig. 3-6. Two separate duct systems at the right and left branch toward a central focus of nodule formation. (H&E, ×70)

5). Interestingly, these nodules often originate as branches from two or more adjacent ducts that converge on each other with scant intervening stroma (Fig. 3-6). Small ducts at the periphery of the growing nodule may contribute additional branches, with these branches growing toward the center of the nodule (Fig. 3-7).

This architectural pattern violates two consistent principles of normal biology. First, formation of new ductal and acinar architecture is generally a forbidden process in adult organs. For example, the adult lung and kidney are unable to replace lost alveoli and nephrons. This ability is limited to embryonic development, disappearing at birth or during early childhood. The lung, a late developer, continues to form new alveoli until about age 8; in contrast, the prostate completes its acinar development during puberty. In the adult prostate, testosterone and other hormones can induce epithelial proliferation and glandular enlargement, but will not cause new ducts and acini to form.

Second, in normal organogenesis, developing duct systems follow a divergent pattern, with branches spreading away from pre-existing ducts and acini to allow a uniform orderly spacing of glandular elements. In nodular hyperplasia, the *convergence* of new formed ductal and acinar elements is unique, causing an extraordinary focal increase in the density of glands (Figs. 3-8 and 3-9).

These characteristic morphologic features of glandular nodules suggest a model for the pathogenesis of nodule formation. If a clone of stromal cells reverted to its embryonic state, it might act as an inductive focus to reactivate the capacity of nearby ducts for budding and branching, and also direct the growth of these new branches toward the inductive center. As this clone of stromal cells grew to encase the new epithelial branches, the epithelium might reciprocate by inducing the new stromal cells to mature into normal adult smooth muscle stroma. If epithelial induction failed to occur, both the proliferation and maturation of embryonic stromal cells could be inhibited. Such a hypothesis could account for the stromal appearance of most periurethral

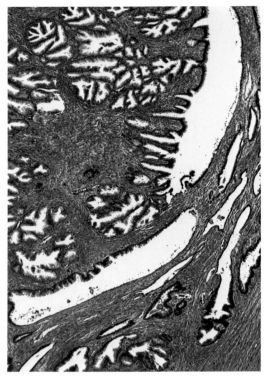

Fig. 3-7. A somewhat larger nodule shows two ducts at the nodule periphery with selective epithelial hyperplasia confined to the wall of the duct facing the nodule center. The duct at top also shows multiple small branches from its wall exclusively on the nodule side. (H&E, ×70)

nodules owing to the paucity of glandular elements at that site.

Studies by Cunha et al.[3] indicate that embryonic processes can be reawakened in the adult prostate. After combining adult rat bladder epithelium with embryonic prostatic mesenchyme, the adult epithelium migrated into the mesenchyme and matured into functional prostatic glandular tissue, apparently as a result of embryonic induction by the prostatic mesenchyme.

Other morphologic clues suggest the presence of a diffusible embryonic inducer in the formation of nodular hyperplasia. The selective hyperplasia of ductal epithelium at the periphery of hyperplastic nodules implies the presence of a stimulus originating within the nodules.

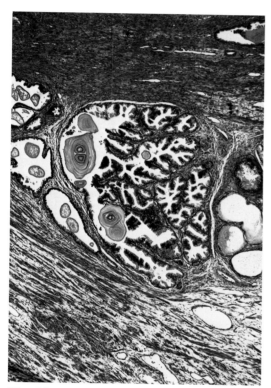

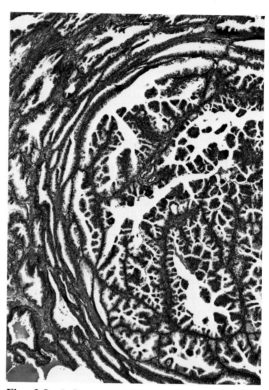

Fig. 3-8. Convergence of new branches of a duct containing corpora amylacea producing focal increased gland density in the early stage of nodule genesis. (H&E, ×70)

Fig. 3-9. A larger nodule exhibiting continuation of the duct convergence process seen in Figure 3-8. (H&E, ×70)

PATHOGENESIS OF NODULAR HYPERPLASIA

The pathogenesis of BPH nodule formation is probably the result of changes at the local tissue level. Nodular hyperplasia can occur without any detectable abnormality in serum levels of steroid hormones. Furthermore, abnormal hormonal stimulation of most target organs usually produces diffuse changes in the target tissue. Dramatic focal responses with intervening unaffected areas such as nodular hyperplasia would not be expected unless there had been a localized change in tissue responsiveness to the hormone.

Within the transition zone, nodules show a strong predilection for the medial portion, precisely the area in which there is the densest intermingling of transition zone glands and preprostatic sphincteric smooth muscle. It is proposed that the sphincteric stroma provides the growth stimulus for nodule formation, thus accounting for the origin of nodular hyperplasia in a limited area of the prostate, and explaining the fact that most transition zone nodules are embedded in the sphincter.

Judging from detailed autopsy studies,[1] there is a linear increase in the number of hyperplastic nodules, starting in the fourth decade, with little increase in nodule mass in subsequent years.

In the seventh and eighth decades, the average size of nodules in many men abruptly increases, perhaps owing to some alteration in endocrine status. However, no dramatic change in the levels of steroid hormones has been identified in this age group, so it is possible that nonsteroidal hormones may be involved.

The natural history of BPH is probably complex and multifactorial. An early localized tissue change probably plays a dominant role in nodule genesis. Subsequently, an independent endocrine change or changes may variably accelerate the rate of nodule growth. The early local tissue alteration seems to occur in most men, but the second change occurs less commonly and may be characteristic of those men who develop large-mass (more than 50 g) BPH.

REFERENCES

1. McNeal JE: Origin and evolution of benign prostatic enlargement. Invest Urol 15:340, 1978
2. McNeal JE: Normal histology of the prostate. Am J Surg Pathol 12:619, 1988
3. Cunha GR, Lung B, Reese B: Glandular epithelial induction by embryonic mesenchyme in adult bladder epithelium of BALB/c mice. Invest Urol 17:302, 1980

4

Premalignant Lesions

David G. Bostwick and John R. Srigley

Precancerous lesions of the prostate can be divided into two main categories: prostatic intraepithelial neoplasia and atypical adenomatous hyperplasia. In this report, we evaluate the diagnostic criteria, differential diagnosis, and clinical significance of these lesions.

DIAGNOSTIC CRITERIA

PROSTATIC INTRAEPITHELIAL NEOPLASIA

Cellular proliferations within prostatic ducts and acini form a morphologic continuum, ranging from benign growths devoid of architectural and cytologic atypia to proliferations in which the degree of atypia is such that they are recognized as dysplastic. At widely spaced points of this spectrum, the proliferations are distinguished easily; however, no abrupt changes in morphologic pattern are apparent along this continuum. PIN represents the putative precancerous (dysplastic) end of this continuum, characterized by proliferation and anaplasia of cells.

The term *prostatic intraepithelial neoplasia* (PIN) was adopted by Bostwick and Brawer[1] to include all forms of atypical and malignant lesions of epithelial cells confined to the lumens of ducts and acini, as well as similar lesions accompanied by microinvasion (Table 4-1).

In the earliest stages of this lesion (PIN 1), the cells within ducts and acini are heaped up, crowded, and irregularly spaced, with marked variation in nuclear size (anisonucleosis) (Fig. 4-1). Small conspicuous nucleoli and elongate hyperchromatic nuclei may also be observed,

but these are not prominent features. The diagnosis of PIN requires a combination of both architectural and cytologic features, and foci displaying only some of these features are considered atypical but not diagnostic. It should be noted that there may be occasional difficulty in distinguishing PIN 1 from reactive atypia in selected cases without additional clinical and pathologic information (see *Differential Diagnosis,* below). Higher grades of PIN show similar features as PIN 1, although cell crowding and stratification are usually more pronounced. In PIN 2, the majority of nuclei are enlarged, accounting for less variability in nuclear size (Fig. 4-2). Occasional prominent nucleoli are observed, and there is greater hyperchromasia. Cytoplasmic eosinophilia may also be prominent.

In the highest grade of PIN (PIN 3), the cells display large prominent nucleoli, similar to invasive carcinoma (Fig. 4-3). In addition to the architectural features of PIN 2, PIN 3 may also show occasional foci of lumenal bridging, creating a sieve-like pattern reminiscent of cribriform carcinoma. Nucleoli are markedly enlarged and hyperchromatic, with some anisokaryosis. Chromatin margination is frequently observed. PIN 3 may also appear as a single layer of markedly atypical cells with large nuclei and prominent nucleoli displaying apical cytoplasmic blebs (apocrine snouts). PIN 3 corresponds to what others have called *carcinoma in situ.*

PIN spreads through prostatic ducts in three different patterns, similar to prostatic carcinoma.[1,2] The first pattern involves replace-

Table-4-1. Premalignant Lesions of the Prostate: Diagnostic Features

	Prostatic Intraepithelial Neoplasia			Atypical Adenomatous Hyperplasia (AAH)
	PIN 1	PIN 2	PIN 3	
Architecture	Epithelial cell crowding, stratification, with irregular spacing	Similar to PIN 1; more crowding and stratification	Similar to PIN 2; occasional luminal bridging	Localized proliferation of small, round glands
Cytology				
Nuclei	Enlarged, with marked size variation	Enlarged; some size variation	Marked enlargement; some size variation	Normal
Chromatin	Normal	Increased	Markedly increased	Normal
Nucleoli	Infrequent	Occasionally large and prominent	Frequently large; similar to invasive carcinoma	Normal or infrequent
Basal cell layer	Intact	Intact	May show some disruption	Absent
Basement membrane	Intact	Intact	May show some disruption	?
Adjacent prostatic epithelium	Usually proliferative	Usually proliferative	Usually proliferative	Usually atrophic
Architectural pattern of associated carcinoma[a]	Tubular-scirrhous endometrioid	Tubular-scirrhous endometrioid	Tubular-scirrhous endometrioid	Alveolar-medullary
Gleason grade of associated carcinoma[b]	3,4,5	3,4,5	3,4,5	1,2

[a] Architectural patterns of carcinoma described by McNeal[14,15] (alveolar-medullary and tubular-scirrhous) and by Bostwick[66] (endometrioid).
[b] Gleason grading system.
(From Bostwick,[73] with permission.)

ment of the normal lumenal secretory epithelium by neoplastic cells, with preservation of the basal cell layer and basement membrane; in advanced cases, foci of high-grade PIN may be indistinguishable from ductal spread of carcinoma and cribriform carcinoma.[3] The second pattern is *pagetoid* spread along ducts, characterized by invagination of neoplastic cells between the basal cell layer and the columnar secretory cell layer. The third pattern of spread of PIN is direct invasion through the ductal or acinar wall, with disruption of the basal cell layer and basement membrane.[1, 4]

ATYPICAL ADENOMATOUS HYPERPLASIA

Atypical adenomatous hyperplasia (AAH), or *adenosis,* is a tightly packed cluster of small acinar structures lined by cuboidal to low-columnar cells[5, 6] (Fig. 4-4 and 4-5; Table 4-1). The glands are single, small, and discrete, with round to oval outlines. Size is usually uniform, with some glands appearing twice the diameter of the smallest glands; tangential sectioning may create rare enlarged elongate tubular glands, usually at the periphery. The small acinar structures push into the stroma, occasionally impart-

Fig. 4-1. PIN 1–2. There is cell crowding and nuclear enlargement. (×200.)

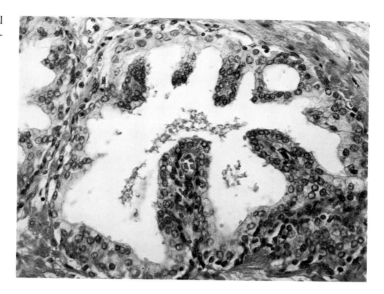

ing a back-to-back arrangement. The glands can also appear loose at the periphery, apparently infiltrating into the adjacent stroma.

AAH may arise at duct branches, with budding of newly formed acini identical in size and appearance to the duct itself. As these glands extend away from the apparent site of origin, they lose some of their uniformity and orderly arrangement. Although these foci are frequently circumscribed and form rounded nodules, at the periphery there may be focal irregularity, suggesting a limited degree of invasiveness. No compression of the surrounding tissues is observed.

The cells within AAH are virtually identical to those of the normal prostate, appearing as cuboidal to columnar cells with pale to clear cytoplasm, round basal nuclei, and uniform granular chromatin. Small lumenal corpora amylacea may be observed. Sharp pointed crystalloids are occasionally found. Frequently, AAH may have an involutional atrophic appearance, similar to adjacent prostatic ductal epithelium. The basal cell layer may be inconspicuous or absent by light microscopy. Mild nuclear pleomorphism may be observed.

AAH is distinguished from well-differentiated

carcinoma by the absence of prominent nucleoli, with the nucleoli in carcinoma appearing larger than 1 μm in diameter.[7, 8] An occasional small basophilic nucleolus may be observed after diligent search in AAH. In cases with diagnostic difficulty, serial sections of the tissue block should be obtained to search for prominent nucleoli. Consequently, an atypical glandular proliferation within the prostate should be evaluated carefully for the presence or absence of nucleoli in order to distinguish AAH from well-differentiated carcinoma. Although lumenal mucin may be observed in AAH, the presence of acid mucin[9–12] and crystalloids[13] would suggest well-differentiated adenocarcinoma.

EVIDENCE FOR THE ASSOCIATION OF PREMALIGNANT LESIONS WITH CARCINOMA

PROSTATIC INTRAEPITHELIAL NEOPLASIA

Putative premalignant epithelial changes were first described by McNeal[14, 15] in 1965. His work is notable for the demonstration of PIN and

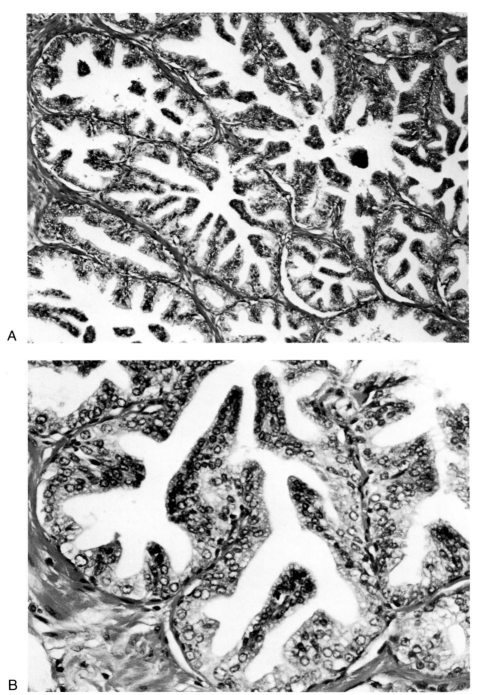

Fig. 4-2. PIN 2. (**A**) Proliferative changes involve adjacent ductules. (×115.) (**B**) At higher magnification, the dysplastic cells are disordered, and occasional prominent nucleoli are present. (×250.) (*Figure continues.*)

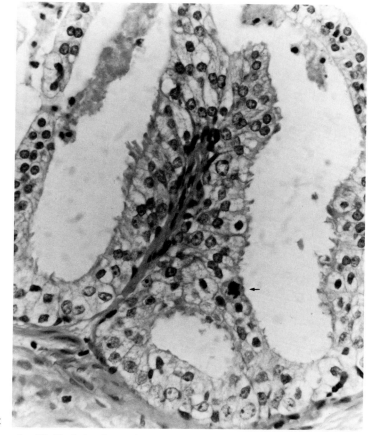

C

Fig. 4-2 (*Continued*). (**C**) Variation in nuclear size, scattered prominent nucleoli up to 2 μm in diameter, and rare mitotic figures (arrow), features diagnostic of PIN 2–3, despite the absence of significant cell crowding. (×560.)

prostatic carcinoma arising from active proliferative epithelium and not from atrophic epithelium, as previously thought.[16] He also noted that premalignant lesions and carcinoma were usually found in the peripheral zone of the prostate, and multifocality was frequently observed.

Other investigators have noted the architectural and cytologic similarity of PIN and invasive carcinoma.[1, 7, 17–23] In the European literature, Helpap and Kastendieck confirmed the existence of atypical epithelial proliferations of the prostate and their close association with adenocarcinoma. Helpap[17] noted that "atypical primary hyperplasia" had more than three times the proliferative activity of benign glands, an

increase similar to that seen with invasive carcinoma. Kastendieck[19] demonstrated foci of dysplasia in 60 percent of radical prostatectomies with carcinoma, and he described four different patterns of dysplasia: cribriform, papillary, tubular, and adenomatous. His morphologic criteria included varying degrees of cytologic atypia, irregular glandular architecture, and disorganization of the interface between glands and stroma. Unfortunately, Kastendieck did not include a control group of prostates without carcinoma, and he and Helpap did not share a common histologic nomenclature. The lesions that these two European investigators studied encompassed a variety of histologic patterns for

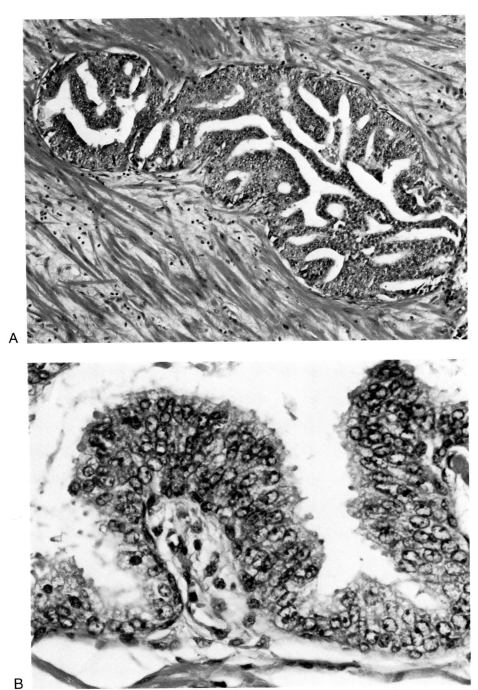

Fig. 4-3. (A & B) PIN 3. Large prominent nucleoli are present in the majority of cells. (Fig. A, ×125; Fig. B, ×425.)

Fig. 4-4. AAH. This circumscribed unencapsulated proliferation of small round glands may be confused with well-differentiated adenocarcinoma. (×45.)

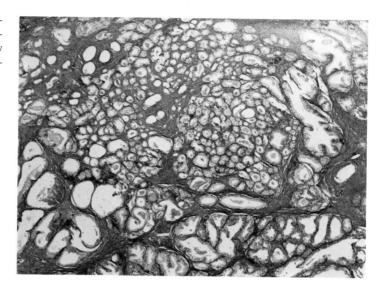

which the diagnostic criteria were not precisely defined.[17–19]

McNeal and Bostwick[20] refined the criteria for PIN (intraductal dysplasia), identifying three grades of increasing severity and providing additional evidence that these lesions were precancerous (Table 4-2). In their report, they noted foci of PIN in 82 percent of prostates with carcinoma, but in only 43 percent of benign prostates. This work was confirmed by Troncosco et al.[21] and Kovi et al.,[22] who showed a statistically significant increase in the frequency of PIN in prostates with cancer when compared with prostates without cancer after step sectioning of entire prostates (Table 4-3). Kovi et al. demonstrated that the prevalence of PIN in malignant glands increased with age, and that these intraepithelial lesions appeared to predate the onset of carcinoma by more than 5 years. Srigley et al.[23] observed foci of PIN in 2 percent of prostates with nodular hyperplasia.

The area of the prostate showing PIN was

Fig. 4-5. AAH (same case as Figure 4-4). Although scattered chromocenters are present within many of the nuclei, none are prominent (larger than 1 μm in diameter). (×280.)

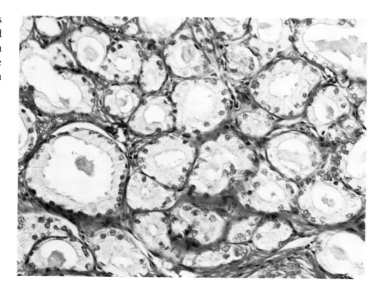

Table 4-2. Evidence for the Association of Prostatic Intraepithelial Neoplasia (PIN) and Prostatic Carcinoma

Histology[1,2,7,8,14,20–22]
 Similar architectural and cytologic features.

Location[14,20]
 Both are located in the peripheral zone.

Correlation with proliferative activity[17]
 Both have more than 3 times the proliferative activity
  of benign glands.

Loss of basal cell layer[1]
 Highest grade of PIN has loss of basal cell layer,
  similar to carcinoma.

Increased frequency of PIN in the presence of
  carcinoma[1,14,17,19,20]
 With higher grades of PIN, there is a statistically significant increase in the frequency of carcinoma.

Increased extent of PIN in the presence of carcinoma[20]
 With higher grades of PIN, there is a statistically significant increase in the frequency of carcinoma.

Increased severity of PIN in the presence of carcinoma[1,20]
 With higher grades of PIN, there is a statistically significant increase in the frequency of carcinoma.

Immunophenotype[24–27]
 Both are immunoreactive for cytokeratins 14, 15, 16,
  and 19, unlike nodular hyperplasia.
 Both show Ulex europeus binding, unlike normal epithelium and nodular hyperplaisa.
 Both show loss of vimentin immunoreactivity, unlike
  nodular hyperplasia.
 Both show loss of blood group A, B, Le[a] and Le[b]
  expression, unlike normal epithelium.

Origin[1,14,20]
 Carcinoma found to arise in foci of PIN.

Age[22]
 Age incidence peak precedes carcinoma.

Prostate-specific antigen (PSA)[35]
 Serum PSA levels intermediate between normal and
  invasive carcinoma.

(Modified from Bostwick,[74] with permission.)

increased in the presence of carcinoma; PIN was present in more than 1 low-power microscopic field in 41 percent of prostates containing carcinoma, but in only 9 percent of prostates without carcinoma.[20] Also, the grade (or severity) of PIN was greater in prostates with carcinoma; PIN 3 was found in 33 percent of prostates with cancer but in only 4 percent of benign prostates.

PIN is closely related to carcinoma according to immunophenotypic studies.[24–27] Both showed intense cytoplasmic immunoreactivity for cytokeratins 14, 15, 16, and 19 in more than 90 percent of luminal cells, unlike nodular hyperplasia, which showed reactivity in only 6 percent. *Ulex europaeus* showed a similar pattern of staining.[24] Other lectin binding studies have shown defective glycosylation of proteins in foci of PIN,[25] indicating impairment of differentiated cell function, although this work has been refuted.[24, 26] Vimentin immunoreactivity is absent in PIN and carcinoma, but is present in 93 percent of luminal cells of nodular hyperplasia. Expression of A, B, and Lewis blood group antigens is also absent in PIN and carcinoma, but is observed in up to 15 percent of normal prostatic epithelium.[26] McNeal et al.[27] demonstrated progressive reduction of cytoplasmic immunoreactivity for prostate specific antigen, prostatic acid phosphatase, and Leu-7 with increasing severity of PIN, suggesting that loss of biochemical differentiation appears early during the preinvasive phase of prostatic carcinoma. However, this work was performed on formalin-fixed paraffin-embedded tissues, and other investigators[18] have not been able to reproduce these results using frozen sections of prostate.

Table 4-3. Prostatic Intraepithelial Neoplasia (PIN): Incidence in Step-Sectioned Whole Prostates

	Number of Prostates Examined	Prostates Without Carcinoma (% PIN)	Prostates With Carcinoma (% PIN)
McNeal and Bostwick,[20] 1986[a]	200	43	82
Troncoso et al.,[21] 1988	30	60	100
Kovi et al.,[22] 1988[b]	429	46	59.2

[a] PIN referred to as *intraductal dysplasia*.
[b] PIN referred to as *large acinar atypical hyperplasia*.
(From Bostwick,[73] with permission.)

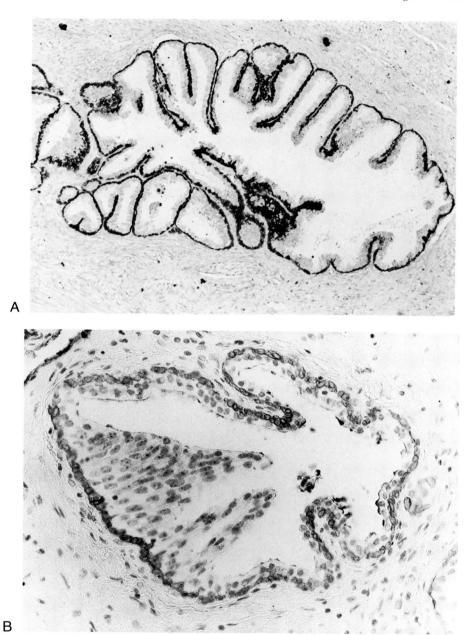

Fig. 4-6. The keratin-immunoreactive basal cell layer is invariably intact in PIN 1–2 (**A**), and is frequently intact in PIN 3 (**B**). (Immunoperoxidase keratin and hematoxylin.)

McNeal[14, 15] had originally described carcinoma arising in foci of PIN, and this was demonstrated immunohistochemically by Bostwick and Brawer.[1] Employing an antikeratin monoclonal antibody directed against the basal cell layer of the prostate, these investigators identified progressive disruption of the basal cell layer with increasing grades of PIN (Fig. 4-6). Early invasive carcinoma was shown to occur at sites of glandular outpouching and basal cell disrup-

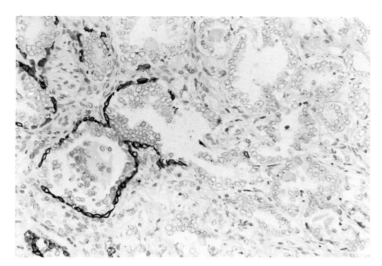

Fig. 4-7. Focus of PIN 3 with partially disrupted basal cell layer and invasive carcinoma. Note the absence of an immunoreactive basal cell layer around the malignant glands. (Immunoperoxidase keratin and hematoxylin.)

tion (Fig. 4-7). Barsky et al.[28] and Beckman et al.[4] had previously shown loss of the basement membrane in invasive carcinoma, and Bostwick and Brawer included these findings in construction of a morphologic continuum for PIN and early carcinoma (Fig. 4-8).

The term *prostate intraepithelial neoplasia* was proposed as an alternative to McNeal's[1] *intraductal dysplasia*, similar to the terminology of premalignant lesions in other organs. This proposal was based on the conclusions of Rywlin[29] and others[30] that the term *dysplasia* was ambiguous and should be retained only for

its classical meaning as a malformation resulting from abnormal embryonic anlage. Also, because the precise location within the prostate is not known for the origin of these lesions, the terms *intraglandular, intraductal,* and *intra-acinar* were considered inappropriate. Other synonymous terms have been proposed, including *large acinar atypical hyperplasia,*[22] *atypical primary hyperplasia,*[6] *hyperplasia with malignant change,*[31] *marked atypia,*[32] and *duct-acinar dysplasia,*[27] but these are considered awkward and have the same deficiencies as *intraductal dysplasia.* Replacement of all of these terms by PIN

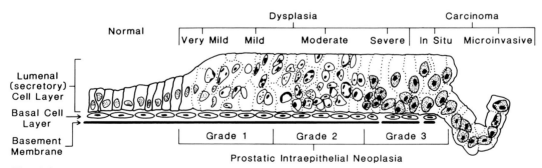

Fig. 4-8. Diagram of carcinogenesis in the human prostate. According to the disease continuum concept, Grade 1 PIN corresponds to very mild to mild dysplasia, Grade 2 to moderate dysplasia, and Grade 3 to severe dysplasia–carcinoma in situ. The precursor stage ends when malignant cells invade the stroma; this invasion occurs where the basal cell layer is disrupted and the basement membrane is fragmented. Notice that the dysplastic changes occur in the superficial (lumenal) secretory cell layer, perhaps in response to lumenal carcinogens. The basal cell layer and basement membrane are disrupted with high-grade dysplasia or early invasive carcinoma. (From Bostwick and Brawer,[1] with permission.)

has been endorsed by consensus at a recent international conference.[30]

Heatfield and associates[33] have concluded that neoplastic transformation in the prostate occurs directly from columnar secretory cells, in contrast with their previous suggestion of a role for basal cells in transformation.[34] These investigators noted that in human prostate explant cultures, a stratified metaplastic epithelium was regenerated by the basal cells, with absence of all columnar secretory cells. This basal cell regeneration was hormone-independent, and appeared to maintain the integrity of the epithelium, similar to the basal cell proliferation seen in vivo at the periphery of foci of prostatic infarction. In these cases, there appeared to be no replenishment of the columnar secretory cell layer. These investigators also showed that the basal cells displayed a stable phenotype in vivo and in vitro, with no evidence of metaplastic or neoplastic transformation of the columnar secretory cells. Heatfield and associates believed that these observations supported direct neoplastic transformation of columnar secretory cells, similar to the morphologic continuum proposed by Bostwick and Brawer.

Serum levels of prostate-specific antigen (PSA) were frequently elevated in patients with PIN, ranging from 0.3 to 22.3 mg/ml (mean 4.0).[35] It was suggested that PSA may be useful in the early detection of these lesions.[35] In addition, 11 percent of hypoechoic lesions identified by transrectal ultrasound are PIN.[36]

It is expected that DNA ploidy analysis of tissue sections showing PIN will reveal DNA content intermediate between normal and cancerous tissues; such results should be available in the next few years.

Atypical Adenomatous Hyperplasia

In a large series of autopsy prostates, McNeal[14, 15] recognized atypical glandular proliferations that he termed *atypical adenomatous hyperplasia* (AAH). He noted that these distinct lesions shared some but not all of the features of well-differentiated adenocarcinoma. This histologic similarity has been confirmed by other investigators[5, 7, 19, 23] (Table 4-4).

Brawn[5] described a similar atypical glandular proliferation that he termed *adenosis*. He noted that *adenosis* could be confused with *adenocarcinoma*, but also stated that there were "no absolute histologic criteria to separate these two entities." Brawn demonstrated that 6.4 percent of patients with adenosis developed prostatic carcinoma in a follow-up period of 5 to 15 years, compared with 3.7 percent of patients with nodular hyperplasia; no statistical analyses were performed by that investigator, and he did not refer to the previous work by McNeal. Also, other authors[7] have interpreted Brawn's moderate and severe adenosis (noted in Figure 4 of his article) as well-differentiated adnocarcinoma, and his mild adenosis as AAH. Despite the differences in diagnostic criteria and nomenclature, Brawn's conclusions were in agreement with those of McNeal and others that atypical proliferations are associated with prostatic carcinoma. Kastendieck's[19] "adenomatous pattern" of primary atypical hyperplasia appears to be similar to AAH, although the investigator included cellular atypia in his description.

Gleason[7] verified the existence of both AAH and PIN, having noted similar lesions during the Veterans Administration study of over 2,000 human prostates that resulted in the Gleason grading system of prostatic carcinoma. Srigley et al.[23] observed foci of AAH in 20 percent of prostates with nodular hyperplasia.

AAH is found most frequently in the periph-

Table 4-4. Evidence for the Association of Atypical Adenomatous Hyperplasia (AAH) and Prostatic Carcinoma

Histology[5–7,14]: Similar architectural features.

Location[14]: Both are located in the peripheral zone.

Loss of basal cell layer.[1,18]

Increased frequency of AAH in the presence of carcinoma.[5,14,20]

Correlation with proliferative activity[17]: Both have greater proliferative activity than benign glands.

Carcinoma found to arise in foci of AAH.[14]

Age incidence peak precedes carcinoma.[37]

(Modified from Bostwick,[74] with permission.)

eral zone of the prostate, but may also be seen in the central zone, similar to adenocarcinoma. European investigators[17] showed that the ^{3}H-thymidine labeling index of small acinar lesions was significantly higher than that of benign nodular hyperplasia and similar to that of small acinar carcinoma. Also, the age for peak incidence of AAH preceded that of carcinoma.[37]

Basal cell-specific antikeratin monoclonal antibodies may be useful in distinguishing AAH from well-differentiated adenocarcinoma. Hedrick and Epstein[38] reported intense discontinuous staining of the basal cell layer in 60 to 90 percent of glands with AAH, and complete absence of immunoreactivity in well-differentiated carcinoma. Other studies[1, 18] reported that AAH exhibited no immunoreactivity; these differences in results may be due to variations in the diagnosis of AAH. Further studies are necessary to determine the status of the basement membrane and basal cell layer in AAH.

The increased frequency of AAH in the presence of carcinoma suggests that this lesion has some predictive value for malignancy, although this has not been tested statistically. Carcinoma has been shown to arise in foci of AAH, but there may be some difficulty in precisely defining the point of transition. One could argue that the presence of AAH in association with carcinoma is an epiphenomenon. Only long-term prospective follow-up studies of patients with AAH using a variety of tissue sampling techniques would provide proof that AAH is truly premalignant. Nonetheless, at the present time, most investigators consider AAH as a marker for the development of adenocarcinoma.[6]

DIFFERENTIAL DIAGNOSIS AND DIAGNOSTIC PITFALLS

NORMAL ANATOMIC STRUCTURES

Seminal Vesicles and Ejaculatory Ducts

The seminal vesicles and ejaculatory ducts are anatomically and histologically heterogenous. The seminal vesicles display variability in size and location between individuals, and may be located partly within the prostatic substance, merging into the ejaculatory ducts. Both of these normal anatomic structures can be confused with AAH or small acinar carcinoma (Table 4-5), particularly in limited tissues samples such as needle biopsies[6, 39] (Fig. 4-9). The small glands from these structures appear to bud off of adjacent larger glands, and may be haphazardly arranged in the stroma, simulating malignancy. The cytologic features, particularly in the aging seminal vesicle, may also suggest malignancy, and are of significant concern in needle biopsies and in cytologic preparations of prostatic aspirations.[40, 41] Lipofuscin may be scanty, although the presence of this golden pigment is the single most useful feature in distinguishing seminal vesicle from adenocarcinoma. Coyne et al.[39] reported that the absence of immunoperoxidase staining for PSA is the most specific method for identifying seminal vesicular epithelium. The incidence of seminal vesicle epithelium in prostatic needle-biopsy

Table 4-5. Differential Diagnosis of Premalignant Lesions of the Prostate

Normal anatomic structures
    Seminal vesicles and ejaculatory ducts
    Cowper's glands
    Paraganglionic tissue

Hyperplasia
    Florid benign papillary/cribriform hyperplasia
    Basal cell hyperplasia
        Complete
        Incomplete (acinar)
    Atrophy and atrophy-associated hyperplasia
        Simple lobular atrophy
        Sclerotic atrophy
        Postatrophic hyperplasia
        Sclerosing adenosis

Metaplasia and reactive atypia
    Transitional metaplasia
    Infarction-induced atypia
    Inflammation-induced atypia
    Radiation-induced atypia

Carcinoma
    Small-acinar carcinoma
    Transitional cell carcinoma
    Cribriform carcinoma
    ''Endometrioid'' carcinoma

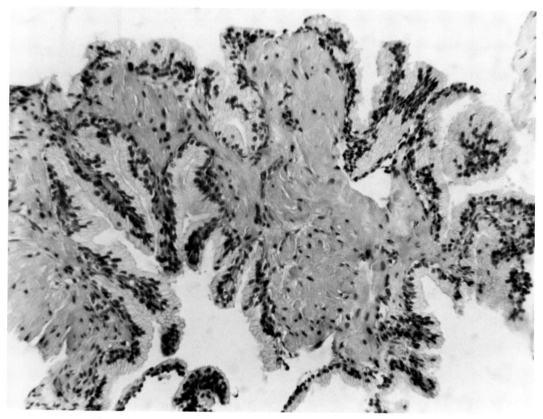

Fig. 4-9. Fragment of seminal vesicle found in a needle biopsy. (×220.)

specimens is approximately 5 percent. Adenocarcinoma arising from the seminal vesicles is rare, and, when present, usually displays a papillary or anaplastic pattern with mucin production.[42]

Cowper's Glands

Cowper's glands should be considered in the differential diagnosis of glandular proliferations. These glands are present lateral to the distal prostatic urethra, with their ducts opening into the proximal membranous urethra. They are composed of lobules of closely packed uniform acini lined by cytologically bland cells with abundant apical mucinous cytoplasm. Nuclei are inconspicuous. Fragments of these glands may be observed in sectioned specimens or needle biopsies, especially in those obtained transperineally. Recognition of these glands will avoid misdiagnosis. Carcinoma of Cowper's gland is rare, and is characterized by frank anaplasia of tumor cells.

Paraganglionic Tissue

Rarely, normal paraganglionic tissue may be observed in protatic tissue specimens.[6] It shows tightly packed uniform cells without glandular lumina arranged in an organoid pattern.

HYPERPLASIA

Epithelial hyperplasia exhibits a variety of histologic patterns that may be confused with PIN and AAH.

Florid Papillary-Cribriform Hyperplasia

Florid benign papillary-cribriform hyperplasia appears as papillary fronds or grows in a sieve-like (cribriform) pattern, usually in the setting of nodular hyperplasia (Fig. 4-10). These exuberant growths are distinguished from PIN by the uniform proliferation of large cells with pale cytoplasm. Some variation in size and shape of nuclei is seen, but this is not a prominent feature. Nucleoli are conspicuous only in the deeper layers. Ayala and colleagues[43] described the clear-cell variant of cribriform hyperplasia, characterized by preservation of a nodular configuration with bland cytology and double cell layer. Cribriform hyperplasia is distinguished from intraductal cribriform carcinoma by the absence of nuclear and cytologic anaplasia.[3]

Basal Cell Hyperplasia

Basal cell hyperplasia appears as circumscribed clusters of small uniform cytologically bland cells with scant cytoplasm forming acinar structures and solid nests (Fig. 4-11). These nests may be closely packed or separated by fibrous bands, and commonly merge with areas of nodular hyperplasia. When solitary, basal cell hyperplasia has been referred to as *basal cell adenoma*. Others[44-48] have noted the resemblance of this lesion to the fetal prostate owing to the presence of nests of basaloid cells within a cellular stroma. Basal cell hyperplasia is clinically benign and is thought to be a histologic variant of nodular hyperplasia.

In the complete form of basal cell hyperplasia, the proliferation is composed of only basaloid cells, with no secretory (lumenal) differentia-

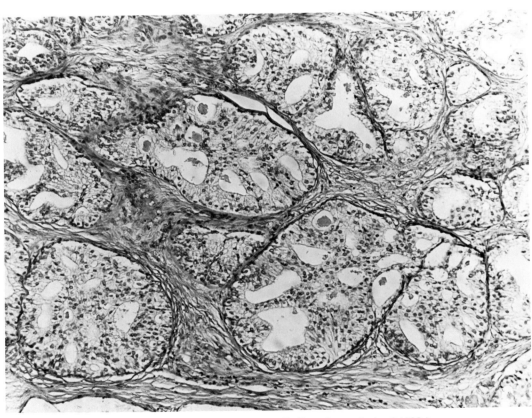

Fig. 4-10. Clear cell pattern of cribriform hyperplasia. (×120.)

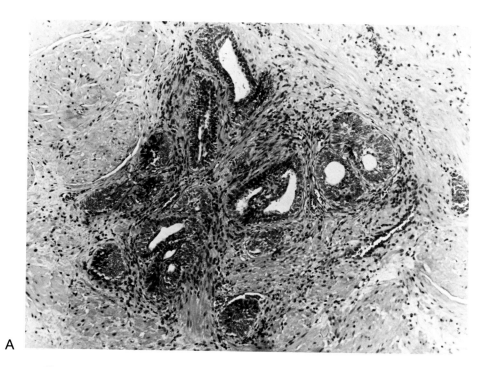

A

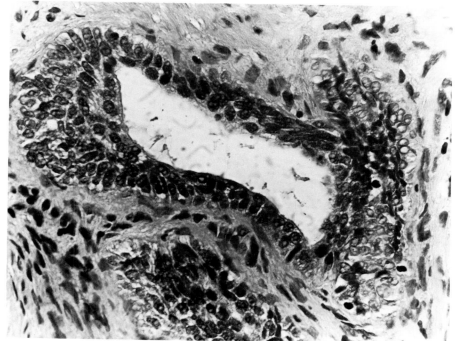

B

Fig. 4-11. (**A & B**) Basal cell hyperplasia. (Fig. A, ×40; Fig B, ×360.)

tion. In the incomplete form of basal cell hyperplasia, two cell types are observed, with the basaloid nests containing small lumina lined by cuboidal secretory cells.[6]

Basal cell hyperplasia must be distinguished from AAH, transitional cell carcinoma, and well-differentiated adenocarcinoma. Basal cell-specific antikeratin monoclonal antibodies are useful in making this distinction.[49, 50]

Atrophy and Atrophy-Associated Hyperplasia

Atrophic changes in the normal aging prostate are a normal finding, and frequently exhibit secondary hyperplastic changes. The histologic features are variable, and may be confused with AAH. Patchy lobular atrophy frequently coexists with hyperplasia, and both have been noted in prostates of young adults.[51] Atrophy is characterized by small condensed closely packed hyperchromatic glands that retain their distinctive lobular configuration. The basal cell layer is usually identifiable, and the intralobular stroma appears atrophic with shrunken fibromuscular elements. Nucleoli are inconspicuous.

When atrophic glands are associated with stromal sclerosis (sclerotic atrophy), the atrophic acini are widely separated by intervening stroma, and appear elongated and distorted by proliferative periacinar collagen (Fig. 4-12). The glands retain their double cell layer, although the flattened and attenuated darkly staining basal cells may be difficult to appreciate. Nuclei are hyperchromatic, but no prominent nucleoli are observed, and the cells within the glands are cuboidal, flattened, and darkly staining. The greatest diagnostic difficulty is distinguishing sclerotic atrophy from tumor-induced desmoplasia, particularly in needle-biopsy specimens.

Atrophic glands may become proliferative, a change referred to by some investigators as *postatrophic hyperplasia*. Although Franks[52] considered this change as an evolutionary stage of early adenocarcinoma, this has been convincingly disputed by more recent investigators.[14, 15, 53] Postatrophic hyperplasia may coexist with simple lobular atrophy and sclerotic atrophy. The hyperplastic changes usually involve the entire lobule, and tightly packed new acini appear to bud off pre-existing small atrophic ducts. The double cell layer is maintained, and nuclei appear uniform and bland without prominent nucleoli. The atrophic stroma

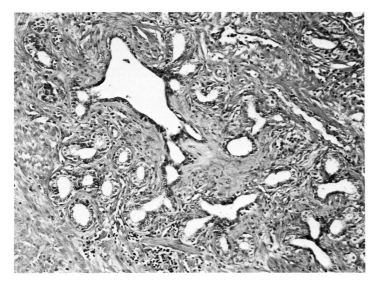

Fig. 4-12. Sclerotic atrophy of the prostate. (×100.)

is usually still apparent, and this may be a useful diagnostic clue. When occurring in association with sclerotic atrophy, secondary hyperplasia mimics small-acinar adenocarcinoma. In this setting, small acini bud off atrophic ducts and appear to push into adjacent dense sclerotic stroma, becoming separated from one another. The lack of back-to-back arrangement and acinar separation with pseudoinvasion can cause considerable diagnostic difficulty. The lumina are usually small and may be empty or contain small amounts of secretion. The double-layered epithelium is present, but may be inconspicuous. Nucleoli are small, but the nuclear hyperchromasia may make this evaluation difficult. It is interesting to note that small-acinar carcinoma is less likely to cause an irregular stromal desmoplastic response.

Sclerosing adenosis of the prostate is a recently described entity that is morphologically analogous to sclerosing adenosis of the breast.[54, 55] It may represent one end of the histologic spectrum of postsclerotic hyperplasia, characterized by small irregular distorted glands embedded in a stromal matrix of immature fibroblasts and abundant ground substance. One investigator[6] has suggested calling these *pseudoadenomatoid tumors*.

METAPLASIA AND REACTIVE ATYPIA

Transitional Metaplasia

Transitional metaplasia consists of transitional epithelium within ducts and acini of the prostate beyond the normal transitional-columnar junction, arising apparently as a result of metaplastic change. In fragmented specimens such as transurethral sections, difficulty may be encountered in distinguishing metaplasia from normal urothelium, and the diagnosis of metaplasia may be overused. Transitional metaplasia is clinically benign and readily distinguished from PIN by its characteristic architectural and cytologic features.

Infarction-Induced Atypia

Infarction-induced atypia consists of replacement of normal prostatic epithelium by flattened squamous or transitional epithelium (Fig. 4-13). Prostatic infarcts are present in 25 percent of prostates with nodular hyperplasia, and may occur in the central, transitional, or peripheral zone. These foci may be confused with PIN or invasive carcinoma owing to the presence

Fig. 4-13. Infarction-induced atypia. Note the presence of prominent nucleoli and rare mitotic figures (arrow) at the edge of an infarct. (×360.)

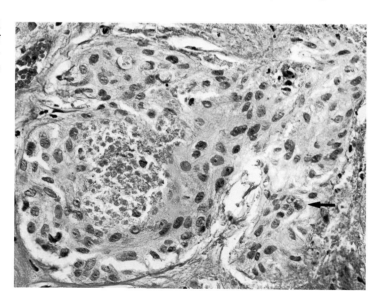

of prominent nucleoli within cells, particularly in areas of recent infarction.

Inflammation-Induced Atypia

Inflammation-induced atypia may simulate PIN, and caution is warranted in diagnosing PIN in this setting. Granulomatous prostatitis is a known source of diagnostic concern, and may be mistaken for PIN or invasive carcinoma. In less-involved areas at the periphery, there may be reactive atypia of the epithelium with hyperplasia and prominent nucleoli. Recognition of the histologic features of granulomatous prostatitis and consideration of it in the differential diagnosis will usually avoid this pitfall.

Radiation-Induced Atypia

Radiation-induced atypia comprises a variety of morphologic changes, including atrophy,

squamous metaplasia, and cytologic changes of prostatic glands and urothelium.[56] There may also be stromal fibrosis with atypical fibroblasts, myointimal proliferation of vessels, and atrophy and fibrosis of seminal vessels. Cytologic atypia of glands was present in the majority of irradiated samples according a recent study, and may be indistinguishable from PIN.[56]

CARCINOMA

Small-Acinar Carcinoma

Small-acinar carcinoma is one of many growth patterns of prostatic adenocarcinoma, and is the most difficult to distinguish from AAH[6] (Table 4-6). AAH is more frequent in the central zone, in contrast with small-acinar carcinoma. Architecturally, a variety of features are useful in distinguishing these two lesions. At low power, AAH tends to be well circumscribed, conforming to Gleason's pattern 1 to 2, displaying pushing borders at the periphery.

Table 4-6. Atypical Adenomatous Hyperplasia (AAH) and Small-Acinar Carcinoma: Histologic Features

	Atypical Adenomatous Hyperplasia (AAH)	Small-Acinar Carcinoma
Most frequent location	Central zone	Peripheral zone
Architectural features		
Low-power appearance	Well-circumscribed (Gleason pattern 1, sometimes 2)	Less-circumscribed (Gleason pattern 1,2, and sometimes 3)
Peripheral borders	Pushing	Often infiltrative, splitting fibromuscular bundles
Relation to parent duct	Yes, with budding acini	Often not related
Acinar size and shape	Usually variable	Usually uniform
Cytologic features		
Nuclear configuration	Similar to cells of parent	Different from adjacent benign glands
Chromatin pattern	Uniform distribution	Frequently irregular with clumping and clearing
Nucleoli	Usually absent; may be minute and similar to those of adjacent benign glands	Often prominent, irregular, and acidophilic
Cytoplasm	Clear	Acidophilic or clear
Other features		
Luminal crystalloids	Rare	Frequent
Luminal corpora amylacea	Occasionally present	Acidophilic or clear
Basophilic (mucinous material)	Rare	Frequent

(Modified from Srigley,[6] with permission.)

Rarely, an infiltrating pattern similar to Gleason's pattern 3 may be noted. The acini are frequently arranged around a benign "parent" gland. Small-acinar carcinoma is a proliferation of small glands that may be back-to-back with pushing borders, or appear looser and show infiltration into the stroma with splitting of muscle fibers. Interestingly, small-acinar carcinoma tends to have greater uniformity in size and shape of glands than does AAH.

The nuclei of small-acinar carcinoma frequently show a subtle degree of pleomorphism, chromatin clumping, and chromatic rim thickening, and at least a few of the cells contain significantly enlarged nucleoli (greater than or equal to 1 μm). Nuclear changes may be focal or widespread, and are best appreciated on thin sections with light to moderate hematoxylin staining. These enlarged nucleoli are often eosinophilic and display some pleomorphism and variation in size. The cytoplasm of small-acinar carcinoma may be vacuolated, but is more often eosinophilic, granular, or slightly basophilic.

Other histologic features may be useful in distinguishing AAH and small-acinar carcinoma. Lumenal crystalloids are more frequent in adenocarcinoma, but have been observed in atypical hyperplasia.[57-59] Crystalloids were initially thought to be related to Bence Jones proteins, but subsequent ultrastructural and immunohistochemical studies have shown that this is not the case; instead, they are thought to represent some form of altered lumenal secretion.[13] Lumenal corpora amylacea are not observed in small-acinar carcinoma, but may be seen in atypical adenomatous hyperplasia. Mucin histochemistry may be of some value, with acidic mucins present in adenocarcinoma and not in uninvolved glands.[9-11] The presence of abundant luminal mucin on alcian blue staining (acid mucin) can sometimes confirm a diagnosis of adenocarcinoma. Immunoperoxidase stains for prostate specific antigen (PSA) and prostatic acid phosphatase (PAP) appear to be of little value in making the differential diagnosis of small-acinar carcinoma and atypical adenomatous hyperplasia, because cells of both stain intensely with these markers.[6]

Transitional Cell Carcinoma

Prostatic ducts and acini with transitional cell carcinoma may be confused with PIN. Transitional cell carcinoma of the prostate is usually associated with synchronous or metachronous carcinoma in the bladder, although primary prostatic and urethral involvement have been described.[60-65] These tumors are clinically distinguished from adenocarcinoma by the lack of responsiveness to hormonal therapy, normal levels of serum PAP, and lack of a palpable prostatic nodule.[64] The histologic features of transitional cell carcinoma of the prostate are identical to those of the bladder. Hardeman and Soloway[64] noted that transitional cell carcinoma of the bladder extending into the prostate can easily be missed cystoscopically, and random biopsies of the prostate were recommended. Although terms such as *ductal carcinoma* and *carcinoma in situ* have been used to describe this entity, we prefer the name *transitional cell carcinoma in situ.*[61-63] Some confusion may arise from the use of the term *ductal carcinoma* because this has also been used to describe some cases of prostatic adenocarcinoma with endometrioid features.[66]

Cribriform Carcinoma and Endometrioid Carcinoma

Other histologic variants of prostatic adenocarcinoma may also be confused with premalignant lesions. *Cribriform* carcinoma consists of large epithelial cell masses punctuated by multiple small lumens, imparting a sieve-like appearance.[3] It is usually present within ducts, frequently displaying lumenal necrosis, and may arise adjacent to foci of PIN. *Endometrioid* carcinoma consists of malignant glands and papillae growing within the prostatic urethra, usually near the verumontanum, and giving rise to obstructive symptoms.[66] When appearing within ducts, both of these variants of adenocarcinoma may mimic PIN 3 (carcinoma in situ). It is important to search for evidence of stromal invasion in making this distinction.

CLINICAL SIGNIFICANCE

NATURAL HISTORY OF PROSTATE CANCER

One of the first steps in understanding the natural history of cancer is the identification of premalignant lesions. The multifocality of PIN and AAH in the peripheral zone suggests a "field" effect similar to multifocality of transitional cell carcinoma of the bladder, and supports the concept of carcinogens within the fluids bathing the prostatic epithelium.[1]

As premalignant lesions increase in size, there appears to be a progressive increase in aggressiveness. It has been shown that only tumors that have grown larger than 1 cc in volume have the ability to metastasize, and that larger tumors acquire poorly differentiated areas as a manifestation of tumor progression.[67] In the early stages of development of prostate cancer there appears to be a constant sequence of progression, although the chronology of this progression is not understood. It should be noted that studies to date have not determined whether PIN and AAH remain stable, regress, or progress, although the implication is that these lesions can progress. Leav et al.[68] recently reported induction of prostatic hyperplasia, dysplasia, and carcinoma in the Noble rat by administration of testosterone and 17-β-estradiol. This report in an animal model indicates that dysplasia may progress to carcinoma, and that long-term hormonal stimulation plays a significant role in the genesis of these lesions. Prospective studies are needed to assess the natural history of PIN and AAH.

REPORTING OF PREMALIGNANT LESIONS

As emphasized by McNeal and Bostwick,[20] the diagnosis of high-grade PIN (PIN 3) on biopsy warrants further search for concurrent invasive carcinoma. Lower grades of PIN were present too frequently in prostates without carcinoma to be useful for predicting the likelihood of invasive carcinoma elsewhere in the prostate. The high predictive value of PIN 3 as a marker for adenocarcinoma was considered the most important and clinically useful conclusion of their study.[20]

In view of the difficulty distinguishing minimal-deviation small-acinar carcinoma from AAH, pathologists may differ in their diagnostic threshold for low-grade acinar carcinoma.[6] Some pathologists may be influenced by treatment practices in the local urologic community, and may be reluctant to diagnose small-acinar carcinoma for fear of subjecting a patient to aggressive treatment that may or may not be indicated.

The pathologist must have an understanding of the criteria for distinguishing PIN and AAH from benign and malignant mimics, and should report the presence, severity, and extent of these lesions when present. Only by identifying and reporting premalignant lesions can further investigations be ensured and periodic re-examinations be undertaken. In difficult and borderline situations, it is wise for the pathologist to communicate closely with the urologist and to report as much information as possible.

It is important to recognize the cytologic features of PIN and AAH in order to avoid confusion with carcinoma in evaluating fine-needle aspirates of the prostate. Carcinoma was observed in 39 percent of 104 follow-up aspiration biopsies of patients with an original diagnosis of PIN 3, according to Park et al.[69] An additional 35 percent had recurrent PIN. Of 48 patients with clinical suspicion of carcinoma but with negative aspiration biopsy, follow-up aspiration revealed PIN in 15 (31 percent) and carcinoma in 8 (17 percent). These data indicate a strong association of PIN and adenocarcinoma, and suggest that vigorous diagnostic procedures are needed in patients suspected of having carcinoma. Oyasu et al.[70] noted that fine-needle aspiration specimens that rely on cytologic features may not allow dysplastic changes to be distinguished from prostatic carcinoma.

CLINICAL EVALUATION

Most investigators agree that the identification of premalignant lesions in the prostate should not influence therapeutic decisions. However, regular and long-term follow-up is warranted[71] (Table 4-7).

When PIN or AAH are encountered in prostatic specimens, all tissue should be embedded and made available for examination. Serial sections of suspicious foci may be useful. Antikeratin antibodies can be employed to determine the presence of basal cells, and this procedure can be applied to cytologic specimens as well as histologic sections. On transrectal ultrasound (TRUS), PIN and AAH appear as hypoechoic lesions, indistinguishable from carcinoma.[36, 72] In a series of 248 hypoechoic lesions reported by Torp-Pedersen et al.,[72] 11 percent consisted of PIN measuring 1.0 ± 0.39 cm in diameter. TRUS-directed biopsy, whether core biopsy or fine-needle aspiration biopsy, allows precise localization of the needle and the tissue being sampled. Repeat biopsy is suggested by some investigators if the first attempt is unrevealing. Serum PSA should be obtained, and may be elevated in patients with PIN.[35] If all procedures fail to identify coexistent carcinoma, then close surveillance and follow-up appears to be indicated.

REFERENCES

1. Bostwick DG, Brawer MK: Prostatic intra-epithelial neoplasia and early invasion in prostate cancer. Cancer 59:788, 1987
2. Kovi J, Jackson MA, Heshmat MY: Ductal spread in prostatic carcinoma. Cancer 56:1566, 1985
3. McNeal JE, Reese JH, Redwine EA, et al: Cribriform adenocarcinoma of the prostate. Cancer 58:1714, 1986
4. Beckman WC Jr, Camps JL Jr, Weissman RM, et al: The epithelial origin of a stromal cell population in adenocarcinoma of the rat prostate. Am J Pathol 128:555, 1987
5. Brawn PN: Adenosis of the prostate: a dysplastic lesion that can be confused with prostate adenocarcinoma. Cancer 49:826, 1982
6. Srigley JR: Small-acinar patterns in the prostate gland with emphasis on atypical adenomatous hyperplasia and small-acinar carcinoma. Semin Diagn Pathol 5:254, 1988
7. Gleason DF: Atypical hyperplasia, benign hyperplasia and well-differentiated adenocarcinoma of the prostate. Am J Surg Pathol 9:53, 1985 (suppl)
8. Helpap B: Observations on the numbers, size and localization of nucleoli in hyperplastic and neoplastic prostatic disease. Histopathology 13:203, 1988
9. Franks LM, O'Shea JD, Thomson AER: Mucin in the prostate: a histochemical study in normal glands, latent clinical and colloid cancers. Cancer 17:983, 1964
10. Hukhill PB, Vidkone RA: Histochemistry of mucous and other polysaccharides in tumors: carcinoma of the prostate. Lab Invest 16:395, 1967
11. Taylor NS: Histochemistry in the diagnosis of early prostatic carcinoma. Hum Pathol 10:513, 1979
12. Ro JY, Grignon DJ, Troncoso P, Ayala AG: Mucin in prostatic adenocarcinoma. Semin Diagn Pathol 5:273, 1988
13. Ro JY, Ayala AG, Ordonez NG, et al: Intraluminal crystalloids in prostatic adenocarcinoma: immunohistochemical, electron microscopic, and x-ray microanalytic studies. Cancer 57:2397, 1986
14. McNeal JE: Morphogenesis of prostatic carcinoma. Cancer 18:1659, 1965
15. McNeal JE: Origin and development of carcinoma in the prostate. Cancer 23:24, 1969
16. Franks LM: Atrophy and hyperplasia in the prostate proper. J Pathol Bacteriol 68:617, 1954
17. Helpap B: The biological significance of atypical hyperplasia of the prostate. Virchows Arch [A] 387:307, 1980
18. Helpap B: Dysplasia—terminology, histopathology, pathobiology, and significance. Urology 1989 (in press)
19. Kastendieck H: Correlations between atypical

primary hyperplasia and carcinoma of the prostate. Pathol Res Pract 169:366, 1980

20. McNeal JE, Bostwick DG: Intraductal dysplasia: a premalignant lesion of the prostate. Hum Pathol 17:64, 1986

21. Troncoso P, Ro J, Grignon D, et al: Prostatic intraepithelial neoplasia and invasive prostatic adenocarcinoma in cystoprostatectomy speciments. Lab Invest 58:95A, 1988

22. Kovi J, Mostofi FK, Heshmat MY, et al: Large acinar atypical hyperplasia and carcinoma of the prostate. Cancer 61:555, 1988

23. Srigley J, Toth P, Hartwick RWJ: Atypical histologic patterns in cases of benign prostatic hyperplasia. Lab Invest 60:90A, 1989

24. Nagle R, Brawer J, Clarke V: Immunophenotypic study of prostatic hyperplasia (BPH), dysplasia (PD) and carcinoma (CA). Lab Invest 60:65A, 1989

25. McNeal JE, Leav I, Alroy J, et al: Differential lectin staining of central and peripheral zones of the prostate and alterations in dysplasia. Am J Clin Pathol 89:41, 1988

26. Perlmen EJ, Epstein JI: Blood group antigen expression in dysplasia and adenocarcinoma of the prostate. Lab Invest 60: 72A, 1989

27. McNeal JE, Alroy J, Leav I, et al: Immunohistochemical evidence for impaired cell differentiation in the premalignant phase of prostate carcinogenesis. Am J Clin Pathol 90:23, 1988

28. Barsky SH, Siegal GP, Jannotta F, et al: Loss of basement membrane components by invasive tumors but not by their benign counterparts. Lab Invest 49:140, 1983

29. Rywlin AM: Terminology of premalignant lesions in light of the multistep theory of carcinogenesis. Hum Pathol 15:806, 1984

30. Workshop on Prostatic Intraepithelial Neoplasia: Significance and correlation with PSA and ultrasound urology. 1989 (in press)

31. Mostofi FK: Precancerous lesions of the prostate. p. 304. In Carter RL (ed): Precancerous States. Oxford University Press, New York, 1984

32. Miller A, Seljelid R: Cellular atypia in the prostate. Scand J Urol Nephrol 5:17, 1971

33. Heatfield BM, Sanefuji H, Trump BF: Role of basal cells in epithelial repair following ischemic injury in human prostate. Lab Invest 54:25A, 1986

34. Heatfield BM, Sanefuji H, Trump BF: Studies on carcinogenesis of human prostate. IV. Comparison of normal and neoplastic prostate during long-term explant culture. p. 659. In Trump BF: Scanning Electron Microscopy. Vol. III. AMF, SEM, Inc., O'Hare, IL, 1979

35. Brawer MK, Nagle RB: Prostatic intraductal dysplasia (intraepithelial neoplasia) and serum prostate specific antigen. Urology 1989 (in press)

36. Lee F, Torp-Pedersen ST, Carrol JP, et al: The use of transrectal ultrasound and prostate-specific antigen in the diagnosis of prostatic intraductal dysplasia. Urology 1989 (in press)

37. Altenahr E, Kastendieck H, Siefret H: Coincidence of prostatic carcinoma and dysplasia in total prostatectomies and in autopsies. Verh Dtsch Ges Pathol 63:415, 1979

38. Hedrick L, Epstein JI: Use of keratin 903 as an adjunct in the diagnosis of prostatic carcinoma. Lab Invest 58:38A, 1988

39. Coyne JD, Kealy WF, Annis P: Seminal vesicle epithelium in prostatic needle biopsy specimens. J Clin Pathol 40:932, 1987

40. Arias-Stella J, Takano-Moron J: Atypical epithelial changes in the seminal vesicles. Arch Pathol 66:761, 1958

41. Kuo T, Gomez LG: Monstrous epithelial cells in human epididymis and seminal vesicles: a pseudomalignant change. Am J Surg Pathol 5:483, 1981

42. Benson RC, Clarke WR, Farrow GN: Carcinoma of the seminal vesicle. J Urol 132:475, 1984

43. Ayala, AG, Srigley JR, Ro JY, et al: Clear cell cribriform hyperplasia of prostate. Am J Surg Pathol 10:665, 1986

44. Dermer GB: Basal cell proliferation in benign prostatic hyperplasia. Cancer 41:1857, 1978

45. Lin JI, Cohen EL, Villacin AB. Basal cell adenoma of the prostate. Urology 11:409, 1978

46. Cleary KR, Choi HY, Ayala AG: Basal cell hyperplasia of the prostate. Am J Clin Pathol 80:850, 1983

47. Reed R: Consultation case. Am J Surg Pathol 8:699, 1984

48. Srigley JR, Dardick I: Basal epithelial cells of prostate are not myoepithelial cells. Lab Invest 58:87A, 1988

49. Brawer MK, Peehl DM, Stamey TA, et al: Keratin immunoreactivity in benign and neoplastic human prostate. Cancer Res 45:3665, 1985

50. Grignon D, Ro J, Ordonez N, et al: Basal cell hyperplasia of the prostate gland: an immunohistochemical study of 10 cases. Lab Invest 58:36A, 1988

51. Gardner WA Jr., Culberson DE: Atrophy and

proliferation in the young adult prostate. J Urol 137:53, 1987

52. Franks LM: Atrophy and hyperplasia in the prostate proper. J Pathol Bacteriol 68:616, 1954
53. Kovi J: Microscopic differential diagnosis of small acinar adenocarcinoma of prostate. Pathol Annu 20:157, 1985
54. Young RH, Clement BB: Sclerosing adenosis of the prostate. Arch Pathol Lab Med 111:363, 1987
55. Chen KTK, Schiff JJ: Adenomatoid prostatic tumor. Urology 21:88, 1983
56. Bostwick DG, Egbert BM, Fajardo LF: Radiation injury of the normal and neoplastic prostate. Am J Surg Pathol 6:541, 1982
57. Holmes EJ: Crystalloids of prostatic carcinoma: relationship to Bence-Jones crystals. Cancer 39:2073, 1977
58. Bennett B, Gardner WA Jr: Crystalloids in prostatic hyperplasia. Prostate 2:31, 1980
59. Jensen PE, Gardner WA Jr, Piserchia PV: Prostatic crystalloids: association with adenocarcinoma. Prostate 1:25, 1980
60. Schujman E, Mukamel E, Slutzker D, et al: Prostatic transitional cell carcinoma: concept of its pathogenesis and classification. J Med Sci 19:794, 1983
61. Ende N, Woods LP, Shelley HS: Carcinoma originating in ducts surrounding the prostatic urethra. J Clin Pathol 40:183, 1963
62. Ullmann AS, Ross OA: Hyperplasia, atypism, and transitional cell carcinoma in situ in prostatic periurethral glands. Am J Clin Pathol 17:497, 1967
63. Rhamy RK, Buchanan RD, Spalding MJ: Intraductal carcinoma of the prostate gland. J Urol 109:457, 1973
64. Hardeman SW, Soloway MS: Transitional cell carcinoma of the prostate: diagnosis, staging, and management. World J Urol 6:170, 1988
65. Wood DP, Montie JE, Pontes JE et al: Transitional cell carcinoma of the prostate in cystoprostatectomy specimens removed for bladder cancer. J Urol 141:346, 1989
66. Bostwick DG, Kindrachuk RW, Rouse RV: Prostatic adenocarcinoma with endometrioid features. Am J Surg Pathol 9:595, 1985
67. McNeal JE, Bostwick DG, Kindrachuk RA, et al: Patterns of progression in prostate cancer. Lancet 1:60, 1986
68. Leav I, Ho S-M, Ofner P, et al: Biochemical alterations in sex hormone-induced hyperplasia and dysplasia of the dorsolateral prostates of noble rats. J Natl Cancer Inst 80:1045, 1988
69. Park C, Galang C, Johenning P, et al: Follow-up aspiration biopsies for dysplasia of the prostate gland. Lab Invest 60:70A, 1989
70. Oyasu R, Bahnson RR, Nowels K, Garnett JE: Cytologic atypia in the prostate gland: frequency, distribution and possible relevance to carcinoma. J Urol 135:954, 1986
71. Garnett JE, Oyasu R: Urological evaluation of atypical prostatic hyperplasia (APH). Urology 1989 (in press)
72. Torp-Pedersen S, Lee F, Littrup PJ, et al: Transrectal biopsy of the prostate guided with transrectal US: longitudinal and multiplanar scanning. Radiology 170:23, 1989
73. Bostwick DG: Origins of prostatic carcinoma. In Damjanov I (ed): Progress in Reproductive and Urinary Tract Pathology. WW Norton, New York, 1989 (in press)
74. Bostwick DG: Premalignant lesions of the prostate. Semin Diagn Pathol 5:240, 1988

5

Stage A Carcinoma of the Prostate

John N. Eble and Jonathan I. Epstein

Throughout history, urinary obstruction caused by prostatic hyperplasia has made the lives of many elderly miserable. Benjamin Franklin had a special carriage built to make driving over cobbled streets comfortable, and Thomas Jefferson died of obstruction after years of suffering.[1] Presently, the treatment for prostatic hyperplasia is surgical: transurethral resection or, for larger glands, open surgical enucleation. In 1986, there were 374,882 transurethral prostatectomies performed in short-term, general, nonfederal hospitals in the United States.[2] Since this statistic excludes Veterans Administration and military hospitals, both of which have many elderly male patients, the true number of transurethral resections done annually in the United States probably exceeds 400,000.

Stage A carcinoma is clinically inapparent, confined to the prostate, and found incidentally during the pathologic examination of tissues removed for relief of obstruction thought clinically to be caused by hyperplasia or other benign conditions, or when removed as part of radical cystoprostatectomy for cancer of the urinary bladder.[3-6] These carcinomas are the subject of this chapter.

Stage B carcinoma is localized and detected clinically by rectal examination; the general scheme for staging in the United States is summarized and compared to the TNM system of the UICC in Table 5-1.[7] These systems are not completely consistent, although stage A corresponds to stage t_1.[4, 8]

The importance of stage A cancer is underscored by the findings of the American College of Surgeons in 1974 and 1983, which reported that more than 55 percent of prostatic carcinomas were first diagnosed in transurethral resection (TUR) specimens.[9] Studies at Finnish and Scottish cancer centers found 20 to 25 percent of patients had incidental prostate cancer, diagnosed during the examination of tissue removed for nodular hyperplasia.[10, 11]

PREVALENCE OF STAGE A CARCINOMA OF THE PROSTATE

AUTOPSY STUDIES

Clinically undiagnosed (stage A) carcinoma is common in men over age 50, present in up to 46 percent of cases, according to autopsy studies (Table 5-2).[12-20] Variations in prevalence among autopsy series are due to differences in examination techniques: studies that were more thorough showed higher prevalence of carcinoma. Submission of the entire prostate for microscopic examination (*step sectioning*) yielded the highest prevalence. Scott and associates[19] noted that complete microscopic examination doubled the observed prevalence in their study. While the compiled results suggest higher prevalence with increasing age, statistical tests were not usually employed. Edwards and associates[17] found no statistically significant difference between the incidence of carcinoma within individual age groups and the incidence of the population as a whole. The discrepancy between the observed death rate of prostate cancer in men over 50 (1 to 5 percent) and the high autopsy prevalence prompted some investi-

Table 5-1. Comparison of American and UICC Staging Systems for Prostate Cancer

Features	American	UICC
Clinically inapparent	A	T1
Focal	A1	T1a
Diffuse	A2	T1b
Palpable, confined to prostate	B	T2
Focal	B1	T2a
Diffuse	B2	T2b
Local extension beyond the prostatic capsule	C	
Without invasion of seminal vesicles	C1	T3
With invasion of seminal vesicles	C2	T3
With fixation of pelvic wall	C2	T4
Metastatic spread	D	N or M

cally recognized prostate cancer.[21–27] Black and white American men are among those with the highest prevalence,[22] as well as men from Western Europe and Scandinavia.[23, 25] These populations have prevalences in the range of 25 to 32 percent for men over 45 years old. In contrast, the prevalence in Chinese and Japanese men is much lower, in the range of 12 to 15 percent.[23–28] There is evidence that the prevalence has increased in Japan since World War II.[28] Populations in Africa and South America have not been adequately studied. These studies suggest that the prevalence of unsuspected carcinoma at autopsy parallels the incidence of clinical cancer in different populations.

gators to conclude that the lesions found at autopsy were biologically different from those that were clinically manifest, and to call them *latent carcinomas*.[18]

GEOGRAPHIC AND RACIAL EPIDEMIOLOGY

The prevalence of clinically unsuspected carcinoma of the prostate in populations throughout the world varies considerably, similar to clini-

SURGICAL PATHOLOGY STUDIES

Since TUR and enucleation specimens do not include the entire prostate, it is not surprising that the prevalence of stage A carcinoma in these specimens differs from the prevalence observed at autopsy. Sampling technique for histologic examination is also important in determining prevalence. Table 5-3 summarizes the results of six large studies of TUR specimens with total or subtotal sampling.[24, 30–34] The prevalence of stage A carcinoma varied from 13 to 22 percent (mean 16 percent). In another series,

Table 5-2. Prevalence of Clinically Inapparent Prostatic Carcinoma in Nine Autopsy Studies

	Patient Ages (By Decades)				
	Fifties	Sixties	Seventies	Eighties	Total (%)
Rich[12]	7/130	8/98	12/59	0/5	27/292 (9)
Moore[13]	9/65	18/77	13/63	7/24	47/229 (20)
Kahler[14]	—	—	—	—	69/491 (14)
Baron and Angrist[15]					
Random sectioning	12/140	18/124	19/81	5/19	54/364 (15)
Complete sectioning	8/19	8/21	6/9	1/1	22/50 (46)
Andrews[16]	2/38	7/39	7/22	—	16/99 (16)
Edwards et al.[17]	3/31	10/54	12/48	3/17	28/150 (19)
Franks[18]	38/241	53/312	70/237	17/93	178/883 (20)
Scott et al.[19]					
Complete sectioning	—	—	36/100	26/58	62/158 (39)
Holund[20]	2/23	7/56	24/87	13/34	46/200 (23)
Totals (%)	93/687 (14)	129/781 (17)	199/706 (28)	72/251 (29)	493/2425 (20)

**Table 5-3. Prevalence of Stage A Prostatic Carcinoma in
Transurethral Resection Specimens**

Study	Number of Specimens	Number of Carcinomas	Prevalence (%)
Newman et al.[30]	500	71	14
Moore et al.[31]	143	31	22
Murphy et al.[33]	386	66	17
Yamabe et al.[24]			
Japan	191	24	13
Netherlands	452	57	13
Rohr[32]	457	65	14
Eble and Tejada[34]	700	132	19
Totals	2829	446	16

Vollmer[35] reported only 49 unsuspected carcinomas in 699 specimens; however, that investigator included an unspecified number of prostatic enucleation specimens, which may account for the apparent discrepancy.

Studies of open enucleation specimens have shown a lower prevalence of incidental carcinoma, probably owing to incomplete histologic examination. Labess[36] found carcinoma in 9 of 98 suprapubic prostatectomy specimens (9.2 percent), and Treiger[37] found carcinoma in 12.6 percent of 108 cases. Bauer and associates[38] reviewed 847 suprapubic prostatectomies, and found 55 cases of clinically unsuspected carcinoma (6.5 percent). This low prevalence may be due to incomplete sampling (mean of 3.6 blocks examined per specimen). In a recent study of 468 prostatic enucleations in which at least eight representative slices were examined histologically, Stillwell and associates[39] reported 28 cases of unsuspected carcinoma (6 percent). By examining additional sections from 490 autopsy specimens that had been considered benign grossly and at initial microscopic examination, Kahler[14] found 54 additional carcinomas. Battaglia and associates[40] found that complete histologic examination of subtotal prostatectomy specimens doubled the number of carcinomas detected.

Pritchett and associates[3] extensively sampled 165 prostates from radical cystoprostatectomy specimens, identifying 45 clinically unsuspected prostatic carcinomas (27 percent); carcinoma was found in 5 of 36 men in their fifties, 23 of 64 in their sixties, and 13 of 47 in their seventies. Thirty-seven carcinomas were stage A, and the others were stage C or D. After submitting entire prostates for histologic examination, Montie and associates[41] found clinically undetected adenocarcinoma in cystoprostatectomy specimens of 33 of 72 patients (46 percent) treated for carcinoma of the urinary bladder.

The aggregate data indicate that the prevalence of clinically inapparent prostatic adenocarcinoma in men over 50 years old is roughly 30 percent, and the prevalence increases with age through the eighth decade of life. In TUR specimens from many centers throughout the United States, the prevalence averages 16 percent when complete histologic examination is done.

CLINICAL IMPORTANCE OF STAGE A CARCINOMA

For many years, adenocarcinoma of the prostate was regarded as an "individual and unpredictable tumor . . . aggressive in the younger age groups but slow growing and potentially harmless in elderly men."[42] Montgomery and associates[43] followed 35 patients with stage A carcinoma for at least 8 years or until death, and found that none succumbed to their cancer. Munsie and Foster[44] found that only 2 of 20 stage A carcinomas progressed in patients followed for at least 10 years or until death. However, in both of these studies patients received varying types of therapy that may have affected their rates of progression. Clinical studies like these, combined with autopsy data, led to considerable controversy over the clinical significance of stage A carcinoma. By the early 1970s, treatment for stage A carcinoma varied from radical resection to hormonal therapy with estrogens, or simple observation.[45]

In addition to the expected mortality from intercurrent disease, the use of estrogens to treat stage A carcinoma of the prostate caused significant excess mortality owing to cardiovascular disease.[46, 47] In 1972, Byar and associates[48] summarized results from 262 patients with stage A carcinoma, and found only five deaths from prostatic carcinoma, although some patients received therapy. However, in their own series of 148 cases, the 6-year survival rate was only about 30 percent. Data from these early studies, which suggested that stage A carcinoma carried little risk of progression or mortality, encouraged adoption of a conservative "watch and wait" strategy. Although there was some evidence that radical prostatectomy enhanced survival, the use of radical prostatectomy for stage A carcinoma declined by 66 percent from 1974 to 1983.[9, 48, 49]

During this period, data emerged that suggested that patients with stage A carcinoma are not a homogeneous group, but that risk of tumor progression was low in patients with *focal* cancer and high in patients whose carcinoma was *diffuse*.[45, 50, 51]

In an influential review article in 1975, Jewett[52] concluded that stage A tumors should be divided into substages A_1 and A_2 according to whether the lesions were focal or diffuse, and that patients with stage A2 cancer required additional treatment. This view was supported by the work of Khalifa and Jarman[50] and of Barnes and associates,[51] which showed that, among stage A cancers, those with multiple foci or diffuse spread were associated with increased recurrence rates and excess mortality, particularly beyond 5 years after diagnosis. Thus, subdivision of stage A tumors based upon the extent of the cancer within the prostate caught on rapidly.

The prognosis of stage A carcinoma relative to that of stage B carcinoma was also studied. In 1974, Gleason and the VACURG[53] reported on outcome for patients with stage A (66 patients) and B (83 patients) carcinoma treated with estrogens, and found 5-year survivals of 69 and 79 percent, respectively; there were no cancer deaths in either group. It should be noted that the recognition of estrogen therapy as the cause of excess mortality owing to cardiovascular disease led to the decline in its use in treating low stage carcinoma.[47] Consequently, it is difficult to compare survival data prior to 1978 with more recent data.[9, 47, 53]

Golimbu and associates[54] compared 16 stage A2 patients with 17 Stage B1 patients and 16 B2 patients, and found the occurrence of lymph node metastases in the A2 patients to be intermediate between that of the B1 and B2 patients (37 percent versus 18 and 62 percent). Similarly, in a study of 452 patients undergoing staging pelvic lymphadenectomy for clinically localized cancer, Smith and associates[55] found lymph node metastases in 12 percent of stage B1, 24 percent of A2, and 28 percent of B2 patients. None of the 45 patients with stage A1 carcinoma in these two studies had lymph node metastases. Comparing 11 stage A and 73 stage B carcinomas in radical prostatectomy specimens, McNeal and associates[56] concluded that these are biologically similar neoplasms, and that the difference between them is merely their location within the prostate.

Since, by definition, stage A carcinoma is diagnosed only by pathologists, recognition that stage A2 carcinoma was associated with substantial risk of progression and mortality made it imperative that surgical pathologists develop methods for detecting and accurately substaging stage A carcinoma of the prostate.

DETECTION OF STAGE A CARCINOMA OF THE PROSTATE

In 1976, Lefer and Rosier[57] reported that submission of one block for every 5 g of tissue from TUR specimens enabled them to detect unsuspected cancer almost twice as frequently as submission of only two or three blocks, regardless of the size of the specimen. This change raised the mean number of blocks from 2.8 to 5.4 per case in their laboratory.

These results prompted a study by Rismyhr and associates[58] of 52 TUR specimens in which carcinoma had been detected. Twenty-one specimens were from clinically benign prostates and 31 were clinically malignant. No specific sampling protocol was used, but at least two to three plastic cassettes were filled from each case when sufficient material was available. From data on the distribution of carcinoma among the chips and blocks, they determined the probability of sampling at least one malignant chip in samples of one to eight blocks, and concluded that four blocks ensured a detection rate of approximately 99 percent. However, the study was biased by the inclusion of a high proportion of clinically apparent cancers; this probably accounts for the finding that, in 28 of the 52 specimens, 50 percent or more of the chips contained cancer. Also, these investigators did not exclude the possibility that other TUR specimens from that period (not included in the study because carcinoma was not diagnosed) might have contained carcinoma. In essence, Rismyhr and associates showed that when substantial cancer is present, a small sample probably will suffice.

In 1982, Newman and associates[30] reported the results of submitting the entire TUR specimen for histologic examination from a series of 500 cases. They found that complete sampling increased the detection of stage A carcinoma by 65 percent when compared with their previous protocol, which called for submission of the entire specimen if it weighed less than 10 g, or submission of one cassette for each 5 g if the specimen weighed more than 10 g. Further, they found that 76 percent of the additional cancers were stage A2 and concluded that histologic examination of every chip yielded diagnoses that made a clinically significant difference in patient management.

In 1986 and 1987, five large prospective studies on TUR specimen sampling for the detection of stage A carcinoma were published or presented at national meetings.[31–35] All tissue was processed for histologic examination in each and, with the exception of the study of Vollmer[35] (not included in the table), each found essentially the same prevalence of stage A carcinoma as had Newman and associates (Table 5-3). The objective of these studies was to determine the optimal sampling strategy for TUR specimens, allowing for sensitivity, clinical relevance, and cost.

Murphy and associates[33] concluded that 90 percent of incidental carcinomas, including all stage A2 carcinomas, would be detected by applying a strategy of embedding the lesser of all tissue or 12 g, regardless of the size of the specimen. Similarly, Vollmer[35] concluded that a strategy of embedding the lesser of all tissue or five blocks (in his laboratory, one cassette held an average of 2.4 g of tissue) would detect approximately 90 percent of cancers. Rohr[32] concluded that examination of the lesser of the entire specimen or eight blocks (in his laboratory, eight blocks held an average of 12.8 g of tissue) would discover "the large majority" of carcinomas and all A2 carcinomas. The central feature of the approach that these three studies took was to stratify the patient population into two groups: those with small specimens that would be entirely submitted for histologic examination and those with larger specimens that would be partially examined on a sliding scale in inverse proportion to the size of the specimen. The investigators differed only about precisely what the cutoff weight should be. In 1981, Golimbu and associates[59] polled 465 departments of pathology in the United States and found that 82 percent of respondents submitted all of the specimen for histology if it weighed less than 10 g, and that 88 percent submitted less than the entire specimen when it weighed more than 10 g. Thus, the studies of Murphy and associates, Vollmer, and Rohr expanded on this widely used strategy, suggesting that 12 g rather than 10 g be used as the cutoff weight for complete histologic examination.

Moore and associates[31] suggested that sampling should be based upon submission of a constant fraction of the specimen for histologic examination, regardless of the weight of the specimen. From this concept and the data in their series, they developed tables showing the probability of detecting carcinoma if different fractions of the specimen were submitted for histology (Table 5-4). For example, they showed that if carcinoma is present in three fragments of a specimen, approximately 53 percent of the specimen must be processed to achieve a sensitivity of 90 percent, while 78 percent of the specimen must be embedded in order to have a 99 percent probability of detecting the carcinoma. Since their results showed that the necessary sampling fraction for a particular sensitivity is, for practical purposes, independent of the weight of the specimen, once the desired level of sensitivity is determined, the procedure is easily implemented in the surgical pathology gross room. The specimen is weighed and the fraction of the chips indicated for the desired sensitivity is submitted for histology. Examination of the entire specimen, as suggested by Newman and associates,[30] represents the most extreme application of this strategy.

All of the studies concluded that, short of processing the complete sample for histology, some small carcinomas would remain unde-

tected. This point of view was echoed by Mostofi[60] in an editorial in 1986.

With two radically different kinds of sampling strategy proposed, both of which can detect 90 percent or more of stage A carcinomas and almost 100 percent of stage A2 carcinomas, the surgical pathologist is faced with choosing which to adopt. At first examination, this might not seem much of a problem since both would seem to give the same result, and the decision could then be based on cost or ease of implementation. However, this is not the case.

The type of strategy proposed by Murphy and associates,[33] Vollmer,[35] and Rohr[32] divides patients into two groups according to the weights of their specimens and offers them different qualities of examination. Those with specimens weighing up to approximately 12 g receive the benefit of histologic examination of every chip, which is the most thorough examination currently offered by any of the strategies; those with specimens weighing more than 12 g receive histologic examination of only a fraction of their specimen and that fraction diminishes as the size of the specimen increases. If small specimens were more likely to contain carcinoma, or if carcinoma in large specimens were of less clinical significance than carcinoma in small

Table 5-4. Percentage of Fragments That Must be Sampled Versus Number of Cancerous Fragments Present for Several Probabilities of Detection

Carcinomatous Chips in Specimen (No.)	Chips (%) Sampled to Assure Probability (P_m) of Detecting Carcinoma		
	$P_m = 90\%$	$P_m = 95\%$	$P_m = 99\%$
1	90.0	95.0	99.0
2	68.4	77.7	90.0
3	53.6	63.1	78.4
4	43.8	52.7	68.3
5	36.9	45.0	60.1
6	31.8	39.3	53.5
7	28.0	34.8	48.1
8	25.0	31.2	43.7
9	22.5	28.2	39.9
10	20.5	25.8	36.8
15	14.2	18.0	26.3
20	10.8	13.8	20.4
25	8.7	11.2	16.7

(From Moore et al.,[31] with permission.)

specimens, it would be logical to concentrate diagnostic efforts and resources on small specimens in this way. Expanding the series of Eble and Tejada[34] to 872 consecutive TUR specimens submitted completely for histologic examination, we found that the prevalence of carcinoma was higher in specimens over 12 g than in specimens less than 12 g (23 percent versus 16 percent). Also, there is no evidence that carcinoma in large specimens has different clinical significance than in small specimens. If the sampling strategy proposed by Murphy and associates, Vollmer, and Rohr cannot be justified on clinical or biologic grounds, the issue of cost must be addressed. Table 5-5 shows the results of applying the two sampling strategies to the expanded series of Eble and Tejada. Using the 12 g strategy of Murphy and associates, Vollmer, and Rohr, 8,853 g of the total of 15,098 g (59 percent of the tissue) would have been submitted for histologic examination. For 90 percent sensitivity, using the proportional strategy of Moore and associates, 8,002 g (53 percent) of the tissue would have been processed. The difference in overall cost between the two strategies appears to be minor. The cost per case would be more variable with the protocol of Moore et al., since the number of blocks would increase in direct proportion to the size of the specimen. The protocol of Murphy et al., Vollmer, and Rohr would cost more for specimens under 12 g, but cost less for larger specimens. At a detection rate of 90 percent, both protocols would save approximately one third of the cost of submitting all of the tissue for histologic examination. This estimate is slightly inflated: when stage A1 carcinoma was found in partially sampled specimens, all investigators advocated processing the remainder in order to ensure that the carcinoma was not stage A2. Among 173 stage A carcinomas in the series of Eble and Tejada, 107 were stage A1, and 66 of these were in specimens weighing more than 12 g. Processing the remainder of those specimens using the 12 g strategy would have required processing another 776 g, raising the fraction examined histologically to 64 percent.

An advantage of the system proposed by Moore et al. is that it enables the surgical pathologist to respond to changing needs imposed by new developments in urologic therapy by choosing the sensitivity level of the sampling protocol. In the strategy proposed by Murphy and associates, Vollmer, and Rohr, it is unclear how large an effect raising or lowering the 12 g threshold would have on the sensitivity of sampling. Those investigators, writing in 1985, tended to discount stage A1 carcinoma as clinically insignificant. However, recent investigations have shown that stage A1 carcinoma is more significant than previously believed (see below), and urologists are increasingly aggressive in their approach to it.[61]

In deciding among sampling strategies, the choices include missing some cancers in larger specimens and detecting all cancers in the smaller specimens while minimizing the variance in cost from case to case; spreading missed cancers evenly throughout the population and having some examinations of low cost and others at high cost; or submitting all tissue for histologic examination, with maximum sensitivity and maximum cost.

DEFINING SUBSTAGES A1 AND A2

Surgical pathologists face the problem of refining the conceptually useful but nebulous notions of *focal* and *diffuse* into working definitions in order to separate patients requiring radical therapy (those with diffuse carcinoma) from those needing conservative treatment or no treatment (those with focal carcinoma). Today, 15 or more years after Jewett's review, four methods for defining substages A1 and A2 of prostatic

Table 5-5. Comparison of Sampling Strategies in the Context of 90 Percent Detection of Carcinomas in 872 Transurethral Resections of Prostate

	Tissue Processed	Blocks[a]
12 g strategy[32,33,73]	8,853 g	4,918
Proportional strategy[31]	8,002 g	4,446

[a] 1.8 g per block in the series.

Table 5-6. Methods of Defining Substages A1 and A2 of Carcinoma of the Prostate

Method	Description	Advantages	Disadvantages
TUR chip counting[54,59,62,63]	Stage A1: Fewer than 3 or 5 chips involved Stage A2: More than 3 or 5 involved	Simplicity Widely used	Lack of supporting studies for 3 or 5 chip thresholds Cannot apply to enucleation specimens
Area ratio estimation[65,67]	Stage A1: 5% or less of specimen area Stage A2: More than 5% of area	Strong empirical support Simplicity	Incompatible with conventional concepts of cancer risk factors Supporting studies are from only one institution.
Volume estimation[69]	Stage A1: 1 cc or less Stage A2: Greater than 1 cc cancer volume	Theoretically sound Modest empirical support	Requires measurement and calculation Based on cubic volume
TUR chip ratio[72,73]	Ratio of malignant to benign chips in TUR specimens correlates with prognosis	Simplicity Low interobserver variation	Does not lend itself to two-tier A1–A2 substaging Cannot apply to enucleation specimens

carcinoma remain in use, although they differ greatly in their premises and methods (Table 5-6).

TUR CHIP COUNTING

In 1981, Golimbu and associates[59] polled the 465 pathology departments listed in the Directory of Residency Training Programs of the Liaison Committee on Graduate Medical Education of the American Medical Association, and asked what the maximum allowable number of malignant TUR chips was for stage A1 carcinoma. Of 293 responses, 96 percent allowed no more than three chips; the rest allowed four or five chips. This classification of prostatic carcinoma in TUR specimens as focal or diffuse based on the number of malignant chips is the most prevalent method for subdividing stage A cancers.

However, the origin of chip counting for substaging prostate carcinoma in TUR specimens is obscure. In 1974, Correa and associates[45] reported that survival of patients with focal carcinoma, most of whom had three or fewer foci, was the same as that of the male population of similar age. This study included patients

treated with varying therapies that may have altered the natural history of the carcinoma or the life expectancy of the patients. Using an unusual variant technique in which the number of foci of carcinoma were counted, Khalifa and Jarman[50] reported that 29 patients with three or fewer foci of carcinoma had 10-year survival of 44.8 percent, while 19 patients with more than three foci had a survival rate of only 21 percent. At 5 years, the technique showed little difference. In 1978, Golimbu and associates,[54] without referencing any source, defined stage A2 as involvement of more than five TUR chips. In a later paper, Golimbu and Morales[62] stated, "since there is no agreement in differentiating focal (A_1) from diffuse (A_2) lesions, we arbitrarily categorized into clinical stage A_2 all clinically unsuspected tumors found in more than five chips at transurethral resection . . . ". The adverb "arbitrarily" must be noted here. In a review in 1980, Sheldon and associates[63] proposed that stage A be divided into three substages: stage Af, in which three or fewer chips contained carcinoma; stage A1, in which more than three chips contained carcinoma, but only one quadrant or two contiguous quadrants were involved; and stage A2, in which there was greater tumor volume, or in which noncontiguous quadrants were involved. These "arbitrary" definitions appear to be the origin of chip counting for substaging, and, by 1981, 96 percent of pathology departments in teaching hospitals had adopted the method.[59]

Notwithstanding the lack of foundation in large controlled studies, this approach of chip counting for substaging carcinoma in TUR specimens has a certain appeal. First, it is conservative: three to five chips or fewer is close to the minimum volume of carcinoma recognizable in a TUR specimen. Thus, this approach minimizes understaging and inadequate therapy. Second, chip counting is simple and reproducible, and does not involve area or volume estimation or measurement as proposed by other methods of substaging. An obvious drawback of chip counting is its inapplicability to suprapubic enucleation specimens. Also, the three-chip threshold for stage A2 carcinoma will result in approximately two thirds of stage A patients being considered stage A2, including a considerable number with small indolent tumors.

RATIO OF AREA OF CARCINOMA TO TOTAL TISSUE AREA

Another approach to substaging stage A cancer is estimation of the area occupied by carcinoma compared with the total area of the chips examined. In 1970, Varkarakis and associates[64] studied 31 stage A carcinomas found in suprapubic and transvesical prostatectomy specimens and found that 11 occupied less than 12 percent of the sectioned area, while the other 20 occupied more than 40 percent. Cantrell et al.[65] performed stepwise discriminant analysis of factors linked to progression in 82 patients with stage A carcinoma followed for at least 4 years without attempt at curative therapy at the Johns Hopkins Hospital between 1961 and 1975. A number of factors were tested, but the most significant ($F=19.90$ and $F=23.22$) were morphometric and naked eye estimates that the area of the sections occupied by carcinoma exceeded 5 percent. Using that estimate as the discriminator

between substages A1 and A2, they found only 1 of 48 stage A1 patients had progression, while 11 of 34 stage A2 patients had progression within 4 years. In contrast, the number of malignant foci was a relatively poor predictor, ($F=7.13$). In 1986, Epstein and associates[66] reported on 50 men with stage A1 carcinoma defined by this method who were followed 8 years or longer after diagnosis. Although eight (16 percent) had progression, including four with tumors that occupied 1 percent or less of the specimen, they concluded that this method was the "best defined and best documented distinction between stages A1 and A2 prostatic cancer."[66] They also noted that patients with stage A1 tumors were less likely to progress than those with stage A2, and those who did, did so later. Recently, the same group compared the volume of cancer with percentage of tissue area on slides, and concluded that both correlated with progression, but the percentage of area involved was more strongly associated, particularly after 4 years of follow-up.[67] The major criticism of this definition of substaging is that the bulk of the specimen in most cases consists of hyperplastic tissue, and there is no explanation for why the ratio of carcinoma to hyperplasia should have prognostic significance. Also the area estimation method of substaging leads to conclusions that are at odds with conventional thinking about cancer. For example, this approach considers carcinoma occupying 6 percent of a 10-g specimen to be stage A2, similar to tumors occupying 6 percent of a 100-g specimen; yet, many would expect the 6-g cancer to be more advanced and have a worse prognosis than the 0.6-g cancer.[67] Nonetheless, empiric evidence to date indicates an excellent correlation with prognosis for the area ratio estimation method.

CARCINOMA VOLUME ESTIMATION

A third method of substaging stage A cancers, the volume estimation method, is based on the results of McNeal[68] in 1969, in which a number of indicators of progression in prostatic carcinoma were correlated with the volume occupied by carcinoma. In that study of 45 malignant prostates from autopsies, loss of differentiation, capsular involvement, local extension, and intraglandular metastasis were more frequent in carcinomas greater than 1 cc. This concept was adopted at the Mayo Clinic and presented in diagrammatic form in 1982.[69] The practical application is simple: the largest dimensions of all foci of carcinoma are summed, and the sum is cubed. If the resulting calculated volume is greater than 1 cc, the lesion is considered to be stage A2.[70] In a study of 320 patients treated with radical prostatectomy at the Mayo Clinic, Benson and associates[71] found (using Kaplan-Meier estimates) that, after 10 years of follow-up, less than 10 percent of carcinomas smaller than 1 cc progressed, while approximately 20 to 25 percent of the larger carcinomas progressed. Although this approach has some empirical support, the drawbacks appear to be the theoretical concern that the largest dimensions may not sum accurately to a length that can be cubed to give an appropriate volume. Also, practical application of this method requires measurement and calculation.

TUR CHIP RATIO

Fan and Peng[72] found that the ratio of malignant chips to the total number of chips in TUR specimens was a good predictor of bone metastasis in 81 patients with prostatic carcinoma who were autopsied. They found that the probability of bone metastasis increased linearly with the percentage of malignant TUR chips. Humphrey and Vollmer[73] applied this method to TUR specimens of 118 patients with stage A carcinoma, and found that approximately 50 percent had ratios less than 0.17, and the rest were distributed almost uniformly between 0.17 and 1.00. They found a strong correlation between the chip ratio and prognosis, and demonstrated that this method had minimal interobserver disagreement. However, their data and that of Fan and Peng suggest a relatively smooth linear relation between chip ratio and prognosis that, al-

though conveying important information, is not conducive to a two-tier substaging system.

INCLUSION OF GRADE IN SUBSTAGE DEFINITIONS

A number of investigators have deviated from the usual practice of defining stage solely in terms of extent by also requiring that stage A1 prostatic carcinoma be low grade. These workers claim that staging and grading are complementary but separate indicators of prognosis for prostate cancer and other cancers. One argument in favor of this unusual mixing of grading and staging is that patients with more aggressive (higher-grade) carcinoma should be followed more closely or given definitive therapy that might otherwise be denied. However, this argument is not convincing since grade is not part of the definition of higher stages of prostate cancer, and urologists are accustomed to considering both grade and stage in planning treatment of stage B prostate cancer, as well as cancers of other organs. In addition to the need for standardization of substaging stage A prostatic carcinoma, there is another benefit to basing substaging solely upon extent: The varied methods of defining tumor extent make comparison of studies done at different institutions difficult enough without introducing variations in grading as an additional source of confusion.

OUTCOME FOR PATIENTS WITH STAGE A1 CARCINOMA

Recent studies indicate an increased long-term risk for development of clinical carcinoma, progression, and death in patients with stage A1 carcinoma of the prostate.

In a study from Johns Hopkins, a series of 94 men with untreated stage A1 tumors and long-term follow-up were reported.[66] Stage A1 carcinoma was defined as clinically unsuspected, occupying 5 percent or less of the TUR specimen, not high grade (less than Gleason score 8), no preoperative observation of nodularity or induration of the prostate, and normal serum prostatic acid phosphatase levels and bone scans. Of 94 patients, 26 died without progression less than 4 years after diagnosis; 18 showed no progression after 4 to 8 years of follow-up; 42 patients showed no evidence of progression after 8 to 18 years (mean and median, 10 years); and 8 patients had clinically evident progression (Fig. 5-1). The average interval from diagnosis to progression in these eight patients was 7 years, with a range of 3.5 to 8 years. In six of the eight men with progression, prostatic cancer was the cause of death. The seventh patient with progression is alive with stage D2 carcinoma, and the last patient died of unrelated causes with B2 carcinoma, both 8 years from diagnosis. Neither volume nor grade predicted progression; of the eight tumors that progressed, four involved less than 1 percent of the resectate, seven had fewer than three tumor foci, and six were of low grade (Gleason score 4 or less).

The rationale for excluding 18 stage A1 patients with 4 to 8 years of follow-up from the calculation of the long-term risk of progression is that these men had an average of only 6 years' follow-up. Since the mean time to progression in the study was 7 years, they had not been followed long enough to determine outcome.

Blute et al.,[70] in a smaller series from the Mayo Clinic, also demonstrated that men with stage A1 carcinomas (defined as less than 1 cc of volume and well differentiated) are at increased risk for progression. Of 15 men less than 60 years old who were followed for a minimum of 10 years, 4 (27 percent) experienced progression of stage A1 carcinoma. Blute et al. were unable to predict progression based on the TUR specimen since all of the carcinomas that progressed had two or fewer foci of cancer and were low grade. The average interval to progression in this series was 10 years.

These reports demonstrate that patients with stage A1 prostate cancer have a significant increase in risk of tumor progression if they do not die of intercurrent disease.

CURRENT CLINICAL APPROACHES TO STAGE A1 CARCINOMA

With the recognition that stage A1 carcinoma has the potential for progression if inadequately treated, new clinical approaches were developed to follow and treat these patients.

Three months after diagnosis of stage A1 carcinoma, 27 patients underwent repeat TUR, and 10 (37 percent) were found to have residual adenocarcinoma.[74] Seven (26 percent) had sufficient additional carcinoma to be restaged as A2, and the authors concluded that follow-up TUR

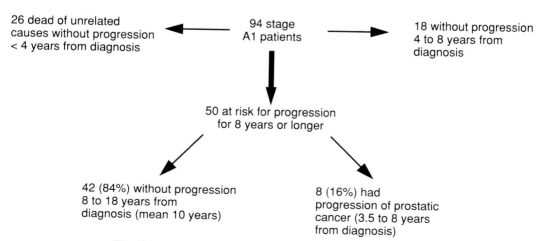

Fig. 5-1. Long-term follow-up of untreated stage A1 patients.

was helpful in obtaining accurate staging and in planning therapy. Similarly, Ford and associates[75] found that 12 of 20 patients (60 percent) had residual carcinoma at repeat TUR, and in 9, carcinoma occupied 6 percent or more of the tissue. Comparing the utility of second TUR with transperineal needle biopsy in 42 patients with stage A1 carcinoma, Carroll and associates[76] found TUR to be more sensitive, with residual carcinoma present in 24 percent of patients. In contrast, Parfitt and associates[77] studied follow-up TUR or radical prostatectomy specimens from 86 patients with stage A1 carcinoma and found only six patients with diffuse residual cancer (7 percent). They concluded that staging based on initial TUR is accurate and repeat TUR was not helpful. Bridges and associates[78] supported this conclusion in their study of repeat TUR in 40 patients with stage A1 carcinoma, 38 of whom remained stage A1 after the repeat TUR. Sonda and associates[79] took an intermediate position, stating that repeat TUR was not routinely necessary, but could be useful in higher-grade carcinoma of minimal extent, in a patient who desired definitive therapy if residual carcinoma was found, or when there was suspicion of incomplete resection.

DeKernion[80] reviewed this controversy, and concluded that patients with stage A1 carcinoma should undergo biopsy 3 months after surgery, and be considered stage A2 if residual carcinoma is found. Catalona and Scott[81] differed, suggesting that further procedures were not necessary in stage A1 patients for whom no immediate treatment was contemplated. While it has been proposed that patients who are not raised to stage A2 by follow-up procedures need no further treatment, most of these studies have not demonstrated the significance of their findings with long-term follow-up data on progression.

RADICAL PROSTATECTOMY FOR STAGE A1 CARCINOMA

Recent developments in the pathology of stage A1 carcinoma and in the surgical technique for radical prostatectomy have combined to make radical prostatectomy an important treatment option for relatively young men with stage A1 carcinoma.

First, as suggested by the studies of follow-up TUR, residual carcinoma is present in a significant percentage of patients with stage A1 carcinoma. This problem has been definitively explored by studies of radical prostatectomy specimens from patients with A1 carcinoma. Parfitt and associates,[77] in a large series of radical prostatectomies for stage A1 carcinoma, reported that 52 percent of 31 prostates contained no residual cancer; 36 percent contained focal residual cancer; and the remaining 13 percent contained diffuse carcinoma. Carcinoma was considered focal if the sum of the foci in the TUR specimen and the foci in the radical prostatectomy specimen was 5 or less. However, they did not embed and histologically examine entire specimens, so that cases with small amounts of residual carcinoma may have been missed. Further, the location of residual cancer was not reported.

Paulson and associates[82] reported their findings in 18 stage A1 prostate cancers treated with radical prostatectomy. After complete histologic examination, three patients had no residual cancer; four had a single focus; and the remainder (61 percent) had more than one focus.

Recently, Epstein and associates[83] reported the volume and anatomic location of residual carcinoma in 21 patients treated with radical prostatectomy for stage A1 cancer. The specimens were sectioned at 3-mm intervals, entirely submitted for histologic examination, and mapped. Three specimens contained no residual cancer, and 13 had cancers of smaller volume than usually seen in specimens resected for early stage B carcinoma. In the 13 cases with small residual cancers, all but one had some cancer at the prostatic apex. In more than two-thirds, the cancer was predominantly in the anterior portion of the specimen, and in all but one, there was carcinoma at the periphery near the prostatic capsule (Fig. 5-2). The five other patients with residual cancer had lesions indistinguishable in size from those found in radical prostatectomies for stage B carcinoma. Although there was a tendency for patients whose TUR specimens contained a low volume of can-

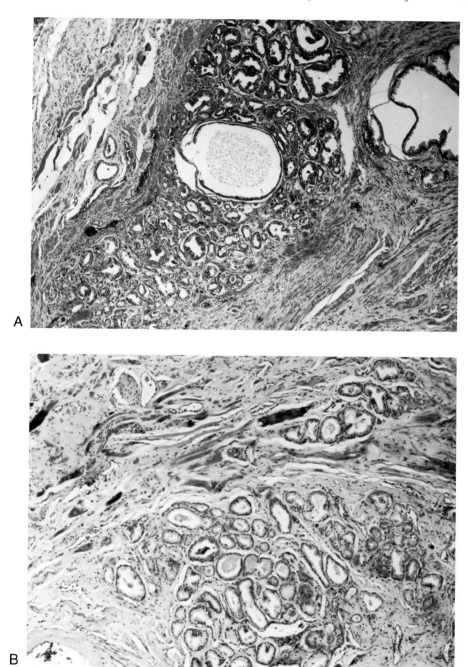

Fig. 5-2. Residual adenocarcinoma of the prostate in radical prostatectomy specimens removed for stage A1 cancer. **(A)** Adenocarcinoma present peripherally just beneath the prostatic capsule (capsule located at top left of field). (×80.) **(B)** Carcinoma at the most apical region of the radical prostatectomy specimen. Skeletal muscle fibers of the urogenital diaphragm are seen in the upper portion of the field. (×130.) (*Figure continues.*)

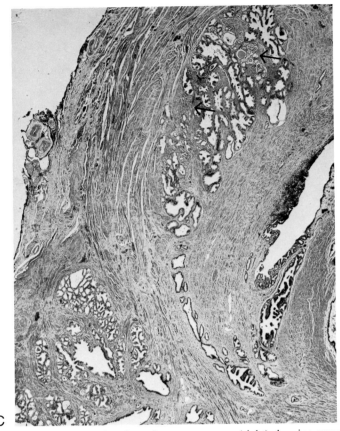

C

Fig. 5-2 (*Continued*). **(C)** Histologic section through verumontanum (right) showing several foci of residual adenocarcinoma (arrows) anterior to verumontanum. (×20.) (From Epstein and Walsh,[61] with permission.)

cer to have radical prostatectomy specimens with a low volume of cancer, enough exceptions occurred to conclude that the volume of cancer in transurethral resectates is not predictive of the volume of residual cancer. The study also found that Gleason grade in the TUR specimen was unreliable in predicting the volume of residual cancer. The implication is that, quite frequently, residual cancer is present at locations within the prostate where it would probably not be completely removed by repeat TUR, including the apex and the periphery. Subsequently, expansion of the study to 40 radical prostatectomies done for stage A1 carcinoma has shown only 3 (8 percent) without residual carcinoma. Lending support to this is the preliminary report by Neerhut et al.,[84] in which residual carcinoma

was found in 10 of 11 stage A1 patients treated with radical prostatectomy; the residual cancer was frequently anterior, peripheral and apical. That residual cancer is present in locations poorly accessible to TUR is important, because earlier studies suggest that focal low-grade carcinoma progresses, given sufficient time.[66, 70]

A second finding from the study of Epstein et al. was that patients with stage A1 carcinoma with substantial residual cancer may not be upstaged by repeated TUR. The mapping component of the study showed that, in two of the five patients with substantial residual cancer, the tumors were located so peripherally that they were probably inaccessible to TUR.

Introduction of the nerve-sparing technique for radical retropubic prostatectomy has greatly reduced the morbidity associated with this operation.[85] In particular, potency may be preserved in more than 90 percent of patients with stage A1 prostate cancer. Also, all of the men operated on for stage A1 carcinoma in a recent study have remained continent.[83]

RADICAL PROSTATECTOMY FOR STAGE A2 CARCINOMA

Studies evaluating pathologic findings in stage A2 carcinoma have primarily investigated the incidence of lymph node metastases, capsular penetration, and seminal vesicle invasion. The incidence of lymph node metastases in large series of A2 carcinomas, using different definitions for staging, range from 22 to 37 percent, with the majority showing less than 25 percent incidence.[54, 55, 86, 87] Stratifying the incidence of lymph node metastases by grade, stage A2 tumors that were well differentiated had a very low incidence of metastases (0 to 2 percent), but higher incidences were observed with moderately differentiated carcinoma (30 percent) and poorly differentiated carcinoma (50 percent).[86, 87] Metastases from stage A2 tumors were almost as common as from stage B2, and more common than from stage B1 carcinomas.[55, 86, 88–90]

Despite using different definitions for stage A2, three of the larger series examining pathologic stage in stage A2 patients undergoing radical prostatectomy showed approximately equal frequency of capsular penetration (12 to 19 percent) and seminal vesicle invasion (4 to 8 percent).[87, 91, 92] One study that undertook complete histologic examination of 39 radical prostatectomies for stage A2 carcinoma found that 26 percent had capsular penetration and 10 percent had invasion of the seminal vesicles. This is comparable to the findings with stage B1 cancers, in which capsular penetration was observed in 32 percent, and seminal vesicle invasion in 12 percent of a series of 129 radical prostatectomy specimens.[90] In the series of Fowler and Mills[91] and Elder et al.,[92] residual carcinoma was found in all but one of the specimens. In another series, no carcinoma was found in 3 of the 26 cases, perhaps owing to random sampling used in that investigation.[87] When Paulson and associates[82] examined entire prostates from 58 radical prostatectomy specimens removed for stage A2 cancer, 96.6 percent had residual cancer; in a recent study of 39 radical prostatectomy specimens examined completely, all contained residual carcinoma.[93]

There are limited data comparing final pathologic stage and tumor grade and volume in TUR specimens. Fowler and Mills[91] found that all carcinomas confined to the prostate had Gleason grades of 7 or less, while those with capsular penetration had Gleason grades greater than or equal to 8. Volume was also predictive of final pathologic stage; all cases with capsular penetration had tumors volume greater than 33 percent in the TUR specimen.[91] Conversely, Parfitt and associates[87] found less correlation; 42 percent of 12 cases with small stage A2 lesions in TUR specimens had diffuse carcinoma at radical prostatectomy, and 2 of 7 well-differentiated small stage A2 carcinomas were diffuse at radical prostatectomy. Paulson and associates[82] reported three patients with 20 to 60 percent involvement of TUR specimens by cancer who had no or only one focus of residual cancer in the radical prostatectomy specimen.

A recent study examined TUR specimens and the subsequent totally submitted radical prostatectomy specimens from 39 patients with stage A2 prostate cancer, comparing morphometrically determined volumes of carcinoma with similar data from 56 patients with stage B carcinoma.[93, 94] Stage A2 carcinomas were much more heterogeneous in grade, location, and volume than were stage B carcinomas. Forty-one percent of stage A2 tumors were low grade (Gleason score less than 4), while only 5 percent of the stage B carcinomas were low grade (Fig. 5-3).

The location of stage A2 carcinoma also differed from stage B carcinoma. Stage A2 cancers were centrally located in 38 percent of cases and central/anterior in 20 percent of cases, making them undetectable by rectal examination (Figs. 5-4 and 5-5). The average volume of

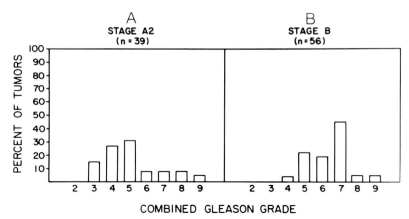

Fig. 5-3. Distribution of tumor grade in stages A2 and B prostatic carcinoma.

tumor resected by TUR was 68 percent (range 6 to 99 percent) of the total tumor, a reflection of the stage A2 carcinoma's central location. Only 20 percent of stage A2 carcinomas were most voluminous in the posterior region of the prostate. The correlation of tumor volume and pathologic stage also differed between stage A and stage B tumors. Stage B tumors with capsular penetration were usually low volume (Fig. 5-6). Because these tumors closely approached

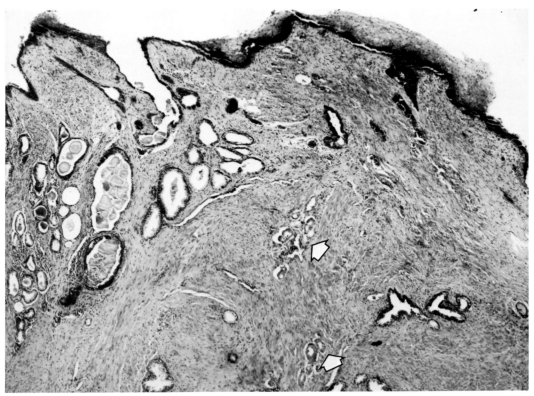

Fig. 5-4. Centrally located tumor with 13.2 cc of carcinoma resected and only several minute foci (total 0.05 cc) in radical prostatectomy specimen (arrows). (×40.)

the prostatic capsule, when they attained a certain size, capsular penetration occurred. In contrast, some stage A carcinomas that were centrally located attained larger volume before capsular penetration occurred (Fig. 5-6). Despite the strong correlation between tumor grade, percent, and volume in TUR specimens and final pathologic stage after radical prostatectomy, the predictive value for the individual patient was unsatisfactory (Fig. 5-7). Of the eight highest volume cancers without capsular penetration, at TUR some were low grade (accounting for their favorable stage). Others were high grade and high volume at TUR, yet were centrally located with minimal residual cancer at radical prostatectomy. Conversely, there were four low-volume carcinomas at TUR with capsular penetration. In each of these, there was substantial residual carcinoma of varying grade in the anterior or posterior regions. Because of the potential for sampling error introduced by tumor location, TUR tumor volume did not always accurately reflect the total volume of carcinoma. Unless all three variables (grade, volume, and location) were known, the final pathologic stage of A2 cancers could not be predicted with confidence. Furthermore, although the generalization of carcinoma arising peripherally and hyperplasia arising centrally is valid, there is a subset of patients with central tumors that

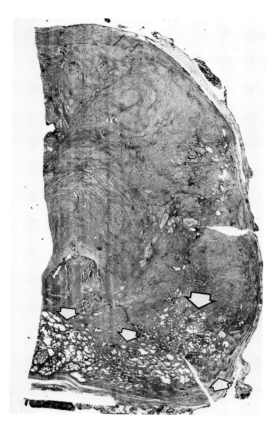

Fig. 5-5. Centrally and anteriorly located tumor with large volume of residual carcinoma located in the anterior region of a radical prostatectomy specimen. Only the posterior peripheral zone is free of carcinoma (arrows) (×4.)

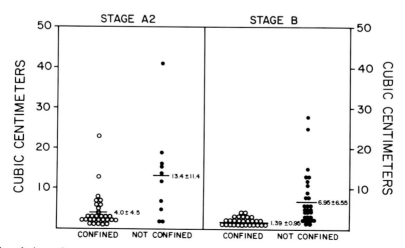

Fig. 5-6. Correlation of confinement of carcinoma within the prostate with tumor volume in stages A2 and B carcinoma.

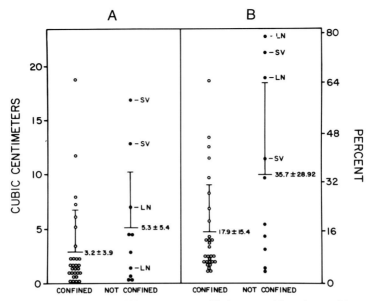

Fig. 5-7. Correlation of tumor volume (**A**) and percent (**B**) in stage A2 patients with carcinoma confined to the prostate (○) and extending outside the prostate (●). *sv,* seminal vesicle.

may cause urinary obstructive symptoms and be diagnosed by TUR.

CONCLUSION

Stage A carcinoma of the prostate remains an important problem for surgical pathologists. The evidence indicating the long-term risks associated with stage A1 carcinomas has persuaded many urologists to actively approach follow-up and therapy.

Surgical pathologists can no longer dismiss these lesions as clinically inconsequential and remain content with sampling strategies that discover all stage A2 lesions but allow many stage A1 lesions to pass unnoticed. Ideally, all TUR and enucleation tissues should be examined histologically, which the editor and one of the authors recommend. Alternatively, in the other author's laboratory, all TUR and enucleation tissues are examined in relatively young men (≤ 65 years of age) in which therapy for stage A1 disease might be pursued. In older men, ten cassettes of tissue are processed which would

identify all stage A2 cancers and over 90 percent of stage A1 tumors.

The issue of substage definition is less clearly resolved than that of sampling. As evidence has accumulated showing that A1 carcinoma is not biologically different from higher-stage carcinoma, and as nerve-sparing prostatectomy has increased acceptance of definitive therapy for stage A1 carcinoma by patients and urologists, there has been less of a need for separating stages A1 and A2 to guide the selection of therapy ("watch and wait" versus radical prostatectomy). Further, the data showing that residual carcinoma is often present after TUR and located in areas inaccessible to repeat TUR indicate that stage A1 carcinoma may be extensive and should be given serious consideration. Nonetheless, because of the high prevalence of stage A carcinoma of the prostate, it seems likely that there always will be utility for stratifying by extent as well as grade. Until more data are accumulated and standards are set, surgical pathologists will have to weigh the advantages and disadvantages of the competing definitions and choose one appropriate for use at their institution.

REFERENCES

1. Prostate operations: neglected gland. The Economist January 10:73, 1987
2. Desktop resource: top 25 most frequently performed surgeries. Health Week 2:23, 1988
3. Pritchett TR, Moreno J, Warner NE, et al: Unsuspected prostatic adenocarcinoma in patients who have undergone radical cystoprostatectomy for transitional cell carcinoma of the bladder. J Urol 139:1214, 1988
4. Murphy GP, Gaeta JF, Pickren J, et al: Current status of classification and staging of prostate cancer. Cancer 45:1889, 1980
5. Whitmore WF Jr: The natural history of prostatic cancer. Cancer 32:1104, 1973
6. Murphy GP: Prostate cancer: continuing progress. CA 31:96, 1981
7. Peeling WB, Griffiths GJ, Evans KT: Clinical staging of prostatic cancer. p. 121. In Blandy JP, Lytton B (eds): The Prostate. Butterworths, Seven Oaks, England, 1986
8. International Union Against Cancer: TNM Atlas. Illustrated guide to the TNM/pTNM-Classification of Malignant Tumors. 3rd Ed. Springer-Verlag, N.Y., 1988
9. Schmidt JD, Mettlin CJ, Natarajan N, et al: Trends in patterns of care for prostatic cancer, 1974-1983: results of surveys by the American College of Surgeons. J Urol 136:416, 1986
10. Haapiainen R, Rannikko S, Makinen J, et al: To carcinoma of the prostate: influence of tumor extent and histologic grade on prognosis of untreated patients. Eur Urol 12:16, 1986
11. Beynon LL, Busuttil A, Newsam JE, et al: Incidental carcinoma of the prostate: selection for deferred treatment. Br J Urol 55:733, 1983
12. Rich AR: On the frequency of occurrence of occult carcinoma of the prostate. J Urol 33:215, 1934
13. Moore RA: The morphology of small prostatic carcinoma. J Urol 33:224, 1935
14. Kahler JE: Carcinoma of the prostate gland: a pathologic study. J Urol 41:557, 1939
15. Baron E, Angrist A: Incidence of occult adenocarcinoma of the prostate after fifty years of age. Arch Pathol 32:787, 1941
16. Andrews GS: Latent carcinoma of the prostate. J Clin Pathol 2:197, 1949
17. Edwards CN, Steinthorsson E, Nicholson D: An autopsy study of latent prostatic cancer. Cancer 6:531, 1953
18. Franks LM: Latent carcinoma of the prostate. J Pathol Bacteriol 68:603, 1954
19. Scott R Jr, Mutchnik DL, Laskowski TZ, et al: Carcinoma of the prostate in elderly men: incidence, growth characteristics and clinical significance. J Urol 101:602, 1969
20. Holund B: Latent prostatic cancer in a consecutive autopsy series. Scand J Urol Nephrol 14:29, 1980
21. Silverberg E: Statistical and epidemiologic data on urologic cancer. Cancer 60:692, 1987
22. Guileyardo JM, Johnson WD, Welsh RA, et al: Prevalence of latent prostate carcinoma in two U.S. populations. J Natl Cancer Inst 65:311, 1980
23. Dhom G: Epidemiologic aspects of latent and clinically manifest carcinoma of the prostate. J Cancer Res Clin Oncol 106:210, 1983
24. Yamabe H, ten Kate FJW, Gallee MPW, et al: Stage A prostatic cancer: a comparative study in Japan and the Netherlands. World J Urol 4:136, 1986
25. Breslow N, Chan CW, Dhom G, et al: Latent carcinoma of prostate at autopsy in seven areas. Int J Cancer 20:680, 1977
26. Karube K: Study of latent carcinoma of the prostate in the Japanese based on necropsy material. Tokohu J Exp Med 74:265, 1961
27. Wynder EL, Mabuchi K, Whitmore WF Jr: Epidemiology of cancer of the prostate. Cancer 28:344, 1971
28. Oota K: Latent carcinoma of the prostate among the Japanese. Asian Med J 4:213, 1961
29. Denton SE, Choy SH, Valk WL: Occult prostatic carcinoma diagnosed by the step-section technique of the surgical specimen. J Urol 93:296, 1965
30. Newman AJ Jr, Graham MA, Carlton CE Jr, et al: Incidental carcinoma of the prostate at the time of transurethral resection: importance of evaluating every chip. J Urol 128:948, 1982
31. Moore GH, Lawshe B, Murphy J: Diagnosis of adenocarcinoma in transurethral resectates of the prostate gland. Am J Surg Pathol 10:165, 1986
32. Rohr LR: Incidental adenocarcinoma in transurethral resection of the prostate, partial versus complete microscopic examination. Am J Surg Pathol 11:53, 1987
33. Murphy WM, Dean PJ, Brasfield JA, et al: Incidental carcinoma of the prostate, how much sam-

pling is adequate? Am J Surg Pathol 10:170, 1986

34. Eble JN, Tejada E: Cost implications of sampling strategies for prostatic transurethral resection specimens: analysis of 549 cases. Am J Clin Pathol 85:382, 1986

35. Vollmer RT: Prostate cancer and chip specimens: complete versus partial sampling. Hum Pathol 17:285, 1986

36. Labess M: Occult carcinoma in clinically benign hypertrophy of the prostate: A pathological and clinical study. J Urol 68:893, 1952

37. Treiger P, Welfeld J, Marx J: Suprapubic prostatectomy: a review of 108 cases. Urol Cutan Rev 52:8, 1948

38. Bauer WC, McGavran MH, Carlin MR: Unsuspected carcinoma of the prostate in suprapubic prostatectomy specimens. A clinicopathological study of 55 consecutive cases. Cancer 13:370, 1960

39. Stillwell TJ, Malek RS, Engen DE, et al: Incidental adenocarcinoma after open prostatic adenectomy. J Urol 141:76, 1989

40. Battaglia S, Barbolini G, Botticelli AR: Early (stage A) prostatic cancer. IV. Methodological criteria for histopathological diagnosis. Virchows Arch [A] 382:245, 1979

41. Montie JE, Wood DP Jr, Pontes JE, et al: Adenocarcinoma of the prostate in cystoprostatectomy specimens removed for bladder cancer. Cancer 63:381, 1989

42. Belt E, Schroeder FH: Total perineal prostatectomy for carcinoma of the prostate. J Urol 107:91, 1972

43. Montgomery TR, Whitlock GF, Nohlgren JE, et al: What becomes of the patient with latent or occult carcinoma of the prostate. J Urol 86:655, 1961

44. Munsie WJ, Foster EA: Unsuspected very small foci of carcinoma of the prostate in transurethral resection specimens. Cancer 21:692, 1968

45. Correa RJ, Anderson RG, Gibbons RP, et al: Latent carcinoma of the prostate—why the controversy? J Urol 111:644, 1974

46. Byar DP: Treatment of prostatic cancer: studies by the Veterans Administration Cooperative Research Group. Bull N Y Acad Med 48:751, 1972

47. Heaney JA, Chang HC, Daly JJ, et al: Prognosis of clinically undiagnosed prostatic carcinoma and the influence of endocrine therapy. J Urol 118:283, 1977

48. Byar DP, VACURG: Survival of patients with incidentally found microscopic cancer of the prostate: results of a clinical trial of conservative treatment. J Urol 108:908, 1972

49. Lehman TH, Kirchheim D, Braun E, et al: An evaluation of radical prostatectomy for incidentally diagnosed carcinoma of the prostate. J Urol 99:646, 1968

50. Khalifa NM, Jarman WD: A study of 48 cases of incidental carcinoma of the prostate followed 10 years or longer. J Urol 116:329, 1976

51. Barnes R, Hirst A, Rosenquist R: Early carcinoma of the prostate: comparison of stages A and B. J Urol 115:404, 1976

52. Jewett HJ: The present status of radical prostatectomy for stages A and B prostatic cancer. Urol Clin North Am 2:105, 1975

53. Gleason DF, Mellinger GT, VACURG: Prediction of prognosis for prostatic adenocarcinoma by combined histological grading and clinical staging. J Urol 111:58, 1974

54. Golimbu M, Schinella R, Morales P, et al: Differences in pathological characteristics and prognosis of clinical A2 prostatic cancer from A1 and B disease. J Urol 119:618, 1978

55. Smith JA Jr, Seaman JP, Gleidman JB, et al: Pelvic lymph node metastasis from prostatic cancer: influence of tumor grade and stage in 452 consecutive patients. J Urol 130:290, 1983

56. McNeal JE, Price HM, Redwine EA, et al: Stage A versus stage B adenocarcinoma of the prostate: morphological comparison and biological significance. J Urol 139:61, 1988

57. Lefer LG, Rosier RP: Increased prevalence of prostatic carcinoma due to more thorough microscopic examination. N Engl J Med 296:109, 1977

58. Rismyhr B, Eide T, Stalsberg H: The diagnosis of carcinoma in transurethral resectates of the prostate. Acta Path Microbiol Scand Sect A 88:211, 1980

59. Golimbu M, Glasser J, Schinella R, et al: Stage A prostate cancer from pathologist's viewpoint. Urology 18:134, 1981

60. Mostofi FK: Prostate sampling. Am J Surg Pathol 10:175, 1986

61. Epstein JI, Walsh PC: Stage A prostate cancer is incidental but not insignificant: data to support radical prostatectomy for young men with stage A1 disease. Prob Urol 1:34, 1987

62. Golimbu M, Morales P: Stage A2 prostatic carcinoma, should staging system be reclassified. Urology 13:592, 1979

63. Sheldon CA, Williams RD, Fraley, EE: Inciden-

tal carcinoma of the prostate: a review of the literature and critical reappraisal of classification. J Urol 124:626, 1980

64. Varkarakis M, Castro JE, Azzopardi JG: Prognosis of stage 1 carcinoma of the prostate. Proc R Soc Med 63:91, 1970

65. Cantrell BB, DeKlerk DP, Eggleston JC, et al: Pathological factors that influence prognosis in stage A prostatic cancer: the influence of extent versus grade. J Urol 125:516, 1981

66. Epstein JI, Paull G, Eggleston JC, et al: Prognosis of untreated stage A1 prostatic carcinoma: a study of 94 cases with extended followup. J Urol 136:837, 1986

67. Epstein JI, Oesterling JE, Walsh PC: Tumor volume versus percentage of specimen involved by tumor correlated with progression in stage A prostatic cancer. J Urol 139:980, 1988

68. McNeal JE: Origin and development of carcinoma of the prostate. Cancer 23:24, 1969

69. Zincke H, Farrow GM, Myers RP, et al: Relationship between grade and stage of adenocarcinoma of the prostate and regional pelvic lymph node metastases. J Urol 128:498, 1982

70. Blute ML, Zincke H, Farrow GM: Long-term followup of young patients with stage A adenocarcinoma of the prostate. J Urol 136:840, 1986

71. Benson RC Jr, Tomera KM, Zincke H, et al: Bilateral pelvic lymphadenectomy and radical retropubic prostatectomy for adenocarcinoma confined to the prostate. J Urol 131:1103, 1984

72. Fan K, Peng C: Predicting the probability of bone metastasis through histological grading of prostate carcinoma: a retrospective correlative analysis of 81 autopsy cases with antemortem transurethral resection specimen. J Urol 130:708, 1983

73. Humphrey P, Vollmer RT: The ratio of prostate chips with cancer: a new measure of tumor extent and its relationship to grade and prognosis. Hum Pathol 19:411, 1988

74. McMillen SM, Wettlaufer JN: The role of repeat transurethral biopsy in stage A carcinoma of the prostate. J Urol 116:759, 1976

75. Ford TF, Cameron KM, Parkinson MC, et al: Incidental carcinoma of the prostate: treatment selection by second-look TURP. Br J Urol 56:682, 1984

76. Carroll PR, Leitner TC, Yen TSB, et al: Incidental carcinoma of the prostate: significance of staging transurethral resection. J Urol 133:811, 1985

77. Parfitt HE Jr, Smith JA Jr, Gliedman JB, et al: Accuracy of staging in A1 carcinoma of the prostate. Cancer 51:2346, 1983

78. Bridges CH, Belville WD, Insalaco SJ, et al: Stage A prostatic carcinoma and repeat transurethral resection: a reappraisal 5 years later. J Urol 129:307, 1983

79. Sonda LP, Grossman HB, MacGregor RJ, et al: Incidental adenocarcinoma of the prostate: the role of repeat transurethral resection in staging. Prostate 5:141, 1984

80. DeKernion JB: Treatment of localized prostatic carcinoma. p. 329. In Kaufman JJ (ed): Current Urologic Therapy. 2nd Ed. WB Saunders, Philadelphia, 1986

81. Catalona WJ, Scott WW: Carcinoma of the prostate. In: Walsh PC, Gittes RF, Perlmutter AD, Stamey TA (eds): Campbell's Urology. 5th Ed. WB Saunders, Philadelphia, 1986

82. Paulson DF, Robertson JE, Daubert LM, et al: Radical prostatectomy in stage A prostatic adenocarcinoma. J Urol 140:535, 1988

83. Epstein JI, Oesterling JE, Walsh PC: The volume and anatomical location of residual tumor in radical prostatectomy specimens removed for stage A1 prostate cancer. J Urol 139:975, 1988

84. Neerhut GJ, Wheeler TM, Dunn JK, et al: Residual tumor after TUR: Pathologic features of stage A prostate cancer in the transurethral and radical prostatectomy specimens. J Urol 139:315A, 1988

85. Walsh PC, Epstein JI, Lowe FC: Potency following radical prostatectomy with wide unilateral excision of the neurovascular bundle. J Urol 138:823, 1987

86. Donohue RE, Mani JH, Whitesel JA, et al: Pelvic lymph node dissection, guide to patient management in clinically locally confined adenocarcinoma of prostate. Urology 20:559, 1982

87. Parfitt HE, Smith JA, Seaman JP, et al: Surgical treatment of stage A2 prostatic carcinoma: significance of tumor grade and extent. J Urol 129:763, 1983

88. Catalona WJ, Stein AJ: Staging errors in clinically localized prostatic cancer. J Urol 127:452, 1982

89. Fowler JE, Whitmore WF Jr: The incidence and extent of pelvic lymph node metastases in apparently localized prostatic cancer. Cancer 47:2941, 1981

90. Oesterling JE, Brendler CB, Epstein JI, et al:

Correlation of clinical stage, serum prostatic acid phosphatase and preoperative Gleason grade with final pathological stage in 275 patients with clinically localized adenocarcinoma of the prostate. J Urol 138:92, 1987

91. Fowler JE Jr, Mills SE: Operable prostatic carcinoma: correlations among clinical stage, pathological stage, Gleason histological score and early disease-free survival. J Urol 133:49, 1985

92. Elder JS, Gibbons RP, Correa RJ, et al: Efficacy of radical prostatectomy for stage A2 carcinoma of the prostate. Cancer 56:2151, 1985

93. Christensen WN, Walsh PC, Epstein JI: Pathologic findings in stage A2 prostate cancer: Relation of tumor volume, grade, and location to pathologic stage. Cancer (in press)

94. Partin AW, Epstein JI, et al: Morphometric measurement of tumor volume and percent of gland involvement as predictors of pathologic stage in stage B prostate cancer. J Urol 141:341, 1989

6

Histologic Grading of Prostatic Carcinoma

Donald F. Gleason

It has been difficult to select the best treatment for prostatic cancer because of its variable and frequently prolonged course. Many patients must be followed for many years to average-out this variability and compare two different treatments.

Compounding the problem, careful autopsy studies reveal many unsuspected prostate cancers, increasing in incidence with age. The increasing incidence with age indicates that many of these tumors were present for many years. For example, if the incidence of unsuspected tumors is about 10 percent at age 55, 20 percent at age 65, and 30 percent at age 75, then two thirds of the tumors in the 75-year-old men must have been present for more than 10 years and one third must have been present for more than 20 years! Most of them had caused no difficulty and obviously did not need treatment.

However, some of these tumors will inevitably be found in presumed-benign prostate tissue resected during life. If they did not need treatment, then any unnecessary and potentially dangerous treatment should be avoided. On the other hand, some stage A tumors do grow and progress, and a few prove to be fatal cancers.

An estimate of the probability that a certain tumor may progress is provided by the microscopic appearance of the tumor—its histologic structure.

HISTOLOGIC GRADING

Prostatic adenocarcinomas have a unique range of biologic and histologic malignancy. They can vary from rapidly growing, fatal cancers to pathologist-certified cancers that never do progress—with a complete spectrum of intermediate behaviors. Similarly, their histologic structure may range from completely anaplastic malignant tumors to uniform, well-differentiated glandular tumors—with a complete spectrum of intermediate structures.

For more than 50 years, there have been many reports of a strong correlation between the histologic structure and the biologic malignancy of these tumors. Poorly differentiated tumors progress rapidly; well-differentiated tumors progress slowly. These reports grouped histologic patterns into *grades* of malignancy, describing them subjectively with words and illustrating them with photomicrographs. However, it proved difficult for other pathologists to adopt the published systems with confidence and most felt obliged to devise their own grading systems.

THE VACURG (GLEASON) GRADING SYSTEM

The Veterans Administration Cooperative Urological Research Group (VACURG) studied prostatic carcinoma in a prospective, controlled, randomized clinical trial of more than 4,000 patients in 20 Veterans Administration (VA) hospitals from 1960 to 1975, and developed yet another (*Gleason*) histologic grading system.[1-4]

The histologic patterns were categorized at relatively low magnification ($\times$10-40) by the extent of glandular differentiation and the pattern of growth of the tumor in the prostatic stroma.

The larger number of carefully studied and

carefully followed patients in the VACURG studies permitted the objective development of a self-defining grading system. That is, histologic patterns were recorded and much later the patterns were ranked in order of biologic malignancy by their cancer-specific death rates—a numerical or statistical taxonomy.

The system was first published in 1966[1,2] and refined in 1974[3] and 1977.[4] It is now used quite widely in the United States. Four factors seem to contribute to this success:

1. The histologic patterns were identified simply by their appearance, with no attempt to fit them into morphogenetic or other models that imply more than we actually know.
2. The feedback of the subsequently expressed degrees of biologic malignancy enabled us to combine nine different patterns into five grades, because some patterns had similar biologic malignancy and also were frequently associated with each other.
3. For teaching purposes, we "froze" the histologic criteria into a simplified, standardizing drawing (Fig. 6-1).
4. We confirmed the familiar observation that many tumors contain more than one histologic grade. We recorded these without preconceived opinions of "worst" or "best" but did identify a primary grade (predominant by area) and secondary grade.

In the subsequent follow-up data, it was found that patients with two different grades of tumor had cancer death rates that were intermediate between the rates for those patients with only the pure form of each of those two grades. Cancer of the prostate was *not* "as bad as its worst part"—its biologic behavior was more closely related to the average histologic grade.

This led us to average the two grades found in one tumor. That is, the two grade numbers were added together, but division by two was omitted, creating a new *histologic score,* which could range from 2 to 10.[3,4] (If only one grade was present, that grade was multiplied by 2.) This histologic score proved to be the strongest single measurement correlated with the subse-

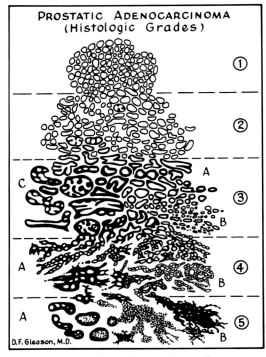

Fig. 6-1. Standardizing drawing for grading prostate cancer.

quently observed total and cancer-specific death rates (Fig. 6-2).

The histologic score was found to correlate to some degree with almost any variable that might relate to the degree of biologic malignancy of the tumors, such as the initial clinical findings—the presence of hydronephrosis, elevation of serum prostatic acid phosphatase, presence of metastases, the amount of pain suffered,[4] etc.—or the incidence of metastases at autopsy many years later.

Byar and Corle[5] found good correlation between the histologic score and the rate of progression from stages I and II to stage IV.

The standardizing drawing enabled others to adopt the grading system. Thus, Corriere et al.,[6] in 1970, confirmed the survival rate correlations. Paulson et al.,[7] Kramer et al.,[8] Thomas et al.,[9] and Pistema et al.[10] found strong correlations between VA histologic scores and the incidence of lymph node metastases in staging laparoto-

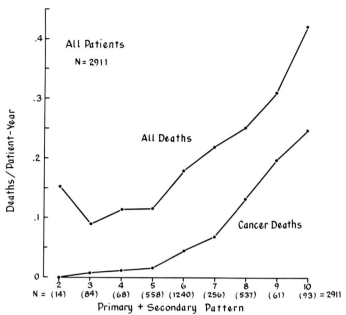

Fig. 6-2. Total and cancer death rates by histologic score.

mies. Some of these investigators even suggested that the correlations were strong enough to forego the risks and complications of laparotomy and lymph node dissection in those patients with the highest and the lowest histologic scores.

Piscioli et al.,[11] in Italy, confirmed the correlation between histologic scores and the incidence of lymph node metastases detected by percutaneous fine-needle aspiration biopsies.

Sogani et al.[12] in New York and Nemoto et al.[13] in Japan confirmed the strength of the VA histologic score in predicting survival, reporting figures quite consistent with each other and with the VACURG data.[3, 4]

In general, the published data of many independent workers confirmed the findings of the VACURG, but a few investigators published differing results, reporting higher rates of metastases for some low grade tumors.[14–16] The general agreement among most workers leads us to suspect that the discrepancies are due to faulty grading, labeling grades 3 and 4 as grades 1, 2, or 3, etc. We have observed such errors when we could review the original material. In this report, we provide a few additional details

for the VA grading system in order to avoid such errors and some other errors we have observed.

SELECTED DETAILS OF THE VA GRADING SYSTEM

The tumor grades are identified by a blending of the degree of glandular differentiation and the growth pattern of the tumors. Neither attribute is completely controlling.

Grade 1. The tumor consists of close-packed, monotonously replicated, simple glands, lined by a single layer of rectangular epithelial cells. These glands are grouped in roughly rounded masses with relatively smooth, "pushing" edges. Since some forms of benign or atypical hyperplasia also fulfill those criteria, the final requirement for grade 1 tumor is the presence of at least a few cells (as few as 1 percent) or many cells, containing very definitely enlarged nucleoli (greater than 1 μm in diameter).

The standard drawing (Fig. 6-1) deliberately overemphasizes the uniformity of the glands,

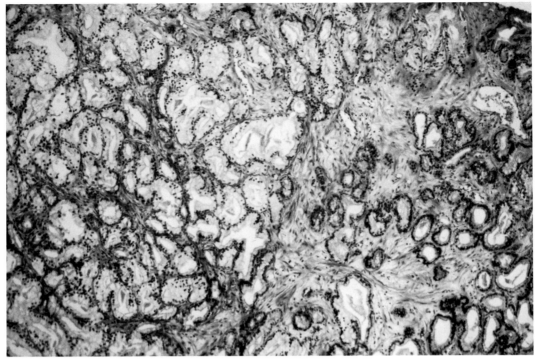

Fig. 6-3. Grade 1 (left); grade 2 (right).

and one must allow for the variation inherent in biologic material. The majority of grade 1 glands will be packed together back-to-back, but more loosely arranged areas may be present, as in Figure 6-3. The size and shape of the glands will be disturbed by plane of section and by other random variations. The outlines of the tumor masses will not be perfectly rounded but must be relatively smooth and abrupt. Definite separation of more than a few glands at the periphery suggests a higher grade. The rounded areas of tumor are usually relatively small, but grade 1 tumor can be quite extensive. Grade 1 tumor can be so well differentiated that some pathologists prefer to call the small areas *adenosis* rather than carcinoma.

Grade 2. The hallmarks of grade 2 tumor are mild but definite separation of the tumor glands by stroma and, usually, more variation in the size and shape of glands (Figs. 6-3 and 6-4) than in grade 1, although not a severe variation, as in grade 3 (Fig. 6-5). The separation of the glands is also seen at the edges of the tumor areas and suggests some limited ability to spread through the stroma. The separation of the tumor glands usually averages less than one average gland diameter, but random variation occurs (Fig. 6-3). Small areas of grade 2 tumor are also called *adenosis* by some pathologists.

Grade 3. The three forms of grade 3 tumor are labeled A, B, and C in the drawing (Fig. 6-1). The hallmarks of grades 3A and 3B are more severe variation in the shape and size and separation of the single, separate glands than in grade 2 (Fig. 6-5 vs Fig. 6-4). Some of the individual grade 3 glands will be angular, or have elongate or twisted forms, some with sharp "corners" (Fig. 6-5). There is often marked variation in the size of the glands and the cytoplasm of the tumor cells tends to be more basophilic than grades 1 and 2, but these changes are variable and of secondary importance. The glands are usually spaced more than one average gland diameter apart, but this may vary markedly from field to field. This separation includes irregular extension of glands into the surrounding prostatic stroma—the tumor areas have

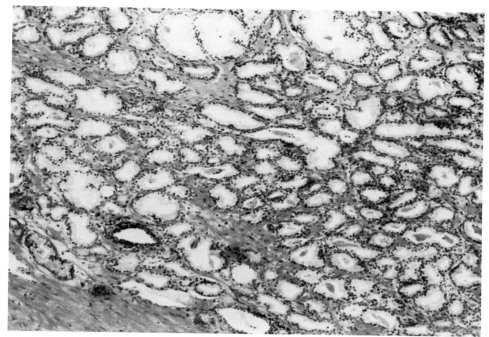

Fig. 6-4. Grade 2.

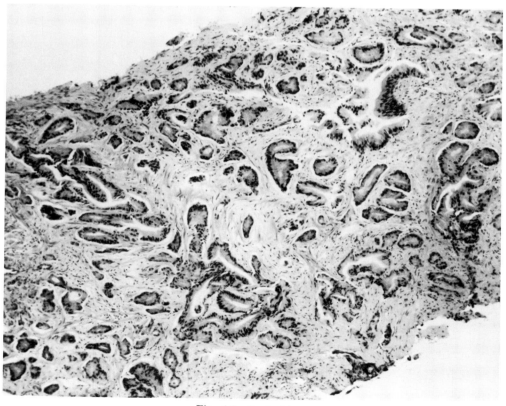

Fig. 6-5. Grade 3A.

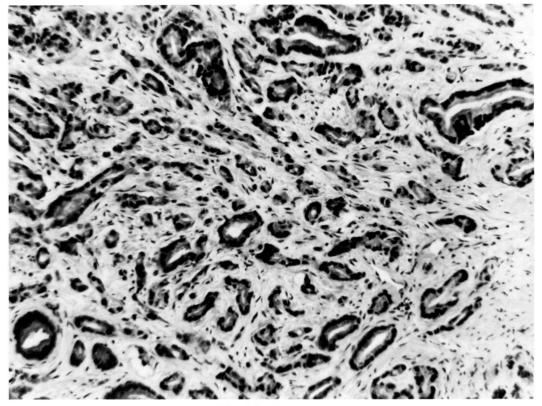

Fig. 6-6. Grade 3B.

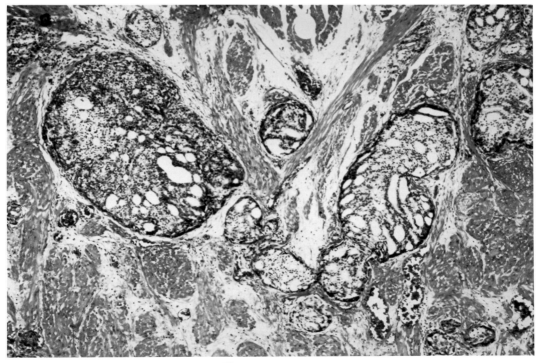

Fig. 6-7. Grade 3C.

"ragged" edges. Rarely, grade 3 tumor glands are closely packed, but then the tumor glands must be very irregular in shape and there must be definite infiltration of glands off into the surrounding stroma. Grades 3A and 3B differ only in the average size of the tumor glands. Grade 3A glands are moderate to large; 3B glands are small, sometimes only tiny clusters of three of more cells, some with tiny lumina or even no lumen (Fig. 6-6) but there must be no linking into cords or chains, as in grade 4, below. Grade 3B tumor is mildly more malignant than 3A.

The third form of grade 3 (3C in the drawing) consists of masses and cords of papillary and/or cribriform tumor, but the edges of the areas of tumor masses have smooth rounded edges with no ragged invasive edges (Fig. 6-7). Some of these tumors have been given morphogenetic names such as *intraductal carcinoma,* and *endometrioid carcinoma,* but in this grading system they are just another growth pattern, often accompanied by and fusing with simple single-gland tumor. Grades 3A, 3B, and 3C are grouped together because they are often found together and have similar cancer death rates. Grade 3C tumor is somewhat more malignant than 3A and 3B.

Grade 4. Grade 4 tumor may also be microacinar, cribriform, or papillary but the masses of tumor have ragged, obviously invading edges, rather than the smooth "pushing" edges of grade 3C. It appears that, in three dimensions, grade 4 tumor grows in a ragged spongework of epithelium, having lost the simple entwined tubular structure of grades 1 and 2 and 3A and 3B, as emphasized in Figure 6-8. The more common form (4A) with dark cells and the *hypernephroid* clear cell form (4B) have approximately the same degree of biologic malignancy and are often found together.

The simpler forms of grade 4 may easily be misgraded as grade 3 or 2. Grade 4 can have quite uniform glandular structure and bland cytology but should be recognized by the fusion of tubules (Figs. 6-9 and 6-10). One form of grade 4 appears to be a transition between grade 3B and anaplastic grade 5B, with tiny glands

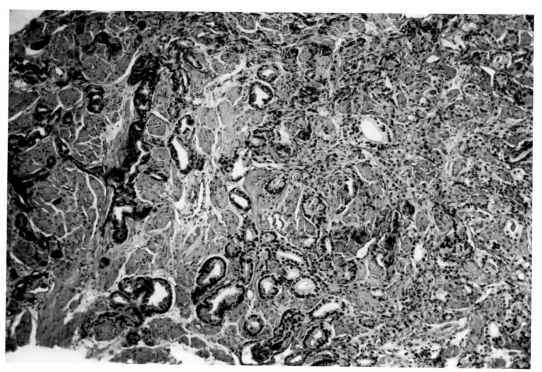

Fig. 6-8. Grade 3A (left); grade 4A (right).

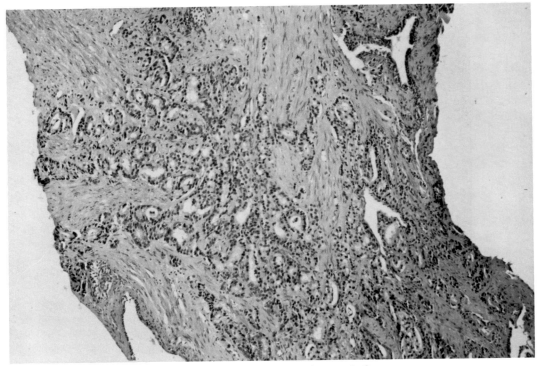

Fig. 6-9. Grade 4, not grade 2 or grade 3.

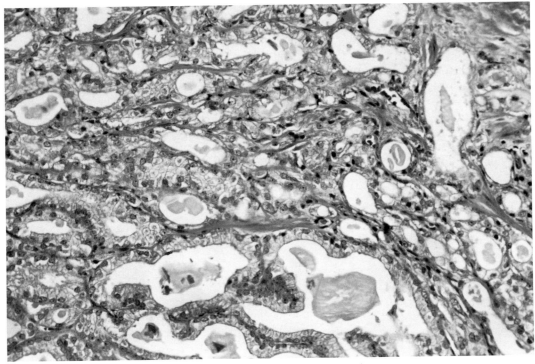

Fig. 6-10. Grade 4, not grade 1, 2, or 3.

linking into chains and cords. Grade 4 is much more malignant than grade 3.

Grade 5. Grade 5 also includes two patterns. Grade 5B in the drawing is raggedly infiltrating, virtually anaplastic tumor, with only scattered gland lumina or vacuoles to remind one that it is an adenocarcinoma. It may be identical to small cell carcinoma of the lung and other organs, histologically and biologically, with various paraneoplastic syndromes.

The other form of grade 5 (5A in the drawing) consists of smooth, rounded, packed, papillary or cribriform cylinders with variable foci of central necrosis—*comedocarcinoma*. Grade 5A may closely resemble grade 3C, but any necrosis of the epithelium overrules that appearance and indicates grade 5 (Fig. 6-11). On the other hand, the tumor cylinders may be so solid that one makes the diagnosis of comedocarcinoma without actual necrosis.

A definite, conscious effort is made to limit the histologic grading to a single grade: Mixtures of 3A, 3B, and 3C are simply grade 3. Minor variations and/or the distortions of inflammation or crushing in otherwise single grade tumors are ignored. Small amounts (less than 3 percent) of a second grade of tumor in the presence of large amounts of pure single grade tumor are ignored. With those exclusions, about half of the VACURG cases had pure single-grade tumor, but half of the cases had a definite second histologic grade that involved more than 5 percent of the total tumor area.

A few tumors contained a third or even fourth or fifth grade, but we limited our reports to two grades. We could never acquire enough three-grade tumors to evaluate their behavior, so we adopted artificial algorithms to deal with three or more grades: The lowest grade is omitted if it is less than 5 percent of the tumor. The middle grade is omitted and the highest and the lowest grades recorded if they each are at least 5 percent of the tumor. If the highest grade is less than 5 percent of the tumor and the other two grades are very extensive, the highest grade is omitted. If the highest grade is more than 5 percent of the tumor and one of the other grades is very extensive, that pre-

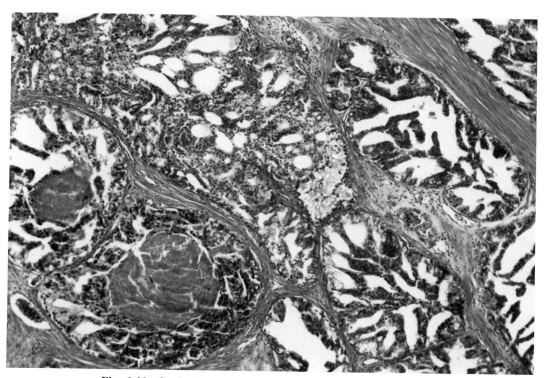

Fig. 6-11. Grade 5A. The presence of necrosis excludes grade 3C.

dominant grade is recorded as the primary grade and the highest grade as the secondary grade. If the three grades are not adjacent numerically, such as 1–2–4, the two highest grades are used (grades 1 and 2 have very little effect on the two higher grades). In needle biopsies or other small samples, the two highest grades are recorded to avoid sampling error.

SOME BIOLOGIC IMPLICATIONS FROM HISTOLOGIC GRADING

The finding that tumors with two grades are *not* as bad as their worst part contradicts a venerable aphorism. The biologic malignancy of prostate cancers is more closely related to their average histologic grade than to their highest grade. The same finding has been noted for breast cancer with objective morphometric data[17] and may be a general phenomenon.

The old aphorism was intuitively satisfying. If tumors are clones of malignant cells and even more malignant cells appear, it seemed logical that the more malignant cells would dominate the growth rate of the tumor, independently of any less malignant cells, and the tumor would be as malignant as its worst part. However, the facts indicate that the presence of lower-grade tumor is somehow associated with less malignant behavior than that of the worst tumor present.

This was puzzling, but some new observations and some very old observations suggest an explanation. Histochemical stains, immunologic stains, flow cytometry, etc., indicate that most tumors are not pure, simple clones. There is substantial heterogeneity in many tumors with varied genetic structure and varying somatic differentiation, including differences in prostatic acid phosphatase and prostate-specific antigen content in adjacent prostatic tumor cells. These somatic differences suggest varying maturation of some cells to better differentiated, less malignant states.

Maturation of tumor cells offers an explanation for the fact that tumors containing two grades of tumor could have degrees of biologic malignancy intermediate between those of the two separate grades. If some fraction of all the newly divided cells matures to a less malignant histologic grade, the overall growth rate of the tumor must be slower than that of the most malignant cells.

This is the concept that Broders[18] presented in 1926, that tumors may "put the brakes on themselves," so to speak, by maturing into slower-dividing or nondividing, postmitotic cells, which produced a correlation between histologic appearance and biologic malignancy.

Maturation of cancer cells was clearly demonstrated by Pierce and Wallace,[19] who traced the apparent migration, with time, of newly formed, labeled DNA from poorly differentiated rapidly dividing cells into the mature squamous cells of a mouse carcinoma. An induced maturation of leukemic cells may explain the favorable effects of some nonspecific agents.[20]

Thus, the better-differentiated areas in malignant tumors probably *become better differentiated* rather than have the less-differentiated areas *become less well differentiated.*

A second implication from histologic grading and follow-up is that most prostate cancers probably maintain their degree of malignancy from inception. This contradicts the more popular hypothesis of "linear progression of malignancy with time," which postulates that most cancers originate as low-grade tumors and gradually grow more malignant with time. It explains the strong correlation between tumor size and degree of malignancy as indicating that the larger tumors had been growing longer and had time to become more malignant. A little awkwardly for this theory, the many small tumors—of long duration—found at autopsy somehow failed to enter an accelerated growth phase.

However, all the relevant observations can be explained just as readily by assuming that the tumors have a relatively fixed degree of biologic malignancy from inception and that they grow at more or less fixed rates predetermined by this innate degree of malignancy—a hypothesis of *biologic determinism.*

This theory suggests that larger tumors are more malignant only because they are more malignant from inception and grow rapidly in size. The less malignant tumors grow more slowly and do not become large. The strong correlations between histologic grade and subsequent tumor growth could not exist if the biologic malignancy of tumors were not relatively stable. Low-histologic-grade tumors very rarely progress rapidly. The many small well-differentiated tumors found at autopsy seem to have been present for many years. There is no strong trend to higher histologic grade or more aggressive malignancy in older men. The poorly differentiated and rapidly growing tumors often seem to have been present for only a short time (causing brief symptoms, having rapid spread after diagnosis, occurring in young men, etc.). The intermediate-grade tumors behave in intermediate fashion.

Thus, prostate cancer may be discovered at any size or stage and will usually pursue a fairly steady course at a rate dictated by its own innate degree of malignancy. Apparently, explosive increases to higher grade are rare exceptions, and their effects are included in the data reported. Subject to the many variables in the battle between the tumor and host, prostate cancers grow at rates correlated, albeit more or less imperfectly, with their histologic grade. The correlations can be accepted and applied at face value, wherever pertinent.

REFERENCES

1. Gleason D: Classification of prostatic carcinomas. Cancer Chemother Rep 50:125, 1966
2. Baillar J, Mellinger G, Gleason D: Survival rates of patients with prostatic cancer, tumor stage and differentiation—a preliminary report. Cancer Chemother Rep 50:129, 1966
3. Gleason, D, Mellinger G, VACURG: Prediction of prognosis for prostatic carcinoma by combined histological grading and clinical staging. J Urol 111:58, 1974
4. Gleason D: Histologic grading and clinical staging of carcinoma of the prostate. p. 171. In Tannenbaum M (ed): Urologic Pathology: The Prostate. Lea & Febiger, Philadelphia, 1977
5. Byar D, Corle D, VACURG: VACURG randomized trial of radical prostatectomy for stages I and II prostatic cancer. Urology suppl. part II, 17:7, 1981
6. Corriere J, Cornog J, Murphy J: Prognosis in patients with carcinoma of the prostate. Cancer 25:911, 1970
7. Paulson D, Piserchia P, Gardner W: Predictors of lymphatic spread in prostatic adenocarcinoma. J Urol 123:697, 1980
8. Kramer S, Spahr J, Brendler C, et al: Experience with Gleason's grading system in prostatic cancer. J Urol 124:223, 1980
9. Thomas R, Lewis R, Sarma D, et al: Aid to accurate staging—histologic grading in prostatic cancer. J Urol 128:726, 1980
10. Pistenma D, Bagshaw M, Freiha F: Extended-field radiation therapy for prostatic adenocarcinoma: status report of a limited prospective trial. p. 229. In Johnson D, Samuels M (eds): Cancer of the Genitourinary Tract. Raven Press, New York, 1979
11. Piscioli F, Leonardi E, Reich A, Luciani L: Percutaneous lymph node aspiration biopsy and tumor grade in staging of prostatic carcinoma. Prostate 5:459, 1984
12. Sogani P, Israel A, Lieberman P, et al: Gleason grading of prostate cancer: a predictor of survival. Urology 25:223, 1985
13. Nemoto R, Uchida K, Harada M, et al: Experience with Gleason histopathologic grading of prostate cancer in Japan. Urology 30:436, 1987
14. Olsson C: Staging lymphadenectomy should be an antecedent to treatment in localized prostatic carcinoma. Urology 25:4, 1985
15. Catalona W, Stein A, Fair W: Grading errors in prostatic needle biopsies: relation to the accuracy of tumor grade in predicting pelvic lymph node metastases. J Urol 127:919, 1982
16. Lange P, Narayan P: Understaging and undergrading of prostate cancer: argument for postoperative radiation as adjuvant therapy. Urology 21:113, 1983
17. Sharkey F: Morphometric analysis of differentiation in human breast carcinoma: tumor heterogeneity. Arch Pathol Lab Med 307:309. 1982
18. Broders A: Carcinoma. Grading and practical application. Arch Pathol 2:376, 1926
19. Pierce G and Wallace C: Differentiation of malignant into benign cells. Cancer Res 31:127, 1971
20. Ross D: Leukemic cell maturation. Arch Pathol Lab Med 109:309, 1985

7

Variants of Prostatic Carcinoma

David G. Bostwick and John N. Eble

Numerous interesting and rare morphologic variants of prostatic carcinoma have been identified in the last two decades. It is important to recognize and accurately diagnose special variants, and understand the criteria that distinguish these from benign mimics. Unusual tumors arising in the prostate raise questions of tumor origin, particularly whether the tumor represents metastasis from another site. Also, the clinical behavior of morphologic variants may differ from usual prostatic adenocarcinoma, carrying a better or worse prognosis. A proposed classification of variants of prostatic carcinoma is presented in Table 7-1.

ADENOCARCINOMA WITH ENDOMETRIOID FEATURES

Adenocarcinoma with endometrioid features, also called *endometrioid carcinoma* or *ductal carcinoma,* occurs within the prostatic urethra and periurethral prostatic ducts, exhibiting a striking histologic similarity to endometrial adenocarcinoma of the female uterus. In the original reports, the morphologic appearance and consistent location of these tumors near the prostatic verumontanum suggested origin from the müllerian (female) remnant of the utriculus masculinus, and the implication was that these tumors might display estrogen dependence.[1, 2] The therapeutic importance of estrogen-dependent prostatic carcinoma would be considerable, since hormonal (estrogen) therapy would be contraindicated. Although the hypothesis of true uterine (endometrial) carcinoma arising in the male is intriguing, there is at present no evidence that these tumors are derived from müllerian epithelium. Recently, investigators have demonstrated that endometrioid carcinoma is an unusual variant of prostatic adenocarcinoma, according to embryonic, morphologic, enzymatic, immunologic, and clinical evidence.[3–29] It has been suggested that the term *endometrial* be abandoned, and these tumors be classified as adenocarcinoma with endometrioid features, or prostatic duct carcinoma with endometrioid features.[3, 20]

CLINICAL FEATURES

Endometrioid carcinoma occurs exclusively in older men, who present with symptoms of

Table 7–1. Variants of Prostatic Carcinoma

Adenocarcinoma and Associated Tumors
    Adenocarcinoma with endometrioid features
    Adenoid cystic carcinoma (adenoid cystic-like tumor)
    Mucinous carcinoma
    Signet ring cell carcinoma
    Squamous and adenosquamous carcinoma
    Sarcomatoid carcinoma
    Neuroendocrine neoplasms (carcinoid and small cell carcinoma)
    Cribriform carcinoma[a]
    Comedocarcinoma[a]

Other Malignant Epithelial Tumors
    Transitional cell carcinoma
    Malignant melanoma
    Mixed tumors
        Malignant phyllodes tumor
        Carcinosarcoma
    Metastatic carcinoma

[a] These histologic patterns should not be considered as distinct clinicopathologic entities (see text).

95

hematuria, urinary urgency and frequency, and rarely with acute retention. In some instances, asymptomatic patients are found to have abnormal digital rectal examinations, and, in such cases, coexistent acinar adenocarcinoma is identified in addition to the endometrioid pattern. Cystoscopically, endometrioid carcinoma consists of multiple friable polypoid "worm-like"

white masses protruding from ducts at or near the mouth of the prostatic utricle at the apex of the verumontanum, with or without infiltration.

The prostate gland is usually enlarged, with palpable induration or nodularity in up to 54 percent of cases.[3] Nodular hyperplasia is occasionally observed.

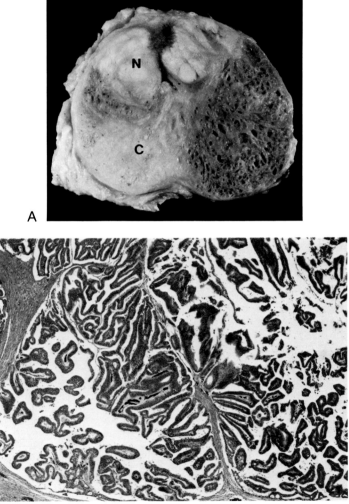

Fig. 7-1. Prostatic adenocarcinoma with endometrioid features. **(A)** Autopsy prostate showing extensive unilateral adenocarcinoma *(C)* and rounded lobulated masses of nodular hyperplasia *(N)* compressing the urethral lumen. Carcinoma involves the large periurethral prostatic ducts, but does not extend into the urethra. **(B)** Papillary pattern of endometrioid carcinoma. (H&E, ×35) *(Figure continues.)*

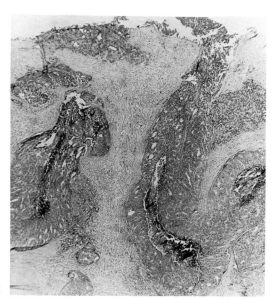

C

Fig. 7-1. (*Continued*). (**C**) Complex ramifying glandular pattern of endometrioid carcinoma. Note the urethral lumen at top. (H&E, ×40).

At the time of presentation, the majority of patients have tumors confined to the prostate or urethra, with concurrent invasive acinar prostatic adenocarcinoma in up to 77 percent of cases.[3] In a recent report, Ro et al. noted that 9 of 35 patients had stage C tumors, and 11 of 35 had stage D tumors.[20]

Serum levels of prostatic acid phosphatase (PAP) are usually normal at the time of diagnosis except in patients with bone metastases.[3] This is in contrast with the usual acinar prostatic adenocarcinoma, which has elevated serum PAP levels in 64 percent of cases.[30] This discrepancy in levels of serum PAP might be due to the early onset of obstructive symptoms and rapid diagnosis of centrally located (periurethral or intraurethral) endometrioid carcinoma as compared with the usual peripheral prostatic carcinoma, and also the smaller tumor volume of endometrioid carcinoma at the time of diagnosis. Numerous reports have stressed the importance of tumor volume rather than histologic differentiation in predicting serum levels of PAP.[31]

PATHOLOGIC FINDINGS

Prostatic adenocarcinoma with endometrioid features usually involves the large periurethral prostatic ducts and verumontanum, with direct spread through the duct-acinar system. The tumors are at least focally indistinguishable from uterine carcinoma, consisting of masses of complex ramified glands lined by variably stratified columnar epithelium. Two architectural patterns have been observed: intraductal papillae and complex ramifying glands (Fig. 7-1). These two growth patterns coexist in about half of the cases, and both usually display nuclear anaplasia and frequent mitoses. The characteristic appearance of endometrioid carcinoma is attributed to exophytic growth into a luminal space such as large ducts or the urethra, in a manner similar to endometrial tumors expanding into the uterine cavity or ovarian tumors growing into cystic spaces or the peritoneal cavity. This accounts for the endometrioid pattern of all intraurethral prostatic adenocarcinomas found in the files of Bostwick et al.[3] The limited space and stromal influences in the peripheral zone of the prostate usually cannot accommodate formation of papillae or complex ramified glands, accounting for the rarity or absence of tumors with endometrioid pattern at that location.

One papillary carcinoma was found in association with a benign-appearing adenomatous polyp, suggesting transition from benign to malignant.[15]

Adenocarcinoma with endometrioid features invariably displays intense cytoplasmic immunoreactivity for PAP or prostate-specific antigen (PSA).[3, 20, 22] Focal carcinoembryonic antigen (CEA) immunoreactivity has also been observed.

Ultrastructural findings include well-developed glands with distinct basal lamina, luminal microvilli, large nuclei with prominent nucleoli, desmosomes, secretory droplets, lysosomes, and abundant rough endoplasmic reticulum.[3] Two types of tumor cells are distinguished on the basis of cytoplasmic differentiation: light cells are most common, containing secretory droplets, lipid-filled vacuoles, and pinocytotic vesicles; dark cells contain electron-dense cytoplasm with abundant endoplasm reticulum and free ribosomes. Transitional forms of each of these cell types are present. In addition, rare basal-type cells are identified adjacent to the basal lamina, with cytoplasmic features similar to those of dark cells. Although Carney and Kelalis[8] described tumor cell cilia, subsequent studies indicated that these probably were microvilli, similar to microvilli observed in usual prostatic carcinoma.[3]

TREATMENT AND PROGNOSIS

Recent reports indicate that endometrioid carcinoma of the prostate is more aggressive than previously thought. Epstein and Woodruff[22] reported a series of 10 patients, of whom three were alive with metastases at 24, 41, and 44 months, and 2 were dead with metastases in less than 4 years. Bostwick et al.[3] reported 13 patients, of whom 7 died of metastases within 6 years of diagnosis. Ro et al.[20] noted that seven of eight patients followed for more than 8 years died of metastases. The 5-year survival rates have ranged from 15 to 43 percent. The pattern of metastasis is identical to that of the usual acinar prostatic adenocarcinoma, with bones, brain, lungs, and lymph nodes the most common sites. Examination of metastases usually reveals tumor histologically similar to the endometrioid carcinoma, even when coexistent acinar carcinoma is present in the prostate, suggesting that the endometrioid pattern is more aggressive. Even if all of the 48 patients reported by Bostwick et al. and Ro et al. had presented with stage C or D tumors, the 5-year survival rates were less than those reported by the Veterans Administration Cooperative Urologic Research Group[32] study for patients with untreated stage C (58 percent 5-year survival) and stage D (20 percent) prostatic acinar carcinoma.

The compiled results indicate that the distinctive endometrioid pattern is highly predictive of invasive carcinoma and subsequent metastases. Adjuvant therapy provides palliative relief in many cases, but does not appear to influence survival. In the study by Ro et al.,[20] seven patients showed a clinical response to orchiectomy or estrogen therapy, with decreased serum levels of PAP and marked symptomatic improvement. Radiation therapy has been used to palliate voiding difficulty or hematuria, as well as to control bone pain, and the cumulative experience suggests that these tumors are sensitive to treatment with radiation.[3, 20, 22] Nonetheless, the prognosis is poor.

DIFFERENTIAL DIAGNOSIS

Primary duct (large duct) and secondary duct prostatic adenocarcinomas[10–11] are histologically indistinguishable from endometrioid carcinoma, and most investigators consider these tumors as a single entity.[20] There are no clinical or pathologic criteria for separation of endometrioid carcinoma into utricular and ductal types.

Endometrioid carcinoma must be distinguished from transitional cell carcinoma of the prostate,[33] ectopic prostatic tissue,[34] benign polyps,[35, 36] nephrogenic adenoma,[37] proliferative papillary urethritis,[38] inverted papilloma, and accentuated mucosal folds. Hoang and associates[39] described a papillary endometrioid carcinoma of the urinary bladder neck that displayed PSA and PAP immunoreactivity.

ADENOID CYSTIC CARCINOMA

Adenoid cystic carcinoma of the prostate is histologically similar to its counterparts in the salivary glands and other sites. This tumor represents the malignant end of a morphologic continuum of basal cell proliferations in the prostate that includes basal cell hyperplasia,[40–43] adenoid cystic-like tumor (adenoid basal cell tumor), and adenoid cystic carcinoma. The criteria distinguishing these lesions have recently been refined, and the malignant nature of cases reported as adenoid cystic carcinoma has been questioned.[40, 43, 44]

Young et al.[44] reclassified four previously reported cases of adenoid cystic carcinoma as adenoid cystic-like tumor following review of the histologic slides, and added two cases from their files. Published cases illustrated in the World Health Organization[45] monograph and the AFIP[46] fascicle have been reclassified as variants of adenoid cystic-like tumor, and other reported cases have been disputed.[43, 44] Young et al.[44] indicated that virtually all cases of adenoid cystic carcinoma of the prostate in the literature resembled basal cell hyperplasia, and should not be considered malignant. There have been no documented reports of extraprostatic spread or metastasis from these tumors. Also, squamous differentiation with keratin production is frequently seen in prostatic tumors, but is rare in adenoid cystic carcinoma arising at other sites.[44] Although perineural invasion has been reported, it is rare. Grignon and associates[43] recently described an adenoid basal cell tumor with extensive perineural invasion that was interpreted as adenoid cystic carcinoma; however, that case lacked significant cytologic atypia, and no extraprostatic spread or follow-up was reported.

The histogenesis of these tumors is uncertain. Although seromucinous gland ectopia has been described in the prostate[47] and is a possible site of origin, this suggestion has been refuted.[44]

CLINICAL FEATURES

The age, presenting symptoms, and clinical findings of adenoid cystic-like tumor are similar to typical prostatic adenocarcinoma. All reported cases have been confined to the prostate at presentation and at follow-up (up to 6 years).[40, 43, 44, 48–56] Serum PAP levels are not elevated.

PATHOLOGIC FINDINGS

All reported cases of adenoid cystic carcinoma are histologically identical to the adenoid cystic-like tumor of Young et al.[44] and adenoid basal cell tumor of Grignon et al.[43] These tumors are characterized by irregular solid nests and cords of basaloid cells (Fig. 7-2). In some areas, the tumor nests are punctuated by small cystic spaces, imparting a prominent adenoid pattern. These spaces are filled with hyaline material and mucous or eosinophilic deposits. Two cells types are present: basaloid cells with delicate stippled chromatin and scant cytoplasm, and an inner lining of cuboidal to columnar duct-type cells with moderate amounts of pale eosinophilic cytoplasm. Rarely, mitotic figures and mild cytologic atypia are present. In some areas, prominent keratinization of the secretory luminal cells is observed; foci of basal cell hyperplasia are invariably present.[40–55] These tumors are expansive, extending into the stroma of the prostate without entrapping glandular elements, and are accompanied by a myxoid matrix. Adenocarcinoma has been found adjacent to foci of adenoid cystic-like tumor, but never in direct contact with it.

The basophilic material within the cystic spaces stains with alcian blue at pH 2.5, but staining is eliminated by hyaluronidase predigestion. PAS stain after diastase predigestion is positive, as is the mucicarmine stain. The myxoid stroma surrounding the tumor nests stains strongly with alcian blue at pH 2.5, weakly with periodic acid-schiff (PAS), and is unstained with mucicarmine.[43, 44]

Immunohistochemical stains reveal weak keratin immunoactivity confined to the basaloid cells. The columnar cells contain PSA and PAP. Variable staining is observed with S-100 protein in both cell types. Actin and vimentin immunostaining is negative.[43, 44]

Ultrastructurally, the basaloid cells form cohesive nests surrounded by prominent basal laminae. Well-formed desmosomes are present, and intercellular spaces are occasionally lined by microvilli or rare cilia. In nests with true lumina, the cells exhibit superficial microvilli and have nuclei with conspicuous heterochromatin. The lumina are filled with abundant vesicles, granular material, and cellular debris. In solid nests, the tumor cells have round nuclei with uniform chromatinic rims and prominent euchromatin. There is no evidence of myoepithelial differentiation.[44]

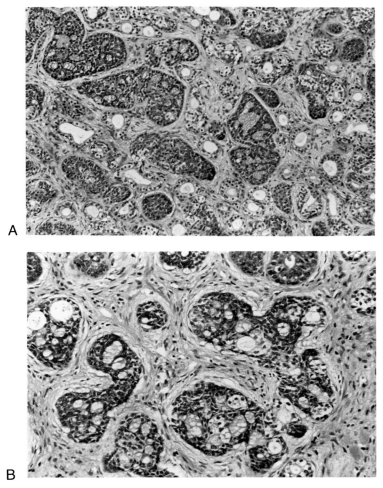

Fig. 7-2. (A & B) Adenoid cystic-like tumor of the prostate. (Fig. A: H&E, ×25; Fig. B: H&E, ×63). (Courtesy of Dr. Robert Young, Boston, MA.)

TREATMENT AND PROGNOSIS

Most patients have been treated by transurethral resection, although other forms of therapy have been employed, including radical prostatectomy and radiation therapy. There is no documented evidence of extraprostatic spread in any case, although the longest follow-up is only 6 years.[43, 44]

We concur with the conclusion of Young et al.[44] that these tumors are of uncertain malignant potential.

DIFFERENTIAL DIAGNOSIS

As discussed by Young et al.,[44] adenoid cystic-like tumor of the prostate should be distinguished from the cribriform type of prostatic adenocarcinoma. The most useful feature in making this distinction is the presence of severe cytologic atypia in cribriform carcinoma.

The case reported by Grignon et al.,[43] which is described as a true adenoid cystic carcinoma of the prostate, displayed extensive perineural invasion, a feature not observed in reported cases of adenoid cystic-like tumor.

To our knowledge, there has been no report of adenoid cystic carcinoma from another organ metastasizing to the prostate.

MUCINOUS CARCINOMA

Fewer than 50 acceptable cases of mucinous carcinoma of the prostate have been reported.[57–69] Although focal mucinous differentiation is frequently observed in prostatic adenocarcinoma, the diagnosis of mucinous carcinoma of the prostate requires that at least 25 percent of tumor be composed of lakes of extra cellular mucin; also, extraprostatic origin of the tumor must be excluded.[57, 69]

The normal prostatic epithelium contains scattered mucin-producing cells, particularly in the periurethral ducts. High-dose estrogen therapy can induce mucin secretion in prostatic carcinoma.

CLINICAL FEATURES

The clinical presentation of mucinous carcinoma is the same as that of prostatic adenocarcinoma, although serum PAP levels are not usually elevated. However, the majority of early reports of patients with normal PAP levels were low-stage tumors[60–68]; a recent report by Ro et al.[57] showed five of eight patients with high-stage mucinous carcinoma and elevated serum PAP levels.

PATHOLOGIC FINDINGS

The diagnosis of mucinous adenocarcinoma requires that more than 25 percent of excised tumor consists of tumor cells and clusters of cells floating in lakes of mucin, similar to mucinous (colloid) carcinoma of the breast (Fig. 7-3). Other histologic patterns of adenocarcinoma are almost always present in association with mucinous carcinoma, including cribriform and comedo patterns. Signet ring cells are usually not seen in these tumors, although Alfthan and Koivuniemi[66] illustrated an interesting case with abundant signet ring cells. In another unusual case, mucinous adenocarcinoma presented as a 10-cm-diameter retrovesicle cyst.[58]

The mucin stains with PAS, alcian blue, and mucicarmine stains. The tumor cells exhibit immunoreactivity for PSA and PAP, but are unreactive with CEA.[57, 69] In one case, neuron-specific enolase immunoreactivity was observed, confirming the Grimelius-positive histochemical staining.[59]

Ultrastructurally, the tumor cells are set in an amorphous background, joined by zonula adherens junctions. Microvilli and cytoplasmic projections are prominent. Nuclei are compressed to one side of the cell, with cytoplasmic organelles and mucinogen granules filling the remainder of the cell.[65]

Prioa and associates[65] identified estrogen receptors in one case.

Fine-needle aspiration may be diagnostically useful.[66]

TREATMENT AND PROGNOSIS

The pattern of metastases of mucinous carcinoma of the prostate is similar to usual prostatic adenocarcinoma. Early reports had suggested that these tumors were less aggressive and of lower stage than other forms of prostate cancer, with no tendency for bone metastasis.[60–68] However, a recent series of eight patients by Ro et al.[57] refuted these impressions. In their study, osteoblastic bone metastases occurred frequently, and six of eight patients presented with stage C or D tumors.

Treatment has included radiation therapy, hormonal therapy, or both. Five of eight patients reported by Ro et al.[57] died of tumor within 7 years, and the remaining three patients are alive

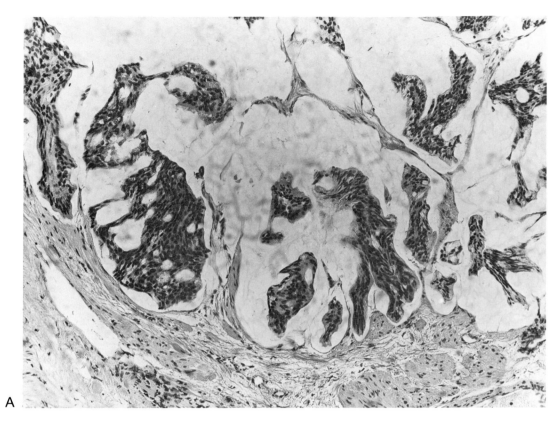

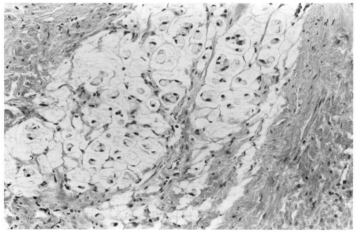

Fig. 7-3. **(A)** Mucinous carcinoma of the prostate. (H&E, ×40.) (Courtesy of Dr. Victor Fazekas, Baltimore, MD.) **(B)** Mucinous carcinoma with numerous signet ring cells. (H&E, ×63.) (Courtesy of Dr. Robert Young, Boston, MA.)

with tumor up to 15 months. The aggregate data indicate that these tumors do not respond well to endocrine or radiation therapy, and are highly aggressive.

DIFFERENTIAL DIAGNOSIS

Mucinous carcinoma of the rectum and urinary bladder may invade the prostate, mimicking mucinous carcinoma of the prostate.[57, 59, 61, 69] Similarly, Cowper's gland carcinoma displays prominent mucinous differentiation.[61] These distinctions are important because of significant differences in treatment and prognosis. Immunohistochemical stains for PSA and PAP are useful in confirming prostatic origin.

SIGNET RING CELL CARCINOMA

Signet ring cell carcinoma of the prostate is rare, and the cytoplasmic clearing is never or almost never mucicarminophilic, in contrast with mucicarmine-positive signet ring cell carcinomas of the bladder/urachus and stomach.[70–73]

CLINICAL FEATURES

Presenting signs and symptoms of signet ring cell carcinoma are similar to usual prostatic carcinoma. Serum PAP levels are frequently elevated. Two reported patients presented with supraclavicular metastases.[70, 71]

Rectal examination of the prostate reveals stony hard induration.

PATHOLOGIC FINDINGS

The diagnosis of signet ring cell carcinoma requires that 50 percent or more of the tumor be composed of signet ring cells, with nuclear displacement by optically clear cytoplasm.[70–73] Almost all reported cases have been associated with other forms of poorly differentiated prostatic adenocarcinoma, including cribriform carcinoma, comedocarcinoma, and solid (Gleason grade 5) carcinoma. The tumor cells diffusely infiltrate the stroma, invading perineural and vascular spaces, and frequently extending through the prostatic capsule.

Histochemical stains have given variable results. Giltman[73] reported pure signet ring carcinoma that was diastase-resistant PAS positive, although other stains for acid mucin and fat (mucicarmine, alcian blue, oil red O) were negative. In another case, tumor cells were shown to stain with sudan black, indicating the presence of intracellular lipid.[72] Ro et al.[70] reported eight cases in which the tumor cells did not stain for alcian blue, mucicarmine, or PAS with or without diastase. However, PSA, PAP, and keratin immunoreactivity was observed within signet ring cells and the non-signet ring cell component. No CEA staining was detected. Conversely, Remmele et al.[71] reported one case with CEA immunoreactivity that was negative for PSA and PAP.

Ultrastructurally, cytoplasmic vacuoles and intracytoplasmic lumina were observed by Ro et al., with no demonstrable mucin or lipid vacuoles. Occasional rod-shaped intraluminal crystalloids were observed in metastatic sites, similar to the crystalloids observed in usual prostatic adenocarcinoma.[70]

The signet ring cell appearance in different cases appears to be due to multiple causes, including cytoplasmic lumina, mucin granules, and fat vacuoles, thus accounting for the contradictory histochemical and immunohistochemical results.

TREATMENT AND PROGNOSIS

All reported patients have presented with stage C or D tumors, and have received hormonal therapy, radiation therapy, or both.

Five of eight patients reported by Ro et al.[70] died between 32 and 60 months after diagnosis, and two patients were alive with less than 12 months follow-up.

DIFFERENTIAL DIAGNOSIS

Signet ring cell carcinoma of the prostate should be distinguished from similar tumors arising in other sites, particularly the gastrointestinal tract and stomach. Prostatic origin should be considered in metastatic signet ring cell carcinoma of supraclavicular lymph nodes that exhibits negative mucin staining; PSA and PAP immunostaining may be useful.

Artifactual changes mimicking signet ring cell carcinoma have been described in transurethral resection specimens, with lymphocytes and vacuolated smooth muscle cells causing diagnostic difficulty (Fig. 7-4).[74] In these cases, PSA and PAP staining was negative, although leukocyte common antigen immunoreactivity was observed within the lymphocyte-like cells.

There have been no reported cases of signet ring cell lymphoma involving the prostate.

SQUAMOUS AND ADENOSQUAMOUS CARCINOMA

Keratinizing squamous cell carcinoma of the prostate usually arises in the periurethral ducts, and is extremely rare.[75–81] Although Kahler[76] identified squamous differentiation in 3 percent of prostate cancers, a lower incidence has been observed in subsequent studies.[79] Three cases of adenosquamous carcinoma of the prostate have been reported, all occurring 4 to 10 years after radiation therapy for usual prostatic carcinoma.[75]

CLINICAL FEATURES

Presenting signs and symptoms are similar to those of prostatic adenocarcinoma. Serum PAP levels were elevated in two cases of adenosquamous carcinoma.[75]

PATHOLOGIC FINDINGS

Evidence of keratinization and squamous differentiation are required for diagnosis (Fig. 7-5).

The adenosquamous carcinoma reported by Moyana[75] displayed keratin immunoreactivity in only the squamous component, but PSA and PAP immunoreactivity in both components. Electron microscopy revealed tonofibrils, tight junctions, desmosomes, and intercellular spaces lined by microvilli. He proposed that adenosquamous carcinoma arises from pluripotent stem cells, probably owing to irradiation.

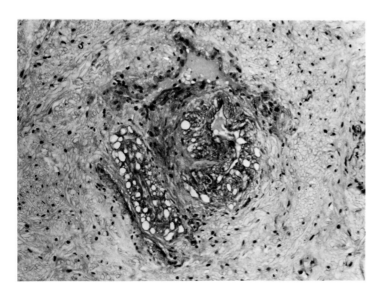

Fig. 7-4. Smooth muscle cell vacuolization following transurethral resection. Vacuolization is present chiefly in the vascular smooth muscle cells. (H&E, ×320.)

TREATMENT AND PROGNOSIS

The number of reported cases of squamous cell carcinoma is too small for any conclusions to be drawn regarding efficacy of treatment. The patient reported by Gray and Marshall[78] underwent radical surgery, but died of perineal recurrence within 1 year of diagnosis. One of three patients reported by Sieracki[77] received surgery, hormonal therapy, and radiation therapy, but died of tumor within 26 months of diagnosis. The three reported patients with adenosquamous carcinoma had metastases at the time of diagnosis.[75]

DIFFERENTIAL DIAGNOSIS

Squamous cell carcinoma of the bladder may invade the prostate. Also, atypical squamous metaplasia following prostatic infarct may simulate carcinoma histologically.

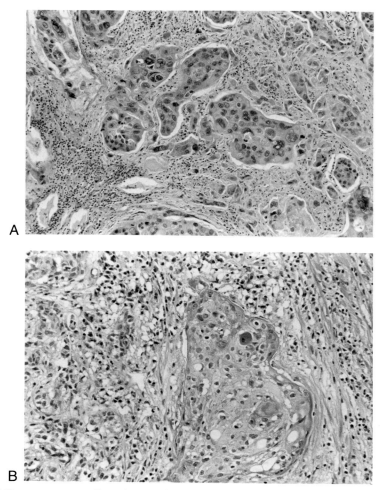

Fig. 7-5. (A) Pure squamous cell carcinoma of the prostate. (H&E, ×63). (Courtesy of Dr. Robert Young, Boston, MA.) **(B)** Adenosquamous carcinoma. Note the large island of keratinizing squamous carcinoma, surrounded by poorly differentiated adenocarcinoma. (H&E, ×63.)

SARCOMATOID CARCINOMA

Sarcomatoid carcinoma of the prostate histologically mimics true sarcoma.[82]

CLINICAL FEATURES

Patients tend to be older men who present with symptoms of urinary outlet obstruction, similar to usual adenocarcinoma. There is no published information on serum PAP levels.

PATHOLOGIC FINDINGS

In the five cases studied by Shannon and associates,[82] three displayed a mixture of sarcomatoid carcinoma and typical acinar adenocarcinoma, with transition from acinar to sarcomatoid morphology observed in two. In another patient, sarcoma was observed following diagnosis of carcinoma. The fifth patient had a long history of prostatic adenocarcinoma, with the sarcomatoid pattern observed by needle biopsy following local recurrence. In all cases, the coexistent adenocarcinoma was high grade (Gleason grades 9 to 10). Immunohistochemistry revealed immunoreactivity for PAP in two of five cases, PSA in one of three, and keratin protein in two of three.

Ultrastructurally, tumor cells within the sarcomatoid areas occasionally display desmosomes and apparent cytokeratin filaments. In two cases of Shannon et al.,[82] there was no ultrastructural evidence of epithelial differentiation.

TREATMENT AND PROGNOSIS

No details of treatment are available. Of the five patients reported by Shannon et al.,[82] three died of tumor within 46 months of diagnosis, one was alive with tumor at 48 months, and one was lost to follow-up after 1 month.

DIFFERENTIAL DIAGNOSIS

The separation of sarcomatoid carcinoma from sarcoma and true carcinosarcoma is difficult, although immunohistochemical stains and electron microscopy may be helpful.

NEUROENDOCRINE NEOPLASMS

Neuroendocrine differentiation in the prostate was first observed by Azzopardi and Evans[83] in 1971, with 10 percent of prostatic carcinomas containing argentaffin-positive cells. Subsequent investigators have confirmed these findings, observing argentaffin and argyrophil-positive cells in up to 33 percent of cases.[84–107] Using the argyrophil stain in association with several immunohistochemical neuroendocrine markers, Di Sant'Agnese and de Mesy Jensen[95] found neuroendocrine differentiation in 47 percent of prostate cancers. Abrahamsson et al.[96] noted at least focal neuroendocrine differentiation in 100 percent of prostatic carcinomas evaluated histochemically and immunohistochemically. Turbat-Herrera et al.[86] identified neuroendocrine differentiation in 12 percent of cancers at autopsy.

CLINICAL FEATURES

Paraneoplastic syndromes are frequently observed in patients with small cell carcinoma and primary carcinoid of the prostate.[100] Ectopic adrenocorticotropic hormone (ACTH) and Cushing's syndrome are most frequently observed, with ACTH immunoreactivity of tumor cells.[84, 88, 99] Antidiuretic hormone secretion and myasthenic (Eaton-Lambert) syndrome have also been observed.[105, 107]

With the exception of paraneoplastic syndromes, the presenting signs and symptoms are similar to those usual of prostatic adenocarcinoma.

Pathologic Findings

A spectrum of neuroendocrine differentiation can be seen in prostatic adenocarcinoma, varying from a carcinoid-like pattern to small cell undifferentiated (oat cell) carcinoma, with the usual patterns of acinar adenocarcinoma present at least focally (Fig. 7-6).[84–107] These tumors are morphologically identical to carcinoid tumors and small cell carcinoma of the lung and other sites.

By immunohistochemistry, a wide variety of secretory products have been observed within the tumor cells, including serotonin, calcitonin, ACTH, human chorionic gonadotropin, thyroid stimulating hormone, bombesin, gene-related peptide, atachalcin, and inhibin. Individual tumor cells may express peptide hormones in addition to PSA and PAP, a finding most frequent in well-differentiated adenocarcinoma with neuroendocrine differentiation and in carcinoid-like tumors.[84, 99, 103]

Ultrastructurally, small cell carcinoma and carcinoid tumors display features similar to their counterparts in the lung.[99] The characteristic finding is variable numbers of round, regular 100-to 400-nm-diameter membrane-bound neurosecretory-like granules. Well-defined cytoplasmic processes are usually present, with approximately 8 to 15 granules per process. The tumor cells are small, with dispersed nuclear chromatin and small inconspicuous nucleoli. No glandular differentiation is present in the neuroendocrine component, and no tonofilaments are observed. Other patterns of differentiation may also be observed within typical prostatic adenocarcinoma. We recently observed two cases of moderately differentiated carcinoma with large numbers of Paneth-like cells (Fig. 7-7).

Treatment and Prognosis

Small cell carcinoma is clinically aggressive, and the degree of aggressiveness may be directly proportional to the extent of neuroendocrine differentiation.[102]

Recent evidence suggests that the neuroendocrine component of prostatic carcinoma may be resistant to hormonal therapy.[84] Stratton et al.[87] noted that typical carcinoma with focal neuroendocrine differentiation recurred as neuroendocrine carcinoma following hormonal

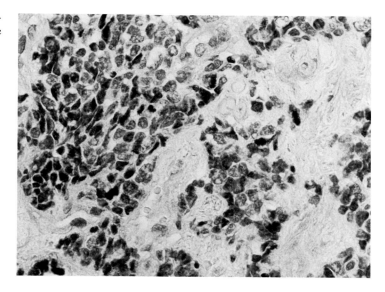

Fig. 7-6. Small cell undifferentiated (oat cell) carcinoma of the prostate. (H&E, ×550.)

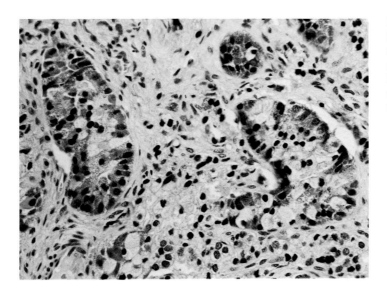

Fig. 7-7. Adenocarcinoma with Paneth-like cells. Note darkly stained granular cytoplasm of many tumor cells. Immunoperoxidase stains for neuron-specific enolase and bombesin were negative. (H&E, ×320.)

therapy. Other investigators have shown that xenografted small cell carcinoma was devoid of estrogen receptors, and also resistant to hormonal manipulation.[102] Di Sant'Agnese suggested a possible autocrine mechanism for stimulation of growth of tumor cells with epithelial and neuroendocrine differentiation.[84]

Differential Diagnosis

Neuroendocrine cells in prostatic adenocarcinoma are more common than previously thought, with an incidence of at least 10 percent.[84] Areas with neuroendocrine differentiation have previously been misinterpreted as poorly differentiated adenocarcinoma. It is important to recognize neuroendocrine components in prostatic carcinoma because of prognostic and therapeutic implications.

Although unusual, metastases to the prostate from other sites may mimic primary carcinoid and small cell carcinoma of the prostate.

CRIBRIFORM CARCINOMA

The cribriform pattern is a histologically distinct form of Gleason grade 3 carcinoma,[108] characterized by large intraductal epithelial cell masses punctuated by multiple small lumens (Fig. 7-8). McNeal et al.[109] have provided evidence that cribriform carcinoma is equivalent to Gleason grade 4 carcinoma growing within pre-existing gland lumens, and that this pattern is associated with high-volume carcinoma. These investigators also showed invasive carcinoma originating from cribriform carcinoma. We consider the cribriform pattern as histologically distinct, but it is invariably present in association with the other patterns of adenocarcinoma, and does not warrant separation as a clinicopathologic entity.

COMEDOCARCINOMA

Comedocarcinoma is characterized by luminal necrosis within ducts expanded by malignant cells, similar to comedocarcinoma of the breast (Fig. 7-9). This morphologic variant of adenocarcinoma was included in the Gleason grading system as poorly differentiated (grade 5) carcinoma based on the degree of glandular differentiation.[108] Currin et al.[110] studied the biologic potential of prostatic comedocarcinoma by flow cytometry, and found a high frequency of aneuploidy, suggesting aggressiveness. PAP and PSA were present in the majority of tumor cells.

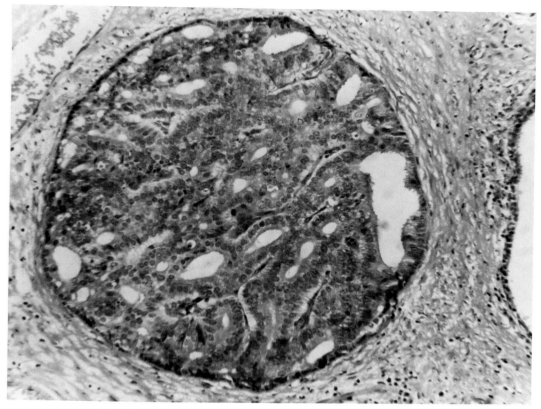

Fig. 7-8. Cribriform (sieve-like) pattern of carcinoma. (H&E, ×40.)

Fig. 7-9. Comedocarcinoma. (H&E, ×200.)

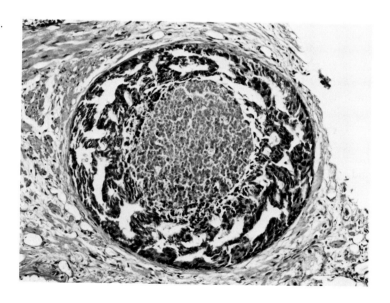

Comedocarcinoma is invariably found in association with other patterns of adenocarcinoma, and does not warrant separation as a clinico-pathologic entity.

TRANSITIONAL CELL CARCINOMA OF THE PROSTATE

Transitional cell carcinoma (TCC) of the prostate may be primary or may be synchronous or metachronous spread from carcinoma in the bladder and urethra.[33, 111–124] TCC involves the prostate in 12 to 40 percent of radical cystoprostatectomy specimens for TCC of the bladder. Primary TCC of the prostate is rare, comprising less than 4 percent of tumors originating in the prostate.[113]

CLINICAL FEATURES

Patients with TCC of the prostate usually present with symptoms of hematuria, urinary obstruction, or prostatitis. Serum PAP levels are not elevated. Clinically these tumors are often mistaken for prostatitis or nodular hyperplasia.

PATHOLOGIC FINDINGS

TCC involves the periurethral prostatic ducts and acini. Diagnostic criteria are identical to those for TCC in the bladder; most cancers are moderately differentiated, and usually associated with prominent chronic inflammation. Squamous metaplasia is infrequent.

TREATMENT AND PROGNOSIS

Radical cystoprostatectomy is the treatment of choice for TCC of the prostate. Estrogen therapy and orchiectomy have not been successful. In a recent study of 21 patients by Hardeman and Soloway,[113] radical surgery was considered the most useful form of therapy. These investigators also noted that TCC of the bladder extending into the prostate can easily be missed cysto-

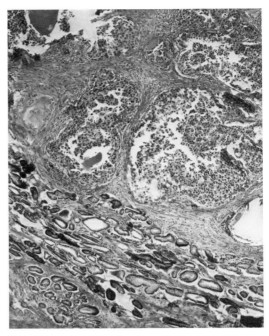

Fig. 7-10. Transitional cell carcinoma of the bladder has filled and expanded ducts and ductules of the prostate (upper half), and is present at the periphery of the gland adjacent to a small focus of adenocarcinoma (lower half). (H&E, ×65.)

scopically, and random biopsies of the prostate were recommended.

DIFFERENTIAL DIAGNOSIS

Transitional cell carcinoma within the prostate usually represents spread from urethral or bladder carcinoma, and only rarely originates in the prostate.

The distinction from adenocarcinoma is clinically important, owing to the estrogen unresponsiveness of TCC. It should be noted that adenocarcinoma and TCC may coincidentally coexist (Fig. 7-10).

MALIGNANT MELANOMA

Melanin pigment has been observed within normal prostatic epithelial cells and in tumor cells of prostatic adenocarcinoma, and rare cases of blue nevus and melanosis of the prostate have been reported (see Ch. 8). A single case of metastatic malignant melanoma presenting with prostatic enlargement has been described.[125, 126]

MIXED TUMORS

Rare prostatic tumors exhibit a mixture of benign epithelium and malignant stroma (malignant phyllodes tumor), and malignant epithelium and malignant stroma (carcinosarcoma) (see Ch. 8).

METASTATIC CARCINOMA

With the exception of leukemia, lymphoma, and cases of contiguous spread from the bladder and rectum, the prostate is infrequently involved by tumors arising in other organs, with metastases comprising only 0.5 to 2.2 percent of all prostatic neoplasms.[127–131] The most common tumors metastasizing to the prostate are lung cancers, accounting for almost half of all metastases. Malignant melanoma accounts for approximately 27 percent of prostatic metastases, with an incidence of prostatic involvement of 1.1 percent of all patients with malignant melanoma at autopsy.[130] Grignon[131] described an unusual case of tumor-to-tumor metastasis of malignant melanoma to prostatic adenocarcinoma. The remaining 25 percent of metastases to prostate are a varied mixture of cancers.

PROSTATIC ADENOCARCINOMA IN CHILDREN AND YOUNG ADULTS

Prostate cancer is rare in patients under age 40.[132, 133] A review of almost 4,000 cases in the surgical pathology files of Stanford University Medical Center between 1969 and 1984 revealed no patients with prostatic adenocarcinoma below the age of 40 years (Bostwick DG: Unpublished data). In the literature, carcinoma has been found in five children less than 12 years old, seven adolescents, and four young

adults between 20 and 25 years old.[132, 133] In all cases, the tumors were poorly differentiated and clinically aggressive. There was no response to hormonal therapy or radiation therapy.

SUMMARY

Many interesting and rare variants of prostatic carcinoma have been described and refined in recent years. Accurate diagnosis of these variants is necessary in order to determine appropriate therapy. Unusual tumors arising in the prostate raise questions of histogenesis, and may carry a better or worse prognosis than usual adenocarcinoma. Virtually the entire spectrum of cellular differentiation has been observed within prostatic epithelium, and rare neoplasms exhibit these unusual forms of differentiation as the chief component of the tumor. Epithelial neoplasms arising in childhood and early adulthood are rare and clinically aggressive.

REFERENCES

1. Melicow MM, Pachter MR: Endometrial carcinoma of prostatic utricle (uterus masculinus). Cancer 20:1715, 1967
2. Melicow MM, ·Tannenbaum M: Endometrial carcinoma of uterus masculinus (prostatic utricle). Report of 6 cases. J Urol 106:892, 1971
3. Bostwick DG, Kindrachuk RW, Rouse RV: Prostatic adenocarcinoma with endometrioid features. Am J Surg Pathol 9:595, 1985
4. August CZ, Oyasu R: Adenocarcinoma of the prostate gland: a spectrum of differentiation. Arch Pathol Lab Med 107:501, 1983
5. Bates HR Jr, Thornton JL: Adenocarcinoma of primary prostatic ducts and utricle. Arch Pathol Lab Med 96:207, 1973
6. Belter LF, Dodson AI Jr: Papillomatosis and papillary adenocarcinoma of prostatic ducts: a case report. J Urol 104:880, 1970
7. Cantrell BB, Leifer G, DeKlerk DP, et al: Papillary adenocarcinoma of the prostatic urethra with clear-cell appearance. Cancer 48:2661, 1981
8. Carney JA, Kelalis PP: Endometrial carcinoma of the prostatic utricle. Am J Clin Pathol 60:565, 1973

9. Drake WM, Burrows S: Papillary carcinoma of prostatic ducts. Urology 3:621, 1974

10. Dube VE, Farrow GM, Greene LF: Prostatic adenocarcinoma of ductal origin. Cancer 32:402, 1973

11. Greene LF, Farrow GM, Ravits JM, et al: Prostatic adenocarcinoma of ductal origin. J Urol 121:303, 1979

12. Merchant RF, Graham AR, Bucher WC Jr, et al: Endometrial carcinoma of prostatic utricle with osseous metastases. Urology 8:169, 1976

13. Satter EJ, Blumenfeld CM: Endometrial carcinoma of the prostatic utricle. J Urol 112:505, 1974

14. Tannenbaum M: Endometrial tumors and/or associated carcinomas of prostate. Urology 6:372, 1975

15. Walker AN, Mills SE, Fechner RE, et al: "Endometrial" adenocarcinoma of the prostatic urethra arising in a villous polyp. A light microscopic and immunoperoxidase study. Arch Pathol Lab Med 106:624, 1982

16. Young BW, Lagios MD: Endometrial (papillary) carcinoma of the prostatic utricle—response to orchiectomy. Cancer 32:1293, 1973

17. Zaloudek C, Williams JW, Kempson RL: "Endometrial" adenocarcinoma of the prostate. A distinctive tumor of probable prostatic duct origin. Cancer 37:2255, 1976

18. Kuhajda FP, Gipson T, Mendelsohn G: Papillary adenocarcinomas of the prostate: an immunohistochemical study. Cancer 54:1328, 1984

19. Cueva C, Urdiales J, Nogales F, et al: Papillary endometrioid carcinoma of the prostate. Br J Urol 61:98, 1988

20. Ro JY, Ayala AG, Wishnow KI, et al: Prostatic duct adenocarcinoma with endometrioid features: immunohistochemical and election miscopic study. Semin Diagn Pathol 5:301, 1988

21. Walther MM, Massar V, Harruff HC, et al: Endometrial carcinoma of the prostatic utricle: a tumor of prostatic origin. J Urol 134:769, 1985

22. Epstein JI, Woodruff JM: Adenocarcinoma of the prostate with endometrioid features: a light microscopic and immunohistochemical study of ten cases. Cancer 57:111, 1986

23. Keith RL, Flegel G: Endometrial carcinoma of the prostatic utricle: report of a case. J Am Osteopath Assoc 82:551, 1983

24. Sufrin G, Gaeta J, Staubitz WJ, et al: Endometrial carcinoma of prostate. Urology 27:18, 1986

25. Rotterdam HZ, Melicow MM: Double primary prostatic adenocarcinoma. Urology 6:245, 1975

26. Scott MB, Goldstein AM, Onofrio RC, et al: Papillary adenocarcinoma of the prostate. Urology 8:227, 1976

27. Walther MM: Endometrial carcinoma of prostate. Urology 27:574, 1986

28. Wernert N, Luchtrath H, Seeliger H, et al: Papillary carcinoma of the prostate, location, morphology, and immunohistochemistry: the histogenesis and entity of so-called endometrioid carcinoma. Prostate 10:123, 1987

29. Witters S, Moerman P, Bussche LV, et al: Papillary adenocarcinoma of the prostatic urethra. Eur Urol 12:143, 1986

30. Kuriyama J, Wang MC, Lee CL, et al: Multiple marker evaluation in human prostate cancer with use of tissue-specific antigens. J Natl Cancer Inst 68:99, 1982

31. Nadji M, Tabei SZ, Castro A, et al: Prostatic origin of tumors. An immunohistochemical study. Am J Clin Pathol 73:735, 1980

32. The Veterans Administration Cooperative Urologic Research Group: Treatment and survival of patients with cancer of the prostate. Surg Gynecol Obstet 124:1011, 1967

33. Schellhammer PF, Bean MA, Whitmore WF Jr: Prostatic involvement by transitional cell carcinoma: pathogenesis, patterns and prognosis. J Urol 118:399, 1977

34. Butterick JD, Schnitzer B, Abell MR: Ectopic prostatic tissue in urethra: a clinicopathological entity and a significant cause of hematuria. J Urol 105:97, 1971

35. Craig JR, Hart WR: Benign polyps with prostatic-type epithelium of the urethra. Am J Clin Pathol 63:343, 1975

36. Eglen, DE, Pontius EE: Benign prostatic epithelial polyp of the urethra. J Urol 131:120, 1984

37. Bhagavan BS, Tiamson EM, Wenk RE, et al: Nephrogenic adenoma of the urinary bladder and urethra. Hum Pathol 12:907, 1981

38. Schinella R, Thurm J, Feiner H: Papillary pseudotumor of the prostatic urethra: proliferative papillary urethritis. J Urol 11:38, 1974

39. Hoang C, Wassef M, Cortesse A, et al: Adenocarcinome papillaire "endometrioide" du col vesical: microscopie optique et électronique et immunohistochimie. Ann Pathol 1985:125, 1985

40. Reed RJ: Consultation case. Am J Surg Pathol 8:699, 1984

41. Cleary KR, Choi HY, Ayala AG: Basal cell

hyperplasia of the prostate. Am J Clin Pathol 80:850, 1983

42. Dermer GB: Basal cell proliferation in benign prostatic hyperplasia. Cancer 41:1857, 1978

43. Grignon DJ, Ro JY, Ordonez NG, et al: Basal cell hyperplasia, adenoid basal cell tumor, and adenoid cystic carcinom of the prostate: an immunohistochemical study. Hum Pathol 19:1425, 1988

44. Young RH, Frierson HF, Mills SE, et al: Adenoid cystic-like tumor of the prostate gland. A report of two cases and review of the literature of ''adenoid cystic carcinoma'' of the prostate. Am J Clin Pathol 89:49, 1988

45. Mostofi FK, Sesterhenn I, Sobin LH: Histological Typing of Prostate Tumors. International Histologic Classification of Tumours. No. 22. World Health Organization, Geneva, 1980

46. Mostofi FK, Price EB Jr.: Tumors of the male genital system, fascicle 8, second series. p. 244. In Atlas of Tumor Pathology. Armed Forces Institute of Pathology, Washington, D.C., 1973

47. Dickman SH, Toker C: Seromucinous gland ectopia within the prostatic stroma. J Urol 109:852, 1973

48. Frankel K, Craig JR: Adenoid cystic carcinoma of the prostate. Report of a case. Am J Clin Pathol 62:639, 1974

49. Gilmour AM, Bell TJ: Adenoid cystic carcinoma of the prostate. Br J Urol 58:105, 1986

50. Karmer SA, Bredael JJ, Krueger RP: Adenoid cystic carcinoma of the prostate: report of a case. J Urol 120:383, 1978

51. Kuhajda FP, Mann RB: Adenoid cystic carcinoma of the prostate. A case report with immunoperoxidase staining for prostate-specific acid phosphatase and prostate-specific antigen. Am J Clin Pathol 81:257, 1984

52. Manrique JJ, Albores-Saavedra J, Orantes A, et al: Malignant mixed tumor of the salivary-gland type, primary in the prostate. Am J Clin Pathol 70:932, 1978

53. Sesterhenn I, Mostofi FK, Davis CJ: Basal cell hyperplasia and basal cell carcinoma. Lab Invest 56:71A, 1987

54. Shong-San C, Walters MNI: Adenoid cystic carcinoma of prostate. Report of a case. Pathology 16:337, 1984

55. Tannenbaum M: Adenoid cystic or ''salivary gland'' carcinomas of prostate. Urology 6:238, 1984

56. Sarma DP, Guileyardo JM: Basal cell hyperplasia of the prostate. J La State Med Soc 134:23, 1982

57. Ro JY, Grignon DJ, Ayala AG, et al: Mucinous adenocarcinoma of the prostate gland. J Urol 141:527A, 1989

58. Krogh J, Lund PG: Mucinous adenocarcinoma of the prostate presenting as a retrovesical cyst. Scand J Urol Nephrol 22:235, 1988

59. Odom DG, Donatucci CF, Deshon GE: Mucinous adenocarcinoma of the prostate. Hum Pathol 17:863, 1986

60. Chica G, Johnson DE, Ayala AG: Mucinous adenocarcinoma of the prostate. J Urol 118:124, 1977

61. Hsueh Y, Tsung SH: Prostatic mucinous adenocarcinoma. Urology 24:626, 1984

62. Patel RS, Dias R, Fernandes M, et al: Adenocarcinoma of the prostate. Mucin secreting. N.Y. State J Med 18:936, 1981

63. Elbadawi A, Craig W, Linke CA, et al: Prostatic mucinous carcinoma. Urology 13:658, 1979

64. Uyama T, Moriwaki S: Papillary and mucus-forming adenocarcinomas of prostate. Urology 13:432, 1979

65. Proia AD, McCarty KS Jr, Woodard BH: Prostatic mucinous adenocarcinoma. Am J Surg Pathol 5:701, 1981

66. Alfthan O, Koivuniemi A: Mucinous carcinoma of the prostate. Scand J Urol Nephrol 4:78, 1970

67. Sika JV, Buckley JJ: Mucus-forming adenocarcinoma of prostate. Cancer 17:949, 1964

68. Bhargava S, Trivedi SK, Agarwal VK, et al: Mucinous adenocarcinoma of prostate. Indian J Cancer 17:64, 1980

69. Epstein JI, Lieberman PH: Mucinous adenocarcinoma of the prostate gland. Am J Surg Pathol 9:299, 1985

70. Ro JY, El-Naggar A, Ayala AG, et al: Signet-ring-cell carcinoma of the prostate. Am J Surg Pathol 12:453, 1988

71. Remmele W, Weber A, Harding P: Primary signet-ring cell carcinoma of the prostate. Hum Pathol 19:478, 1988

72. Kums JJ, van Helsdingen PJ: Signet-ring cell carcinoma of the bladder and the prostate. Report of 4 cases. Urol Int 40:116, 1985

73. Giltman LI: Signet ring adenocarcinoma of the prostate. J Urol 126:134, 1981

74. Alguacil-Garcia A: Artifactual changes mimicking signet ring cell carcinoma in transurethral prostatectomy specimens. Am J Surg Pathol 10:795, 1986

75. Moyana TN: Adenosquamous carcinoma of the prostate. Am J Surg Pathol 11:403, 1987

76. Kahler JE: Carcinoma of the prostate gland. A pathologic study. J Urol 41:557, 1939

77. Sieracki JC: Epidermoid carcinoma of the human prostate. Report of three cases. Lab Invest 4:232, 1955

78. Gray GF Jr, Marshall VF: Squamous carcinoma of the prostate. J Urol 113:736, 1975

79. Sharma SK, Malik AK, Bapna BC: Squamous cell carcinoma of prostate. Indian J Cancer 17:134, 1980

80. Bennett RS, Edgerton EO: Mixed prostatic carcinoma. J Urol 110:561, 1973

81. Saito R, Davis BK, Ollapally EP: Adenosquamous carcinoma of the prostate. Hum Pathol 15:87, 1984

82. Shannon RL, Grignon DJ, Ro JY, et al: Sarcomatoid carcinoma of the prostate. Lab Invest 60:87A, 1989

83. Azzopardi JG, Evans DJ: Argentaffin cells in prostatic carcinoma: Differentiation from lipofuscin and melanin in prostatic epithelium. J Pathol 104:247, 1971

84. Di Sant'Agnese PA: Neuroendocrine differentiation and prostatic carcinoma. Arch Pathol Lab Med 112:1097, 1988

85. Ansari MA, Pintozzi RL, Choi YS, et al: Diagnosis of carcinoid-like metastatic prostatic carcinoma by an immunoperoxidase method. Am J Clin Pathol 76:94, 1981

86. Turbat-Herrera EA, Herrera GA, Gore I, et al: Neuroendocrine differentiation in prostatic carcinomas. A retrospective autopsy study. Arch Pathol Lab Med 112:1100, 1988

87. Stratton M, Evans DJ, Lampert IA: Prostatic adenocarcinoma evolving into carcinoid: selective effect of hormonal treatment? J Clin Pathol 39:750, 1986

88. Ghali VS, Garcia RL: Prostatic adenocarcinoma with carcinoidal features producing adrenocorticotropic syndrome. Immunohistochemical study and review of the literature. Cancer 54:1043, 1984

89. Fetissof F, Bruandet P, Arbeille B, et al: Calcitonin-secreting carcinomas of the prostate: an immunohistochemical and ultrastructural analysis. Am J Surg Pathol 10:702, 1986

90. Schron DS, Gipson T, Mendelsohn G: The histogenesis of small cell carcinoma of the prostate. Cancer 53:2478, 1984

91. Fetissof F, Dubois MP, Arbeille-Brassart B, et al: Endocrine cells in the prostate gland, urothelium and Brenner tumors. Virchows Arch [B] 42:53, 1983

92. Di Sant'Agnese PA, de Mesy Jensen KL: Endocrine-paracrine cells of the prostate and prostatic urethra: an ultrastructural study. Hum Pathol 15:1034, 1984

93. Di Sant'Agnese PA, de Mesy Jensen KL, Churukian CJ, et al: Human prostatic endocrine-paracrine (APUD) cells. Arch Pathol Lab Med 109:607, 1985

94. Di Sant'Agnese PA: Calcitoninlike immunoreactive and bombesinlike immunoreactive endocrine-paracrine cells of the human prostate. Arch Pathol Lab Med 110:412, 1986

95. Di Sant'Agnese PA, de Mesy Jensen KL: Neuroendocrine differentiation in prostatic carcinoma. Hum Pathol 18:849, 1987

96. Abrahamsson PA, Wadstrom LB, Alumets J, et al: Peptide-hormone and serotonin-immunoreactive tumour cells in carcinoma of the prostate. Pathol Res Pract 182:298, 1987

97. Kazzaz BA: Argentaffin and argyrophil cells in the prostate. J Pathol 112:189, 1974

98. Capella C, Usellini L, Buffa R, et al: The endocrine component of prostatic carcinomas, mixed adenocarcinoma-carcinoid tumours and nontumour prostate: histochemical and ultrastructural identification of the endocrine cells. Histopathology 5:175, 1981

99. Ro JY, Tetu B, Ayala AG, et al: Small cell carcinoma of the prostate. II. Immunohistochemical and electron microscopic studies of 18 cases. Cancer 59:977, 1987

100. Matzkin H, Braf Z: Paraneoplastic syndromes associated with prostatic carcinoma. J Urol 138:1129, 1987

101. Almagro UA, Tieu TM, Remeniuk E, et al: Argyrophilic, "carcinoid-like" prostatic carcinoma. Arch Pathol Lab Med 110:916, 1986

102. Dauge MC, Delmas V: APUD type endocrine tumour of the prostate: Incidence and prognosis in association with adenocarcinoma. p. 529. In Murphy GP, Kuss R, Khoury S, et al (eds): Progress in Clinical and Biological Medicine: Prostate Cancer. Part A: Research Endocrine Treatment and Histopathology. Alan R. Liss, New York, 1987

103. Azumi N, Shibuya H, Ishikura M: Primary prostatic carcinoid tumor with intracytoplasmic prostatic acid phosphatase and prostate-specific antigen. Am J Surg Pathol 8:545, 1984

104. Wasserstein PW, Goldman RL: Primary carcinoid of prostate. Urology 13:318, 1979
105. Tetu B, Ordonez NG, Ro JY, et al: Small cell carcinoma of prostate associated with myasthenic (Eaton-Lambert) syndrome Urology 33:148, 1989
106. Manson AL, Terhune D, MacDonald G: Small cell carcinoma of prostate. Urology 33:78, 1989
107. Wenk RE, Bhagavan BS, Levy R, et al: Ectopic ACTH, prostatic oat cell carcinoma, and marked hypernatremia. Cancer 40:773, 1977
108. Gleason DF, Veterans Administration Cooperative Urological Research Group: Histological grading and clinical staging of prostatic carcinoma. p. 171. In Tannenbaum M (ed): Urologic Pathology: The Prostate. Lea & Febiger, Philadelphia, 1977
109. McNeal JE, Reese JH, Redwine EA, et al: Cribriform adenocarcinoma of the prostate. Cancer 58:1714, 1986
110. Currin SM, Lee SE, Walther, PJ: Flow cytometric analysis of comedocarcinoma of the prostate: an uncommon histopathological variant of prostatic adenocarcinoma. J Urol 140:96, 1988
111. Babaian RJ, Troncoso P, Ayala AG, et al: Involvement of prostatic urethra and prostatic ducts by transitional cell carcinoma in patients with bladder cancer. J Urol 141:519A. 1989
112. Wood DP Jr, Montie JE, Pontes JE, et al: Transitional cell carcinoma of the prostate in cystoprostatectomy specimens removed for bladder cancer. J Urol 141:346, 1989
113. Hardeman SW, Soloway MS: Transitional cell carcinoma of the prostate: diagnosis, staging and management. World J Urol 6:170, 1988
114. Mahadevia PS, Koss LG, Tar IJ: Prostatic involvement in bladder cancer: Cancer 58:2096, 1986
115. Taylor HG, Blom J: Transitional cell carcinoma of the prostate: Cancer 51:1800, 1983
116. Schujman E, Mukamel E, Slutzker D, et al: Prostatic transitional cell carcinoma: concept of its pathogenesis and classification. Isr J Med Sci 19:794, 1983
117. Kopelson G, Harisiadis L, Romas NA, et al: Periurethral prostatic duct carcinoma. Cancer 42:2894, 1978
118. Seemayer TA, Knaack J, Thelmo WL, et al: Further observations on carcinoma in situ of the urinary bladder: silent but extensive intraprostatic involvement. Cancer 36:514, 1975
119. Johnson DE, Hogan JM, Ayala AG: Transitional cell carcinoma of the prostate. Cancer 29:287, 1972
120. Rhamy RK, Buchanan RD, Spalding MJ: Intraductal carcinoma of the prostate gland. Trans Am Assoc Genito-Urinary Surgeons 64:61, 1972
121. Rubenstein ARB, Rubnitz ME: Transitional cell carcinoma of the prostate. Cancer 24:543, 1969
122. Ullmann AS, Ross OA: Hyperplasia, atypism, and carcinoma in situ in prostatic periurethral glands. Am J Clin Pathol 47:497, 1967
123. Ende N, Woods LP, Shelly HS: Carcinoma originating in ducts surrounding the prostatic urethra. Am J Clin Pathol 40:183, 1963
124. Franks LM, Chesterman FC: Intra-epithelial carcinoma of prostatic urethra, peri-urethral glands and prostatic ducts ("Bowen's disease of urinary epithelium"). Br J Cancer 10:223, 1956
125. Stein BS, Kendall AR: Malignant melanoma of the genitourinary tract. J Urol 132:856, 1984
126. Berry NE, Reese L: Malignant melanoma which had its first clinical manifestations in the prostate gland. J Urol 69:286, 1953
127. Thompson GJ, Albers DD, Broders AC: Unusual carcinomas involving the prostate gland. J Urol 69:416, 1953
128. Albers DD, Stephenson PL: Metastatic carcinoma of the prostate from silent carcinoma of the stomach. A case report. J Okla Med Assn 55:78, 1962
129. Dowd JB: Carcinoma of the pancreas presenting as obstructing cancer of the prostate. Lahey Clin Bull 13:214, 1964
130. Johnson DE, Chalbaud R, Ayala AG: Secondary tumors of the prostate. J Urol 112:507, 1974
131. Grignon DJ, Ro JY, Ayala AG: Malignant melanoma with metastasis to adenocarcinoma of the prostate. Cancer 63:196, 1989
132. Culkin DJ, Wheeler JS Jr, Castelli M, et al: Carcinoma of the prostate in a 25-year-old man: a case report and review of the literature. J Urol 136:684, 1986
133. Shimada H, Misugi K, Sasaki Y, et al: Carcinoma of the prostate in childhood and adolescence: report of a case and review of the literature. Cancer 46:2534, 1980

8

Soft Tissue Tumors

Bernard Têtu, John R. Srigley, and David G. Bostwick

A wide variety of soft tissue tumors occur in the prostate, including reactive stromal proliferations, benign neoplasms, and sarcomas. Although many of these tumors are distinguished easily, considerable diagnostic difficulty may be encountered with some of the rare and newly identified lesions. This chapter reviews soft tissue tumors and tumor-like proliferations of the prostate, with emphasis on diagnostic criteria and differential diagnosis. The histologic classification of these tumors is shown in Table 8-1.

BENIGN TUMORS AND TUMOR-LIKE PROLIFERATIONS

INFLAMMATORY PSEUDOTUMORS AND TUMOR-LIKE PROLIFERATIONS

Granulomatous Prostatitis

The most common pseudotumor is granulomatous prostatitis. Focally, this lesion may contain a sheet-like proliferation of epithelioid and spindled histiocytes, mimicking anaplastic carcinoma or sarcoma.[1, 2] However, the histiocytes usually do not display significant nuclear or cytologic atypia, and mixed chronic inflammation is invariably present at the periphery. Caution is warranted in interpretation of scant specimens such as needle biopsies, which contain a monotonous cellular infiltrate. The entity is described fully in Chapter 2.

Postoperative Spindle Cell Nodule

This rare lesion occurs within months of surgery, and is composed of a spindle cell proliferation arranged in fascicles with occasional mitoses (Fig. 8-1).[3-5] Tumor cells display central ovoid nuclei, nucleoli, and abundant cytoplasm. Some of these cases have been interpreted as sarcoma, but are distinguished morphologically by the small size of the nodules, the lack of significant nuclear pleomorphism and atypical mitotic figures, and a plexiform pattern of blood vessels with chronic inflammation. Postoperative spindle cell nodules are considered benign, with no evidence of recurrence up to 5 years after surgery, even in patients treated only by TUR.

Stromal Hyperplasia

Pure stromal nodules may occur in the setting of nodular hyperplasia, usually admixed with other typical areas of hyperplasia. Isolated foci of stromal hyperplasia are occasionally observed.

Blue Nevus and Melanosis

Fewer than 25 documented cases of blue nevus and melanosis of the prostate have been reported.[4, 6-17] Patients range in age from 50[7] to 76 years,[4, 8] with a median of 67 years. The

**Table 8–1. Soft Tissue Tumors and Tumor-like Proliferations of the Prostate:
Histologic Classification**

Benign
    Inflammatory pseudotumors and tumor-like proliferations
        Granulomatous prostatitis
        Postoperative spindle cell nodule
        Stromal hyperplasia (nodular hyperplasia)
        Blue nevus and melanosis

    Tumors
        Leiomyoma
        Fibroma
        Hemangioma
        Neurofibroma
        Paraganglioma
        Rhabdomyoma
        Fibroadenoma

Tumors of uncertain malignant potential
    Variants of nodular hyperplasia
        Stromal hyperplasia with atypia
        Phyllodes type of hyperplasia

    Variants of leiomyoma
        Cellular leiomyoma
        Symplastic leiomyoma (''atypical'' leiomyoma)
        Leiomyoblastoma

    Miscellaneous
        Spindle cell proliferation with no prior operation
        Fibromyxoid tumor
        Hemangiopericytoma

Malignant
    Muscular differentiation
        Rhabdomyosarcoma
        Leiomyosarcoma

    Other rare sarcomas
        Fibrosarcoma
        Osteosarcoma
        Malignant fibrous histiocytoma
        Angiosarcoma
        Chondrosarcoma
        Malignant nerve sheath tumor
        Undifferentiated sarcoma

    Mixed tumors
        Carcinosarcoma
        Mixed mesenchymal tumor

    Hematolymphoid differentiation[a]
        Malignant lymphoma
        Leukemic involvement of the prostate

    Other
        Rhabdoid tumor
        Neuroblastoma

[a] Although these are not soft tissue tumors, they are included for historical reasons (''prostatic lymphosarcoma'') and for completeness of the differential diagnosis of tumor-like proliferations of the prostate.

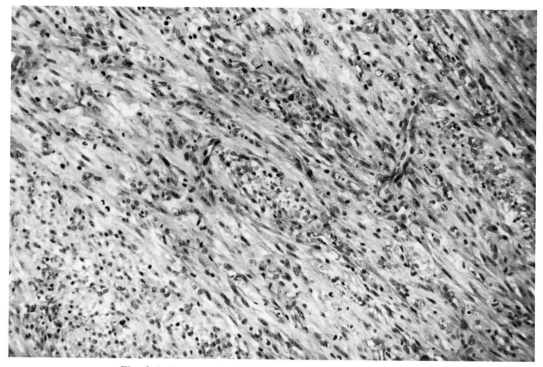

Fig. 8-1. Postoperative spindle cell nodule. (H&E, ×160.)

majority present with urinary retention owing to nodular hyperplasia, and these unusual lesions are discovered incidentally in TUR specimens.

Blue nevus is a stromal spindle cell proliferation with prominent intracellular melanin pigment (Fig. 8-2). Melanosis is histologically identical, but has the additional feature of melanin within the adjacent prostatic epithelium.[11] Blue nevus appears to be more common, comprising approximately two thirds of reported cases.[15] Although some reports have used these terms interchangeably, we prefer to use the definitions stated above.[4, 13]

Three reported cases have been associated with prostatic adenocarcinoma, and melanin pigment was identified within some of the tumor cells.[13, 15]

The histogenesis of prostatic nevus is controversial. Stromal melanocytes are thought to originate from melanoblasts migrating from the neural crest in early embryogenesis.[11, 13] Mela-

nosomes and premelanosomes have been identified at the ultrastructural level in seven cases.[4, 8, 12, 15] Whereas melanosomes at various stages of development were found in a white patient,[8, 15] only stage 4 melanosomes were identified in a black patient.[12, 15] It is uncertain whether prostatic epithelial cells can produce melanin. The exclusive presence of stage 4 melanosomes within prostatic epithelium and tumor cells of rare prostatic carcinomas suggests transfer of pigment from the adjacent stromal cells.[13, 18] However, the identification of melanin within epithelium not associated with pigmented stromal cells indicates that prostatic epithelium can occasionally be melanogenic.[16, 18]

Prostatic blue nevus is considered benign, but may be confused histologically with primary or metastatic malignant melanoma of the prostate.[19, 20] As in the skin, it is thought this lesion does not transform into malignant melanoma.

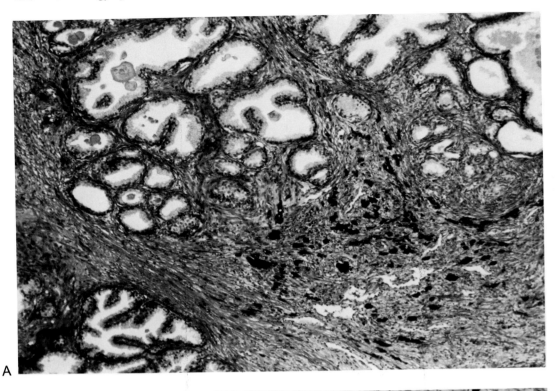

A

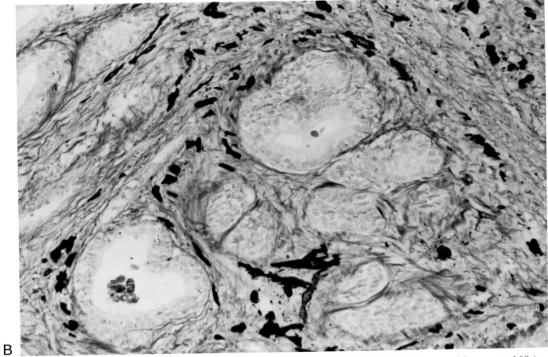

B

Fig. 8-2. (A & B) Blue nevus of the prostate. (Fig. A: H&E, ×100; Fig. B: Fontana-Masson, ×160.)

TUMORS

Leiomyoma and Fibroma

Leiomyoma and fibroma are frequently confused with nodular hyperplasia. Over 50 cases of prostatic leiomyoma have been reported, and are defined as solitary circumscribed proliferations of smooth muscle measuring 1 cm or more in diameter.[21-25] Histologically, prostatic leiomyoma is similar to leiomyomas occurring at other sites, being composed of bland-appearing smooth muscle cells separated by variable amounts of collagen. Fibromas are solitary, circumscribed, unencapsulated masses of collagen (Fig. 8-3) with scant fibroblasts; these tumors may be impossible to distinguish from solitary stromal hyperplasia. The distinction of leiomyoma and fibroma from stromal hyperplastic nodules may be arbitrary, and the existence of such tumors is questioned.

Other Benign Tumors

Other benign soft tissue tumors occurring in the prostate and periprostatic tissues include hemangioma, neurofibroma (Fig. 8-4), and rhabdomyoma. A recent case report described a paraganglioma (pheochromocytoma) of the prostate that secreted high levels of norepinephrine.[26] Magnetic resonance imaging of the pelvis was found to be diagnostically useful prior to surgery.

Fibroadenoma

Benign solitary tumors suggestive of intracanalicular fibroadenoma of the female breast have been described in the prostate.[27-29] These lesions have a moderately cellular fibromuscular stroma with distorted ducts and acini. Fibroadenomas occur in the transition zone and the proximal

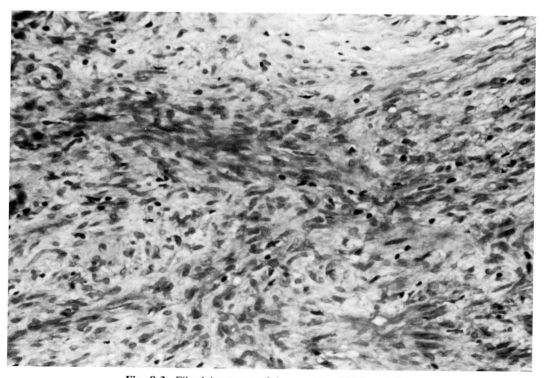

Fig. 8-3. Fibroleiomyoma of the prostate. (H&E, ×160.)

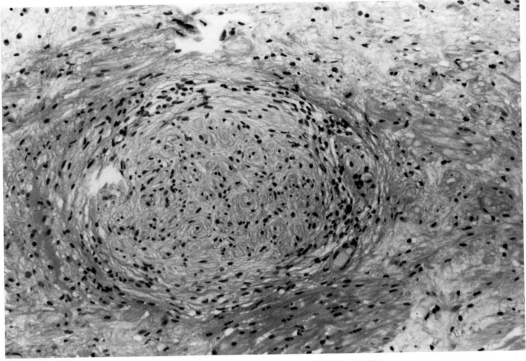

Fig. 8-4. Prostatic neurofibroma. (H&E, ×160.)

periurethral area. Clinically, they appear to be benign.

TUMORS OF UNCERTAIN MALIGNANT POTENTIAL

Although most of these tumors appear to be benign, the small number of reported cases does not allow exact determination of biologic behavior.

VARIANTS OF NODULAR HYPERPLASIA

Stromal Hyperplasia with Atypia

Stromal nodules occurring in the setting of nodular hyperplasia may have areas of increased cellularity and atypical cells. Three cases of stromal hyperplasia with atypia have been described,[4, 30] containing cells with large atypical nuclei, smudged chromatin, and rare nuclear vacuolation (Fig. 8-5). Nucleoli were incon-spicuous, and there were no mitotic figures or areas of necrosis. Most investigators consider the atypical cells to be degenerative, and these lesions are probably within the spectrum of benign nodular hyperplasia. One patient was followed for 6 years after TUR with no evidence of recurrence.[4]

Phyllodes-Type Atypical Hyperplasia

Fibroadenomas with increased stromal cellularity and cytologic atypia have been referred to as phyllodes-type atypical prostatic hyperplasia, with fewer than 12 well-documented cases (Fig. 8-6).[4, 27, 31-36] These rare tumors occur in adults (ages 23 to 74 years), causing urinary retention, hematuria, dysuria, and prostatic enlargement. By computed tomography, phyllodes-type atypical hyperplasia is distinctive, showing enlargement of the prostate without extracapsular extension or retroperitoneal adenopathy, varying degrees of involvement of the bladder base, absence of obstruction of the

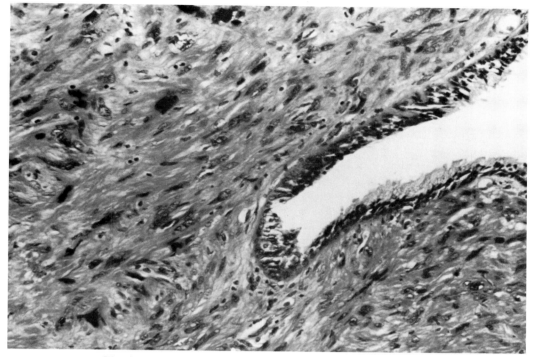

Fig. 8-5. Stromal hyperplasia with nuclear atypia. (H&E, ×160.)

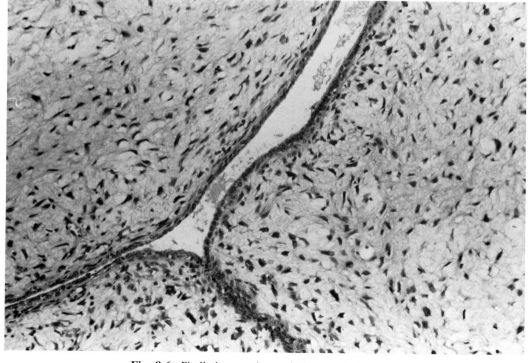

Fig. 8-6. Phyllodes-type hyperplasia. (H&E, ×160.)

ureter, and smoothly marginated collections of fluid within the tumor. These lesions grow up to 15 cm in diameter.[31, 34, 36]

Histologically, phyllodes-type hyperplasia is reminiscent of cellular fibroadenoma and phyllodes tumor of the breast (Fig. 8-6). There is a mixture of epithelium and stroma, with varying degrees of stromal cellularity and cytologic atypia. The epithelial cells are cuboidal to columnar, with a well-formed basal cell layer. The epithelium is arranged in glands or cysts, frequently compressed and distorted by hyperplastic stroma. There may be exuberant epithelial proliferation. Stromal proliferation is the most characteristic component, appearing as a cellular and compact proliferation of smooth muscle cells and fibroblasts, with occasional areas of edema and myxoid change. Focal pure stromal hyperplasia is occasionally observed. In some areas, the atypical stromal cells are present in small numbers, displaying enlarged hyperchromatic nuclei and smudged chromatin. In such low-grade neoplasms, mitotic figures are not present, and there is no evidence of necrosis. In other tumors, there are larger numbers of stromal cells with anaplastic nuclei, but no mitoses are seen. Two reported cases of phyllodes-type hyperplasia were histologically malignant, with nuclear pleomorphism and mitotic figures; both of these tumors recurred after initial therapy.[32, 34]

Prostate-specific antigen has been demonstrated within the epithelial cells, and desmin and vimentin within the stromal cells.[35]

Unlike benign nodular hyperplasia, phyllodes-type atypical hyperplasia is a diffuse proliferative change that displays stromal atypia. It lacks elongate glands at the periphery that are characteristic of nodular hyperplasia. Phyllodes-type hyperplasia is distinguished from malignant phyllodes tumor and leiomyosarcoma by the virtual absence of mitotic figures in stromal cells, analogous to phyllodes tumors in the breast and uterus. Additional cases of phyllodes-type hyperplasia are needed to refine the histologic criteria.

Phyllodes-type hyperplasia is easily distinguished from postoperative spindle cell nodules by the presence of epithelial elements and stromal atypia and the absence of mitotic figures. Also, postoperative spindle cell nodules do not reach the large size seen in phyllodes hyperplasia. Other neoplasms that should be distinguished from phyllodes-type hyperplasia include prostatic cysts, müllerian duct cysts of the utricle,[37] and tumors of the seminal vesicle tumors.

All reported cases of phyllodes-type hyperplasia have been treated surgically, and there is no documentation of metastases. Most investigators advocate surgical treatment similar to nodular hyperplasia. Chemotherapy and radiation therapy have not been used at present.

We concur with the suggestion of Reese and associates[36] that these tumors be termed *phyllodes-type atypical prostatic hyperplasia,* or alternatively, *phyllodes tumors.*

VARIANTS OF LEIOMYOMA

Smooth muscle proliferations of the prostate may vary from the usual pattern by exhibiting increased cellularity (cellular leiomyoma) and atypical cells (symplastic leiomyoma).[4, 27, 38-40] The only important differential diagnosis for these variants of leiomyoma is leiomyosarcoma. Features suggesting that these tumors are benign include the noninfiltrative growth pattern, low or absent mitotic rate, and absence of recurrence following surgery.

Cellular Leiomyoma

Cellular leiomyoma is a solitary smooth muscle proliferation with increased density of cells as the predominant pattern. Mitotic figures are absent, although some cases have been reported as having occasional or infrequent mitoses.[38, 39]

Symplastic Leiomyoma

Smooth muscle tumors that contain multinucleated or hyperlobated giant cells have been referred to as *atypical, bizarre,* or *symplastic leiomyomas* (Fig. 8-7). The nuclear detail is frequently smudged, suggesting degenerative change. Mitotic figures are infrequent or absent. In one case of symplastic leiomyoma originally diagnosed as leiomyosarcoma, there was no recurrence 8 years after diagnosis.[4] Other reported cases of symplastic leiomyoma have had atypical stromal cells admixed with hyperplastic prostatic glands, suggesting that these atypical cells were part of a hyperplastic process and not limited to the pure circumscribed smooth muscle nodules. No strict morphologic criteria separate symplastic leiomyoma from stromal hyperplasia with atypia, so it would be tempting to distinguish these two benign tumors from their malignant counterparts using the same criteria as for smooth muscle tumor at other location (size and histologic features). Because of the small number of published cases and the lack of definitive histologic criteria, these neoplasms should be considered to be of uncertain malignant potential.

Leiomyoblastoma

A single case of leiomyoblastoma of the prostate has been reported.[41]

MISCELLANEOUS TUMORS OF UNCERTAIN MALIGNANT POTENTIAL

Spindle Cell Proliferation with No Prior Operation

Rare cases of pseudosarcomatous spindle cell proliferation similar to postoperative spindle cell nodules have been reported in patients who have not undergone genitourinary tract operations.[4] In one case, a 23-year-old man underwent TUR for urinary obstruction.[4] The prostatic chips contained a loose spindle cell proliferation arranged in fasicles with an admixture of lymphocytes. The lesion was supported by a rich and complex vascular network. Flow cytometery revealed a

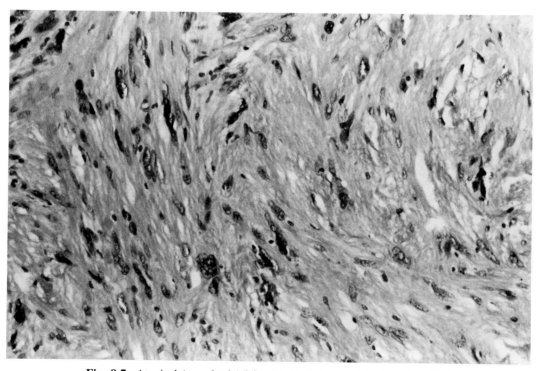

Fig. 8-7. Atypical (symplastic) leiomyoma of the prostate. (H&E, ×160.)

single diploid cell population, supporting its benign nature. In another case, a 67-year-old man underwent TUR for nodular hyperplasia, and a small myxoid nodule containing spindled and stellate cells was found.[4] A capillary network supported the cells, and there was no nuclear atypia or mitotic activity. The patient remained free of recurrence 10 years after surgery.

Fibromyxoid Tumor

Fibromyxoid tumor of the prostate is probably similar to spindle cell proliferation with no prior operation.[42] In the single reported case, a 56-year-old man underwent cystoprostatectomy for a mass in the left side of the prostate that extended into the adjacent bladder wall. The tumor was soft, tan, and elongate, composed of atypical hyperchromatic spindle cells set in an edematous, myxoid background. The cells were variable in size and shape, with irregular nuclei. Some cells were strap-shaped, with eosinophilic cytoplasm and perpheral nuclei, but no cross striations were observed. Although initially considered to be a botryoid sarcoma (rhabdomyosarcoma), there was no cambium layer of cells and no mitotic figures were observed. The tumor was circumscribed, but compressed the adjacent tissues. Ultrastructural examination confirmed the fibroblastic nature of the tumor cells, and immunoperoxidase stains for myoglobulin and S100 protein were unrevealing. The patient remained free of tumor more than 1 year after surgery.[42]

Hemangiopericytoma

Five cases of hemangiopericytoma of the prostate have been reported.[43-45] The light microscopic and ultrastructural features are similar to such tumors arising elsewhere in the body. The biologic behavior of hemangiopericytoma in the prostate is difficult to determine; of the reported cases, one patient is free of tumor 3 years after diagnosis, while two patients have had locally recurrent invasive tumors, and one has had metastases to the bone and skin.

MALIGNANT SOFT TISSUE TUMORS

Sarcomas of the prostate are rare, accounting for less than 0.1 percent of all primary prostatic neoplasms.[46-49] One third occur in children under 10 years of age, and most of these are rhabdomyosarcomas.[47] Sarcomas usually occur in a younger age group than carcinomas, with a median age of 45 years.[49, 50] These are fast-growing neoplasms, with a more rapid clinical progression than adenocarcinoma. Characteristically, patients present with obstructive symptoms, including difficulty in urination, frequency, urgency, dysuria, nocturia, and hematuria.[49] Pelvic pain may also be present. Constipation occurs as a consequence of rectal encroachment.[49, 51] There is usually rapid spread to periprostatic tissues, with lymphatic and vascular invasion. Metastases occur in fewer than half of the cases,[48] with spread to regional lymph nodes, liver, bone, and lung.[47, 51-53] Because of their propensity for causing obstructive symptoms, sarcomas involving the prostate or bladder are usually diagnosed at an earlier stage than other pelvic tumors. Consequently, their response to treatment is more favorable.[52] Unlike prostatic adenocarcinoma, bone metastases from sarcoma are usually osteolytic. Exact site of origin cannot be determined for some large bulky tumors involving the bladder, prostate, colon, and retroperitoneum.

On gross examination, prostates involved by sarcoma are diffusely enlarged, firm, or rubbery in consistency, frequently with soft necrotic areas, in contrast to the characteristic stony hard induration of prostatic carcinoma.[48, 49] Approximately 65 percent of prostatic sarcomas are derived from smooth or striated muscle, and of these, rhabdomyosarcoma is the most frequent (42 percent of sarcomas). Leiomyosarcoma and lymphoma are the second and third most common "soft tissue" tumors.[49, 50] Other types of sarcomas are curiosities.

Muscular Differentiation

Rhabdomyosarcoma

Rhabdomyosarcoma occurs mainly in the first decade of life, with a peak incidence between birth and 6 years, and an average age of 7.2 years.[52] The incidence among childhood tumors is exceeded only by brain tumors, neuroblastoma, and Wilms' tumor. The prostate and genitourinary system account for 21 percent of rhabdomyosarcomas in children, and this site is second in frequency to the head and neck.[52] Occasional cases have been reported in adults over 50 years of age.[48, 56, 60] More than 65 percent are embryonal rhabdomyosarcomas, and the remainder are the alveolar subtype.[52-64]

Rhabdomyosarcoma may be small and apparently limited to the prostate at the time of diagnosis, but can grow rapidly, invading adjacent soft tissues and bladder, accompanied by abundant tumor necrosis. The average tumor measures 5 to 9 cm in diameter.[49, 52, 59]

Histologically, embryonal rhabdomyosarcoma is composed of sheets of round to spindle cells with somewhat uniform hyperchromatic nuclei (Fig. 8-8). Strap cells and "tadpole" cells with abundant eosinophilic cytoplasm and cross striations may be seen. A distinctive cambium layer is frequently present at the periphery, characterized by nuclear condensation around epithelial structures and a delicate myxoid stroma.[60] When the tumor is composed predominantly of round cells, additional studies such as electron microscopy and immunohistochemistry may be necessary to confirm the diagnosis.

Ultrastructurally, two cell types can be identified. Large oval or elongate tumor cells usually contain segments of sarcomere with abundant glycogen and well-formed basement membranes.[55] Smaller round cells contain free ribosomes, rough endoplasmic reticulum, and

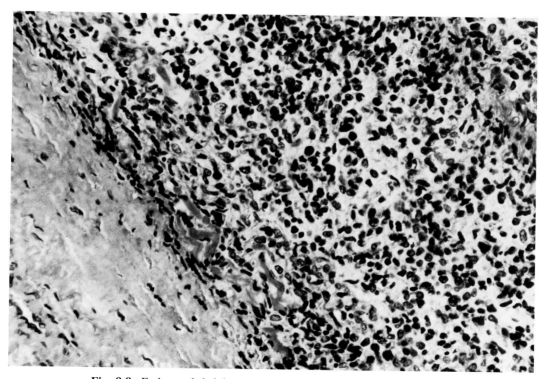

Fig. 8-8. Embryonal rhabdomyosarcoma of the prostate. (H&E, ×160.)

Golgi apparatus, but usually lack myofibrils. These features are similar to embryonal rhabdomyosarcoma arising at other sites. Immunohistochemically, tumor cells may be positive for muscle cell-derived filaments such as myoglobin[59, 61] and desmin.[59]

The main differential diagnostic considerations are small cell undifferentiated carcinoma[65] and lymphoma.[66] Small cell carcinoma usually occurs in adults over age 50, and is often associated with typical prostatic adenocarcinoma.[65] Tumor cells are ovoid, with scant cytoplasm and inconspicuous nucleoli. A cambium layer is lacking. Lymphoma may resemble rhabdomyosarcoma, especially the diffuse large cell or small noncleaved cell subtypes; in such instances, immunohistochemistry and electron microscopy will usually establish a definitive diagnosis.[66]

Patient survival with rhabdomyosarcoma has improved considerably.[53, 57, 59, 62-64] Median survival was 4 months before modern therapy,[49] but the introduction of new treatments, including surgery, multidrug chemotherapy, and complementary radiation therapy has led to a complete response in most patients,[59] and a 3-year survival of greater than 50 percent.[53, 57, 59] Recurrences may occur, usually within a few months after diagnosis.[48] Metastases are less frequent since the advent of combination therapy.

Alveolar rhabdomyosarcoma involving the prostate is rare.[49, 52, 61] It occurs in a somewhat older age group (median, 22 years).[49] Survival is similar to embryonal rhabdomyosarcoma, despite the somewhat worse prognosis for its soft tissue counterpart.[52] Undifferentiated (pleomorphic) rhabdomyosarcoma has also been reported in the prostate, but is rare.[49, 59]

Leiomyosarcoma

Leiomyosarcoma is the second most common sarcoma of the prostate (26 percent of sarcomas),[49, 50] but accounts for the majority of sarcomas occurring in adults. Most patients are between 40 and 71 years of age, with a median

of 58 years.[49, 67] Several patients have been reported under 40 years of age,[46, 67-71] but leiomyosarcoma occurring in patients under 10 years is unusual.[67] In fact, the diagnosis of all reported cases of leiomyosarcoma in pediatric patients has been based on light microscopic study of hematoxylin and eosin (H&E) stained sections, calling into question the validity of smooth muscle derivation of these tumors.

Leiomyosarcoma typically presents as a large bulky tumor diffusely infiltrating the prostate and periprostatic soft tissues.[67, 68, 72–74] Clinically, it may be confused with nodular hyperplasia and prostatitis.[67, 72]

By light microscopy, leiomyosarcoma consists of interlacing bundles of spindle cells with blunted-end nuclei and eosinophilic cytoplasm (Fig. 8-9). Nuclear atypia may be mild, moderate, or severe.[49, 50, 70, 75] Necrosis and hemorrhage frequently accompany these neoplasms.

Smooth muscle differentiation of leiomyosarcoma can usually be demonstrated by routine immunohistochemistry or electron microscopy.[68, 70, 76] Cytogenetic studies have revealed characteristic chromosomal abnormalities, similar to those observed in leiomyosarcomas from other sites.[70]

At present, no strict criteria exist to differentiate leiomyosarcoma of the prostate from cellular or symplastic leiomyoma. Most investigators rely on reproducible criteria from uterine smooth muscle tumors in making this distinction, including cellularity, nuclear atypia, and mitotic rate. The difficulty in assessing biologic behavior of these tumors is compounded by their rarity and incomplete histologic description, including mitotic rates reported as occasional,[75] frequent,[68] high,[76] and moderate.[49] In one article, leiomyosarcoma was noted to have one mitosis per 10 high power fields; despite radiation therapy and chemotherapy, that patient's tumor progressed within 7 months of therapy, indicating that low mitotic rate does not exclude aggressiveness in leiomyosarcomas of the prostate.[73] We recommend a minimum of 1 histologic section per centimeter diameter of tumor.

Most patients with leiomyosarcoma die from

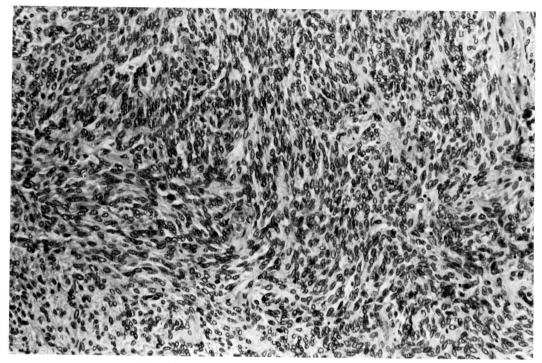

Fig. 8-9. Prostatic leiomyosarcoma. (H&E, ×160.)

their tumor, with a 55 percent 1-year survival, 22 percent 3-year survival, and less than 10 percent 5-year survival.[67] Rare long-term survivors have been reported at 9[49] and 13[67] years. Metastases occur mainly to the lungs, but have also been reported in the liver,[68] bone,[69] adrenals, brain,[67] kidneys,[67, 68] and pleura.[68] Local recurrences are observed up to 6 years after radical surgery,[48] but may occur rapidly within a few months.[74, 76] One case was found in association with incidental carcinoma.[77]

OTHER RARE SARCOMAS

Fibrosarcoma

Other sarcomas involving the prostate are curiosities. Fibrosarcoma has been occasionally reported in the past,[78] but with the advent of immunohistochemistry, most of these tumors have been reclassified as leiomyosarcoma or malignant fibrous histiocytoma.[79]

Osteosarcoma

Osteosarcoma arising in the prostate is exceedingly rare.[80, 81] One case was diagnosed following discovery of adenocarcinoma,[80] and appeared to develop de novo. In another case, osteogenic differentiation appeared 2 years after the onset of radiation therapy for carcinoma.[81] The relationship of this osteogenic change with the radiation therapy is uncertain. Because both of these reported cases of osteosarcoma occurred following adenocarcinoma, the question arises whether these are pure osteogenic sarcomas or mixed carcinosarcomas. It should be noted that the osteosarcoma-like cells did not express prostatic markers.

Malignant Fibrous Histiocytoma

A single documented case of malignant fibrous histiocytoma arising in the prostate was reported in a 63-year-old man.[79] This tumor displayed moderate pleomorphism and rare mitoses, and the patient was free of tumor after 26 months; such features are somewhat unusual for malignant fibrous histiocytoma.

Angiosarcoma

Angiosarcoma rarely occurs in the prostate, usually in adults.[82] Immunohistochemical staining for factor VIII-related antigen has proven useful in one case.[82] The prognosis does not appear to be as poor as angiosarcoma at other sites, but additional cases are needed to verify this impression.

Chondrosarcoma, Malignant Nerve Sheath Tumors, Neuroblastoma

Rare cases of chondrosarcoma, malignant nerve sheath sarcoma, and neuroblastoma have been reported in the prostate.[47]

Undifferentiated Sarcoma

In our experience, sarcomas in the prostate frequently resist all efforts at subclassification. Many sarcomas present as cellular high-grade spindle cell neoplasms with nuclear pleomorphism and increased mitotic rate, often with numerous bizarre atypical forms. Immunohistochemistry and electron microscopy confirm that these are not epithelial neoplasms, but no definite differentiation is observed. We prefer the term *undifferentiated sarcoma* for these tumors. Regardless of the classification, such tumors are aggressive and invariably fatal.

Mixed Tumors

Rare cases of carcinosarcoma, and malignant mixed mesenchymal tumors of the prostate have been reported.[83-87] These are highly malignant neoplasms that may be difficult to distinguish from sarcomatoid carcinoma[88] and other prostatic sarcomas. The diagnosis is based on the identification of both malignant epithelial and mesenchymal components. Immunohistochemistry for prostatic markers and keratin and the presence of desmosomes on electron microscopy are useful in identifying the epithelial component and evaluating the epithelial or mesenchymal nature of the sarcomatoid component.[89]

Hematolymphoid Differentiation

Lymphoma and leukemia are not sarcomas, but are included in this section because of their historic inclusion as lymphosarcoma.[49, 90]

Malignant Lymphoma

Malignant lymphoma involving the prostate, whether presenting as primary extranodular lymphoma or as secondary spread to the prostate from another site, is rare (Fig. 8-10). Difficulty has been encountered in the interpretation of some of the early reported cases, with classification of many as sarcomas, lymphosarcomas, lymphoblastomas, and round cell sarcomas.[66] Fewer than 100 primary and secondary malignant lymphomas involving the prostate have been reported with complete clinical and pathologic documentation.[66, 90-99] The majority of the cases were diagnosed antemortem, and patients ranged in age from 14 to 86 years, with a mean of 61 years.[66]

Patients with prostatic lymphoma usually present with symptoms of urgency and frequency usually attributed to concomitant prostatic hyperplasia or carcinoma.[66] Even in patients with a previous diagnosis of lymphoma, these obstructive symptoms were considered attributable to nodular hyperplasia. Systemic symptoms associated with lymphomas, such as fever, chills, night sweats, and weight loss, were rarely observed, and only in patients with widespread lymphoma.

The prostate was usually diffusely enlarged,

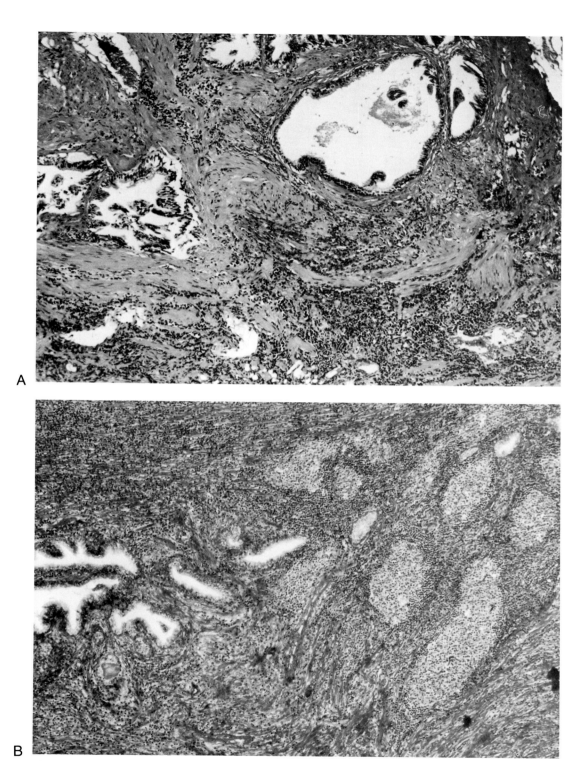

Fig. 8-10. (A & B) Malignant lymphoma involving the prostate. (Fig. A: diffuse; Fig. B: nodular; H&E, ×100.)

and soft and rubbery in consistency. The median furrow, usually present on digital rectal examination, was obliterated.

The distinction of primary prostatic lymphoma from secondary involvement is based on the modified criteria of King and Cox,[66, 90] which includes the following: (1) limitation of lymphoma to the prostate and adjacent tissues; (2) absence of lymph node involvement; (3) major presenting symptoms limited to the prostate; and (4) systemic tumor-free interval of a least 1 month to allow completion of staging procedures. Improved methods of staging, including the use of computed tomography, may aid in the recognition of suspected lymph node involvement. Using these criteria, primary prostatic lymphomas are much less common than secondary lymphomas.[66] Most are diffuse large cell and small cleaved cell types, with rare mixed cell lymphomas. Nodular lymphomas and T-cell lymphomas are exceptional.[66] Small non-cleaved cell lymphomas of Burkitt's[95] and high-grade non-Burkitt's types[66] and Hodgkin's disease[49, 97] have also been rarely observed. A recent case of angiotrophic lymphoma previously misinterpreted as malignant angioendotheliomatosis appeared in the literature.[99]

Malignant lymphoma involving the prostate appears to carry a poor prognosis regardless of stage of presentation, histologic classification, or treatment regimen.[66] Most investigators agree that prostatectomy is not effective in prolonging survival, but it may offer symptomatic relief of urinary obstruction. There is no consensus regarding treating for lymphoma in the prostate, although treatment of systemic tumor may relieve prostatic symptoms, similar to leukemic infiltration of the prostate.

Leukemia Involving the Prostate

Although leukemic infiltration of the prostate may occur, it is usually symptomless. Chronic lymphocytic leukemia is the most common type,[100] and is usually confused with prostatic hyperplasia. Only two cases of symptomatic prostatic granulocytic sarcoma have been reported,[101] and must be considered in the differential diagnosis of patients with urinary obstruction and acute leukemia or myelodysplastic syndrome.

OTHER MALIGNANT TUMORS

Single cases have been reported of prostatic neuroblastoma[47] and prostatic rhabdoid tumor.[103] The rhabdoid tumor occurred in a 14-year-old boy, and displayed immunoreactivity for prekeratin, cytokeratin, epithelial membrane antigen, carcinoembryonic antigen, and vimentin.[102, 103] Electron microscopy showed pleomorphic cells with tonofilaments, microvilli, intracytoplasmic lumina, and rare cell junctions.

REFERENCES

1. Epstein JI, Hutchins GM: Granulomatous prostatitis: distinction among allergic, nonspecific, and posttransurethral resection lesions. Hum Pathol 15:818, 1984
2. Bogomoletz WV: Tumeurs malignes rares et pseudotumeurs de la prostate. Bull Cancer (Paris) 72:423, 1985
3. Proppe KH, Scully RE, Rosai J: Postoperative spindle cell nodules of genitourinary tract resembling sarcomas. A report of eight cases. Am J Surg Pathol 8:101, 1984
4. Tetu B, Ro JY, Ayala AG, et al: Atypical spindle cell lesions of the prostate. Semin Diagn Pathol 5:284, 1988
5. Ro, JY, Ayala AG, Ordonez NG, et al: Pseudosarcomatous fibromyxoid tumor of the urinary bladder. Am J Clin Pathol 86:583, 1986
6. Gardner WA Jr, Spitz WU: Melanosis of the prostate gland. Am J Clin Pathol 56:762, 1971
7. Nigogosyan G, De La Pava S, Pickren JW, Woodruff MW: Blue nevus of the prostate gland. Cancer 16:1097, 1963
8. Jao W, Fretzin DG, Christ ML, Prinz LM: Blue nevus of the prostate gland. Arch Pathol 91:187, 1971
9. Block NL, Weber D, Schinella R: Blue nevi and other melanocytic lesions of the prostate: report of 3 cases and review of the literature. J Urol 107:85, 1972

10. Guillan RA, Zelman S: The incidence and probable origin of melanin in the prostate. J Urol 104:151, 1970
11. Langley JW, Weitzner S: Blue nevus and melanosis of prostate. J Urol 112:359, 1974
12. Kovi J, Jackson AG, Jackson MA: Blue nevus of the prostate: ultrastructural study. Urology 9:576, 1977
13. Aguilar M, Gaffney EF, Finnerty DP: Prostatic melanosis with involvement of benign and malignant epithelium. J Urol 128:825, 1982
14. Simard C, Rognon LM, Pilorce G: Le problème du naevus bleu prostatique. Ann Anat Pathol 9:469, 1964
15. Ro JY, Grignon DJ, Ayala AG et al: Blue nevus and melanosis of the prostate: electron-microscopic and immunohistochemical studies. Am J Clin Pathol 90:530, 1988
16. Goldman RL: Melanogenic epithelium in prostate gland. Am J Clin Pathol 49:75, 1968
17. Tannenbaum M: Differential diagnosis in uropathology. III. Melanotic lesions of the prostate: blue nevus and prostatic epithelial melanosis. Urology 4:617, 1974
18. Rios CN, Wright Jr: Melanosis of the prostate gland: report of a case with neoplastic epithelium involvement. J. Urol 115:616, 1976
19. Berry NE, Reese L: Malignant melanoma which had its first clinical manifestations in the prostate gland. J Urol 69:286, 1953
20. Grignon DJ, Ro JY, Ayala AG: Malignant melanoma with metastasis to adenocarcinoma of the prostate. Cancer 63:196, 1989
21. Kaufman JJ, Berneike RB: Leiomyoma of the prostate. J Urol 65:297, 1951
22. Vassilakis GB: Pure leiomyoma of prostate. Urology 11:93, 1978
23. Regan JB, Barrett DM, Wold LE: Giant leiomyoma of the prostate. Arch Pathol Lab Med 111:381, 1987
24. Michaels MM, Brown HE, Favino CJ: Leiomyoma of the prostate. Urology 3:617, 1974
25. Leonard A, Baert L, Van Praet F, et al: Solitary leiomyoma of the prostate. Br J Urol 60:184, 1988
26. Dennis PJ, Lewandowski AE, Rohner TJ Jr, et al: Pheochromocytoma of the prostate: an unusual location. J Urol 141:130, 1989
27. Cox R, Dawson MP: A curious prostatic tumour, probably a two-mixed tumour (cystadenoleiomyo-fibroma). Br J Urol 32:306, 1960
28. Kafandaris PM, Polyzonis MB: Fibroadenoma-like foci in human prostatic nodular hyperplasia. Prostate 4:33, 1983
29. Attah EB, Powell MEA: Atypical stromal hyperplasia of the prostate gland. Am J Clin Pathol 67:324, 1977
30. Young RH, Scully RE: Pseudosarcomatous lesions of the urinary bladder, prostate gland, and urethra. A report of three cases and review of the literature. Arch Pathol Lab Med 111:354, 1987
31. Kirkland KL, Bale PM: A cystic adenoma of the prostate. J Urol 97:324, 1967
32. Gueft B, Walsh MA: Malignant prostatic cystosarcoma phyllodes. NY State J Med 75:2226, 1975
33. Attah EB, Nkposong EO: Phyllodes type of atypical prostatic hyperplasia. J Urol 115:762, 1976
34. Yokota T, Yamshita Y, Okuzono Y, et al: Malignant cystosarcoma phyllodes of prostate. Acta Pathol Jpn 34:663, 1984
35. Manivel C, Shenoy, BV, Wick MR, Dehner LP: Cystosarcoma phyllodes of the prostate. Arch Pathol Lab Med 110:534, 1986
36. Reese JH, Lombard CM, Krowe K, Stamey TA: Phyllodes type of atypical prostatic hyperplasia: a report of 3 new cases. J Urol 138:623, 1987
37. Lucey DT, McAninch JW, Bunts RC: Genital cysts of the male pelvis: case report of müllerian and ejaculatory duct cysts in the same patient. J Urol 109:440, 1973
38. Rosen Y, Ambiavagar PC, Vuletin JC, Macchia RJ: Atypical leiomyoma of the prostate. Urology 15:183, 1980
39. Persaud V, Douglas LL: Bizarre (atypical) leiomyoma of the prostate gland. Wis Med J 31:217, 1982
40. Karolyi P, Endes P, Krasznai G, Tonkol I: Bizarre leiomyoma of the prostate. Virchows Archiv [A] 412:383, 1988
41. Benassayag E: Leiomyoblastome de la prostate chez un homme jeune. J Urol Nephrol 81:831, 1975
42. Hafiz MA, Toker C, Sutula M: An atypical fibromyxoid tumor of the prostate. Cancer 54:2500, 1984
43. Reyes JW, Shifnozuka H, Garry P, Putong PB: A light and electron microscopic study of a hemangiopericytoma of the prostate with local extension. Cancer 40:1122, 1977
44. Wunsch PH, Muller HA: Hemangiopericytoma

of the prostate, a light microscopic study of an unusual tumor. Pathol Res Pract 172:334, 1982

45. Chen KTK: Hemangiopericytoma of the prostate. J Surg Oncol 35:42, 1987

46. Mackenzie AR, Whitmore WF, Melamed MR: Myosarcomas of the bladder and prostate. Cancer 22:833, 1968

47. Mostofi FK, Price EB Jr: Tumors of the male genital system. p. 177. In Atlas of Tumor Pathology. Armed Forces Institute of Pathology, Washington, DC, 1973

48. Narayana AS, Loening S, Weimar GW, Culp DA: Sarcoma of the bladder and prostate. J Urol 118:72, 1978

49. Smith BH, Dehner LP: Sarcoma of the prostate gland. Am J Clin Pathol 58:43, 1972

50. Kastendieck H, Altenahr E, Geister H: Das Myosarkom der Prostata. Dtsch Med Wschr 99:392, 1974

51. Tannenbaum M: Histopathology of the prostate gland. p 303. In Tannenbaum M (ed): Urologic Pathology: The Prostate. Lea & Febiger, Philadelphia, 1977

52. Newton WA, Soule EH, Reiman HM, et al: Histopathology of childhood sarcomas: intergroup rhabdomyosarcomas studies I and II. Clinicopathologic correlation. J Clin Oncol 6:67, 1988

53. Ghavimi F, Herr H, Jereb B, Exelby PR: Treatment of genitourinary rhabdomyosarcoma in children. J Urol 132:313, 1984

54. Goodwin WE, Mims MM, Young HH: Rhabdomyosarcoma of the prostate in a child: first 5-year survival (combined treatment by preoperative, local irradiation; actinomycin D; intraarterial nitrogen mustard and hypothermia; radical surgery and ureterosigmoidostomy). J Urol 99:651, 1968

55. Sarkar K, Tolnai G, McKay DE: Embryonal rhabdomyosarcoma of the prostate. An ultrastructural study. Cancer 31:442, 1973

56. King DG, Finney RP: Embryonal rhabdomyosarcoma of the prostate. J Urol 117:88, 1977

57. Sarnacki S, Flamant F, Valayer J: Thérapeutiques conservatrices dans les rhabdomyosarcomes génito-urinaires de l'enfant. Chir Pediatr 28:299, 1987

58. Henkes DN, Stein NP: Fine-needle aspiration cytology of prostatic embryonal rhabdomyosarcoma: a case report. Diag Cytopathol 3:163, 1987

59. Raney B Jr, Carey A, Snyder HM, et al: Primary site as a prognostic variable for children with pelvic soft tissue sarcomas. J Urol 136:874, 1986

60. Keenan DJM, Graham WH: Embryonal rhabdomyosarcoma of the prostatic-urethral region in an adult. Br J Urol 57:241, 1985

61. Tamauchi H, Tsutsumi Y, Nishino T, et al: Rhabdomyosarcoma of the prostate—report of a case with an immunohistochemical study of the neoplastic rhabdomyoblast. Tokai J Exp Clin Med 9:323, 1984

62. McDougal WS, Persky L: Rhabdomyosarcoma of the bladder and prostate in children. J Urol 124:882, 1980

63. Fleischmann J, Perinetti EP, Catalona WJ: Embryonal rhabdomyosarcoma of the genitourinary organs. J Urol 126:389, 1981

64. Kaplan WE, Firlit C, Berger RM: Genitourinary rhabdomyosarcoma. J Urol 130:116, 1983

65. Têtu B, Ro JY, Ayala AG, et al: Small cell carcinoma of the prostate. I. A clinicopathologic study of 20 cases. Cancer 59:1803, 1987

66. Bostwick DG, Mann RB: Malignant lymphomas involving the prostate. A study of 13 cases. Cancer 56:2932, 1985

67. Christoffersen J: Leiomyosarcoma of the prostate. Acta Chir Scand, Suppl 433:75, 1973

68. Ohmori T, Arita N, Tabei R: Prostatic leiomyosarcoma revealing cytoplasmic virus-like particles and intranuclear paracrystalline structures. Acta Pathol Jpn 34:631, 1984

69. Mottola A, Selli C, Carini M et al: Leiomyosarcoma of the prostate. Eur Urol 11:131, 1985

70. Limon J, Dal Cin P, Sandberg AA: Cytogenetic findings in a primary leiomyosarcoma of the prostate. Cancer Genet Cytogenet 22:159, 1986

71. Cookingham CL, Kumar NB: Diagnosis of prostatic leiomyosarcoma with fine needle aspiration cytology. Acta Cytologica 29:170, 1985

72. Fitzpatrick TJ, Stump G: Leiomyosarcoma of the prostate: Case report and review of the literature. J Urol 83:80, 1960

73. Witherow R, Molland E, Oliver T, Hind C: Leiomyosarcoma of prostate and superficial soft tissue. Urology 15:513, 1980

74. Aragona F, Serretta V, Marconi A, et al: Leiomyosarcoma of the prostate in adults. Ann Chir Gynaecol 74:191, 1985

75. Muller HA, Wünsch PH: Features of prostatic sarcomas in combined aspiration and punch biopsies. Acta Cytol 25:481, 1981

76. Carmel M, Massé SS, Lehoux JG, Elhilali M: Leiomyosarcoma of prostate. Urology 12:190, 1983

77. Rodrigues Palma PC, Rodrigues Netto N Jr, Ikari O, et al: Leiomyosarcoma in association with incidental adenocarcinoma of the prostate. J Urol 129:156, 1983

78. Tannenbaum M: Sarcomas of the prostate gland. Urology 5:810, 1975

79. Chin W, Fay R, Ortega P: Malignant fibrous histiocytoma of prostate. Urology 27:365, 1986

80. Meeter UI, Richards JN: Osteogenic sarcoma of the prostate. J Urol 81:654, 1960

81. Locke JR, Soloway MS, Evans J, Murphy WM: Osteogenic differentiation associated with x-ray therapy for adenocarcinoma of the prostate gland. Am J Clin Pathol 85:375, 1986

82. Smith DM, Manivel C, Kapps D, Uecker J: Angiosarcoma of the prostate: report of 2 cases and review of the literature. J Urol 135:382, 1986

83. Haddad JR, Reyes E. Carcinosarcoma of the prostate with metastasis of both elements: case report. J Urol 103:80, 1970

84. Hamlin WB, Lund PK: Carcinosarcoma of the prostate: a case report. J Urol 97:518, 1967

85. Quay SC, Proppe KH: Carcinosarcoma of the prostate: case report and review of the literature. J Urol 125:436, 1981

86. Hokamura K, Kurozumi T, Tanaka K, Yamaguchi A: Carcinosarcoma of the prostate. Acta Pathol Jpn 35:481, 1985

87. Ginesin Y, Bolkier M, Moskovitz B, et al: Carcinosarcoma of the prostate. Eur Urol 12:441, 1986

88. Shannon RL, Grignon DJ, Ro JY, et al: Sarcomatoid carcinoma of the prostate. Lab Invest 60:87A, 1989

89. Ordonez NG, Ayala AG, von Eshchenbach AC, et al: Immunoperoxidase localization of prostatic acid phosphatase in prostatic carcinoma with sarcomatoid changes. Urology 11:210, 1982

90. King LS, Cox TR: Lymphosarcoma of the prostate. Am J Pathol 27:801, 1951

91. West WO: Primary lymphosarcoma of prostate gland. Arch Intern Med 109:145, 1962

92. Cartagena R, Baumgartner G, Wajsman Z, Merrin C: Preliminary reticulum cell sarcoma of prostate gland. Urology 5:815, 1975

93. Hampel N, Richter-Levin D, Gersh I: Primary lymphosarcoma of prostate. Urology 9:461, 1977

94. Doll DC, Weiss RB, Shah S: Lymphoma of the prostate presenting as benign prostatic hypertrophy. Southern Med J 71:1170, 1978

95. Boe S, Nielsen H, Ryttov N: Burkitt's lymphoma mimicking prostatitis. J Urol 125:891, 1981

96. Cos LR, Rakshid HA: Primary non-Hodgkin lymphoma of prostate presenting as benign prostatic hyperplasia. Urology 23:176, 1984

97. Sridhar KN, Woodhouse CRJ: Prostatic infiltration in leukaemia and lymphoma. Eur Urol 9:153, 1983

98. Lewi HJE, Whaite A, Cassidy M, et al: Lymphocytic infiltration of the prostate. Br J Urol 56:301, 1984

99. Banerjee SS, Harris M: Angiotrophic lymphoma presenting in the prostate. Histopathology 12:667, 1988

100. Cachia PG, McIntyre MA, Dewar AE, Stockdill G: Prostatic infiltration in chronic lymphatic leukaemia. J Clin Pathol 40:343, 1987

101. Frame R, Head D, Lee R, et al: Granulocytic sarcoma of the prostate. Two cases causing urinary obstruction. Cancer 59:142, 1987

102. Haas JE, Palmer NF, Weinberg AG, Beckwith JB: Ultrastructure of malignant rhabdoid tumor of the kidney. A distinctive renal tumor of children. Hum Pathol 12:646, 1981

103. Ekfors TO, Aho HJ, Kekomaki M: Malignant rhabdoid tumor of the prostatic region. Immunohistological and ultrastructural evidence for epithelial origin. Virchows Arch [A] 406:381, 1985

9

Application of Immunocytochemistry in the Pathology of the Prostate

Nelson G. Ordóñez, Jae Y. Ro, and Alberto G. Ayala

The success of the different modalities of treatment currently available to the patient with cancer of the prostate greatly depends on the accuracy of the histopathologic diagnosis. The vast majority of prostatic malignancies are carcinomas and usually do not present a diagnostic problem, especially when they are well differentiated. However, when they initially present as metastatic disease from an undetected primary prostatic tumor, the diagnosis can become a challenge for the surgical pathologist, who must establish the site of origin on the basis of the histologic characteristics of the neoplasm. In these circumstances, the differential diagnosis may include a wide variety of epithelial tumors and, less frequently, other neoplastic conditions, such as melanoma or some types of sarcomas with which prostatic carcinoma can be confused.

Immunohistochemistry has proven to be a powerful tool in surgical pathology. Results obtained using immunocytochemical methods provide the pathologist with more objective criteria for the diagnosis of tumors that look alike by routine light microscopy. In addition, these methods may provide evidence on the function of the tumor, as well as information on some of the structural aspects of the tumor that may affect the prognosis, such as the presence of lymphovascular invasion, differentiation of carcinoma in situ, or microinvasion from a frankly invasive tumor. In these circumstances, antibodies to components of the basement membrane and endothelial cells may assist in producing more reproducible and interpretable results than those obtained by conventional methods.

In this chapter, we discuss the practical application of various tissue and cell markers in the diagnosis of selected pathologic conditions that affect the prostate. We also comment briefly on recent developments in molecular biology and their potential use in the study of prostate cancer.

PROSTATE-SPECIFIC MARKERS

Prostatic acid phosphatase (PAP) and prostate-specific antigen (PSA) are two distinct tissue-specific antigens present exclusively in the prostatic epithelium and its secretory products; therefore, these are considered markers of prostatic origin. Metastases from tumors whose origin is undetermined are not uncommon,[1] and, since these are often carcinomas, the possibility of prostatic carcinoma may be raised in the differential diagnosis. Measurements of PAP in the serum are often used as indirect evidence of metastatic carcinoma from the prostate. Unfortunately, the value of this marker is limited by the fact that high serum levels of PAP can occur in cases of infarcted nodular hyperplasia of the prostate and prostatitis, and after digital manipulation of the gland.[2] PSA is a more sensitive prostatic serum marker than PAP, but this marker may also be elevated in benign prostatic diseases.[3] Therefore, in patients who present with metastatic disease from an unknown primary tumor, the finding of a serum elevation of PAP or PSA cannot be used as unequivocal evidence for metastasis from the prostate. In addition, not all patients who have prostate carcinoma have PSA and PAP elevations in the serum.

Because of the high specificity and frequent expression of PAP and PSA in prostatic carcinoma, antibodies directed against these markers have proved to be extremely helpful in the histopathologic diagnosis of prostatic tumors in biopsy material showing poorly differentiated cancer of unknown origin.[4-7] At present, there are numerous commercially available monoclonal and polyclonal antibodies to both substances that can be used successfully on formalin-fixed, paraffin-embedded tissue. These antibodies are also useful for cytologic preparations obtained by fine-needle aspiration biopsy, including those that have been previously stained with Papanicolaou stain.[8, 9] Immunocytochemical studies for PAP and PSA can also be performed on previously decalcified specimens. In a recent study of EDTA and formic acid decalcified specimens, Flisch and colleagues[10] found reactivity for PAP in 35 of 40 cases of metastatic carcinomas of the prostate to bone (87.5 percent). The results of the study were very similar to those obtained by other investigators on lymph node specimens (86 to 100 percent).[11, 12] In our experience, failure to demonstrate these tumor markers by immunocytochemical methods can occur when the tissue remains in the fixative for long periods of time (several days or weeks), but the decalcification procedure itself has little or no effect on the demonstration of these antigens.[13]

PROSTATIC ACID PHOSPHATASE

Acid phosphatases are enzymes that hydrolyze phosphoric acid esters at acid pH. These enzymes are found in various tissues, most notably in erythrocytes, spleen, and prostate. Prostate-specific acid phosphatase is an isoenzyme of acid phosphatase with a molecular weight of 100 kDa.[14, 15] In the prostate, acid phosphatase is produced in acinar cells and secreted into the ductal system, where it can be detected in the semen and expressed prostatic secretions, and urine.[16] Under normal conditions, very little PAP is found in the general circulation. Although the reason PAP is elevated in carcinoma of the prostate is not completely understood, it has been postulated that disruption of the normal architecture of the gland, together with occlusion of the prostatic ducts, permits leakage of the enzyme into lymphatics and blood vessels, resulting in an elevation in the patient's serum.[16] Using enzymatic techniques, elevated serum PAP levels are found in 60 to 90 percent of patients with stage C and D carcinoma of the prostate, but in only 5 to 30 percent of those with localized tumor (stages A and B).[17-19]

Thus, up to 30 percent of patients with documented metastases have normal PAP levels.[16] The reason PAP levels are sometimes undetectable in advanced disease is not clear, but it may be due to the increased anaplasia of high-stage tumors, which sometimes lose the capacity to synthesize the enzyme.[20]

Immunohistochemical reactivity for PAP has been demonstrated in 80 to 100 percent of prostatic carcinomas.[11, 21-24] False-positive reactions are very rare but have been reported on occasion in carcinomas of the breast[21, 22, 25] and kidney,[25] islet cell tumors of the pancreas,[23, 26] and adenocarcinoma of the urinary bladder.[27] Epstein et al.[27] demonstrated PAP reactivity in 3 of 11 adenocarcinomas of the bladder, and in 1 of 5 mixed transitional cell carcinomas and adenocarcinomas in males. They also found positive immunoreactivity for this antibody in two of four adenocarcinomas, and two of four mixed adenocarcinomas and transitional cell carcinoma in females. None of the tumors seen in males or females reacted for PSA. Although some controversy still exists about whether the intensity and incidence of reactivity is influenced by the degree of tumor differentiation, most investigators agree that well-differentiated tumors almost invariably stain positively for these markers.

Some of the discrepancies in the results found between some series may be due to differences in the spectrum of antigens detected by the various antibodies or to technical differences between laboratories.[24] In a comparative study, Schevchuk and colleagues[28] found positivity in 83 percent of the cases stained with an antiserum raised in goats against extracts of benign prostatic hyperplasia, in contrast to 70 percent positivity when the same tissue was tested with rabbit antiserum generated against sperm-free ejaculate. The rate of positivity in these tissue specimens dropped to 59 percent when a monoclonal antibody to PAP was used that recognized only one antigenic determinant. It was concluded from this study that, unless pools of several monoclonal antibodies capable of recognizing multiple antigenic determinants are used, polyclonal antibodies are more suitable for screening purposes than monoclonal antibodies.

PROSTATE-SPECIFIC ANTIGEN

In 1979, Wang and associates[29] isolated and purified a 33-kDa single-chain glycoprotein specific for prostatic epithelial cells, designated *prostate-specific antigen* (PSA). PSA is biochemically and immunologically different from PAP, and has no known enzymatic or other function. PSA is an organ-specific marker that is produced by normal and malignant prostatic epithelial cells, but not by any other cells in the body. PSA is also found in prostatic fluid and seminal plasma.[30] Using an immunoperoxidase method, Nadji and colleagues[11] demonstrated PSA reactivity in the acinar and ductal prostatic epithelium and in luminal secretions, but not in the periurethral glands, seminal vesicles, or urothelium. Immunoelectron microscopic studies have demonstrated that PSA is localized in rough endoplasmic reticulum and lysosomal dense bodies in normal, hyperplastic,

and malignant epithelial cells, but not in the acinar basal cells.[31, 32]

When PSA levels were compared with other commonly used markers for prostatic tumors, they appeared to be a more reliable prognostic indicator.[33] Serum levels have been reported to be proportional to the clinical stage of the disease.[3] Unfortunately, PSA is not a useful marker for screening for early prostatic cancer, since it is elevated in 55 percent to 88 percent of the patients with benign prostatic hyperplasia.[3, 34] In spite of this limitation, PSA has proven to be a very sensitive marker after total prostatectomy and, therefore, useful for the detection of metastasis.[3]

Although most primary and metastatic carcinomas of the prostate react for PSA, there is some controversy regarding the percentage of reactive cases for this marker, as well as whether the degree of differentiation correlates with the intensity of the immunostaining. While some investigators[11] have found positive immunostaining in all cases studied, regardless of whether the tumor is primary or metastatic or its degree of differentiation, in our experience, as well as that of others,[5, 35, 36] a small number of tumors may not show reacticity for this marker. Some investigators[37] have suggested that the presence of PSA-negative cells in prostatic tumors correlates with more aggressive behavior, but more information is required before a definitive conclusion regarding the prognostic value of PSA immunostaining can be drawn.

Several studies comparing PSA with PAP immunostaining have shown that the number of cases staining for PAP is larger than that reacting with PSA.[38, 39] In a recent study, Feiner and Gonzalez[40] found that a histologic type of high-grade carcinoma of the prostate, characterized by large cells with large nuclei, moderate amount of cytoplasm, and indistinct cell borders, frequently loses PSA immunoreactivity, but usually retains PAP expression. Because this type of prostate carcinoma may be confused with transitional cell carcinoma, the authors indicated that staining for both PAP and PSA should be performed. Based on their observations, as well as the occasional finding of tumors that may react with only one of these tissue markers, we routinely advise that all poorly differentiated tumors be stained for both PAP and PSA when carcinoma of the prostate is considered in the differential diagnosis (Fig. 9-1).

USE OF IMMUNOCYTOCHEMISTRY IN THE STUDY OF SPECIAL TYPES OF PROSTATIC CARCINOMA

PAPILLARY ADENOCARCINOMA OF THE PROSTATIC DUCTS

Endometrial carcinoma of the prostate is a term introduced by Melicow and Pachter[41] to designate a distinctive morphologic group of prostatic tumors originating centrally in the vicinity of the urethra. Histologically, these tumors consist of a glandular, papillary, and sometimes villiform proliferation of cells having moderate atypia and increased mitotic activity. Owing to their consistent location near the prostatic verumontanum, it was suggested that these tumors originated from the utricle.[41, 42] The concept of an endometrial origin for this tumor was based on morphologic similarities between endometrioid prostatic adenocarcinoma and endometrial adenocarcinoma of the uterus, as well as on embryologic evidence suggesting that the prostatic utricle may be of müllerian origin since vestigial female tissue may persist in the utricle. However, this concept is currently not accepted by most embryologists, who believe that this epithelium is replaced by the urogenital sinus in early life.[43, 44] It is unclear whether the epithelial lining of the utricle is derived entirely from the urogenital sinus; is a mixture of mesonephric, müllerian, and urogenital sinus epithelium; or is entirely müllerian.[43, 45-47]

In order to determine whether endometrial prostate carcinomas were tumors of prostatic or müllerian origin, we recently studied 20 of these tumors by immunocytochemical methods, and compared them with normal prostatic utricles from adults and children.[48] All 20 endometrial prostate carcinomas reacted strongly with both PAP and PSA. In addition, all normal adult utricles and five of nine normal utricles from children stained for PAP and PSA. Furthermore, we were unable to demonstrate any structure suggesting müllerian remnant in the verumontanum areas. These findings are in agreement with those obtained by other investigators,[49, 50] who also found immunocytochemical and electron microscopic evidence indicating that endometrial carcinomas of the prostate are tumors of prostatic ductal origin, and are not müllerian derivatives.

In the practice of pathology, the most common diagnostic problem encountered with this tumor is its differentiation from transitional cell carcinoma of the urethra, prostatic duct, or trigone, or adenocarcinoma of urethral origin. In this situation, the utilization of PAP and PSA is extremely valuable (Fig. 9-2).

SIGNET RING CELL CARCINOMA

Traditionally, the term *signet ring cell carcinoma* has been used to designate a subgroup of mucin-producing adenocarcinomas usually arising in the stomach, colon, pancreas, breast, or urinary bladder. These tumors typically display cells containing nuclei pushed and compressed by mucin-loaded cytoplasm. In recent years, however, this term has also been used to designate other types of neoplasms that do not secrete mucin but present a signet ring-like appearance on hematoxylin and eosin-stained tissue sections. These include some types of thyroid tumors,[51, 52] lymphomas,[53, 54] melanomas,[55] oligodendrogliomas,[56] smooth muscle tumors,[57] and prostate carcinomas. Primary signet ring cell carcinoma of the prostate is a rare variant of poorly differentiated carcinoma that, in our experience, usually is not associated with mucin production, although rare cases of mucinous signet ring cell carcinomas of the prostate have been reported.[58] When this tumor presents as metastatic tumor, it may be confused with

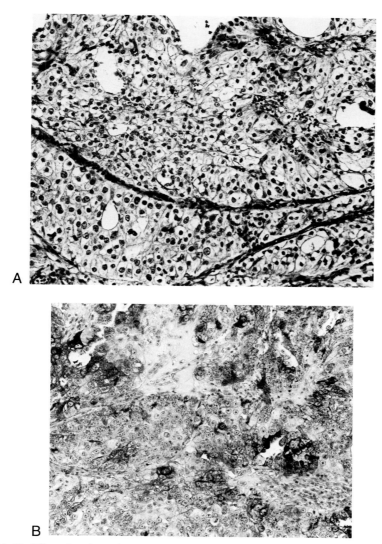

Fig. 9-1. (A) Undifferentiated carcinoma involving the bladder wall. The main differential diagnosis is between prostatic carcinoma and urothelial carcinoma. **(B)** Immunostaining preparation showing focal staining for PSA.

other signet ring cell neoplasms. In a recent immunocytochemical study of eight signet ring cell carcinomas of the prostate, we found re-activity for both PAP and PSA in both signet ring cell and non-signet ring cell tumor cells, including one case that presented as a supraclavicular lymph node metastasis.[59] Unlike other sig-

net ring cell carcinomas, the signet ring cells of prostatic origin are generally negative for mucin; therefore, PAP and PSA immunostudies should always be done in mucin-negative meta-static signet ring cell carcinoma, especially in a man over 45 years old[60] (Fig. 9-3).

On occasion, vacuolated lymphocytes having

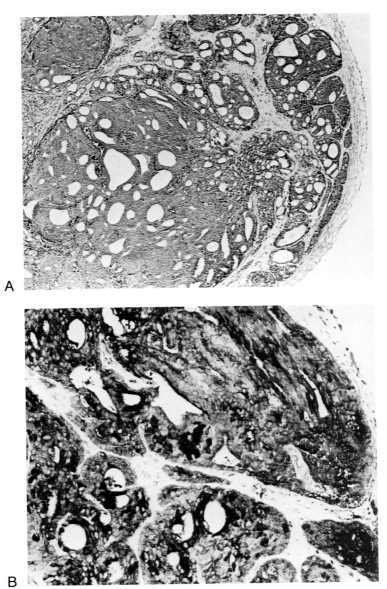

Fig. 9-2. (A) Endometrioid carcinoma containing a solid tumor component and central glandular differentiation. **(B)** Immunohistochemical preparation showing positive staining for PAP.

a signet ring cell-like appearance can be found in prostatic biopsies. In these situations, the dense lymphocytic infiltration, which occasionally permeates the fibromuscular stroma, may mimic carcinoma. The absence of immunostaining for PSA and PAP and the finding of leukocyte common antigen reactivity rules out prostatic carcinoma.[61, 62]

MUCINOUS ADENOCARCINOMA

Primary prostatic mucinous adenocarcinoma is rare. Histologically, these tumors are similar to colloid carcinomas of the breast or colon, and consist of clusters of cells floating in lakes of mucin (Fig. 9-4A). The differential diagnosis includes prostatic invasion by mucinous adeno-

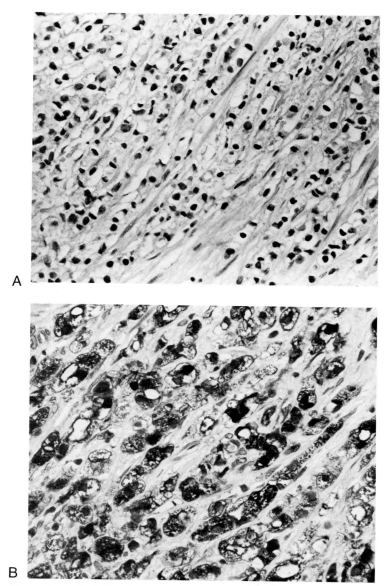

Fig. 9-3. (A) Signet ring cells infiltrating prostate stroma. **(B)** Prostatic signet ring cell carcinoma staining for PSA.

carcinoma of the rectum, urinary bladder, or Cowper's glands. Distant metastasis to lymph nodes, bone, brain, liver, and lung have also been reported.[63-66] In those cases, immunocytochemical studies can be of great help in confirming the prostatic origin of the tumor.[67, 68] Recently, we had the opportunity to study seven of these tumors by immunocytochemical methods. In all seven cases, we were able to demonstrate reactivity for PAP and PSA, but not for carcinoembryonic antigen (CEA) (Fig. 9-4B). The negative staining for the latter indicates that CEA immunostaining can be useful in differentiating a primary prostatic tumor from a carcinoma of the rectum with invasion into the prostate gland.

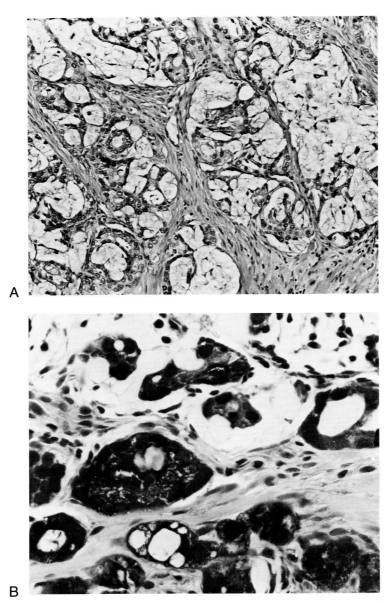

Fig. 9-4. (A) Mucinous prostatic carcinoma. The carcinoma cells are floating in pools of extracellular mucin. **(B)** Immunohistochemical preparation demonstrating intense PSA reactivity in tumor cells.

SARCOMATOID CARCINOMA

Sarcomatoid carcinoma of the prostate, a tumor containing carcinoma and a spindle cell component, is uncommon and can be difficult to differentiate from true sarcomas. In this differ- ential diagnosis, immunocytochemical studies using antibodies against keratin, PAP, and PSA can be helpful in disclosing the epithelial nature of this neoplasm.[69, 70] In our experience, all cases were associated with high-grade prostatic adenocarcinoma of the usual histologic pattern either previous to or simultaneous with the spindle sarcomatoid component. This spindle cell component seldom expressed keratin reactivity, and approximately one third of the cases show focal reactivity for PAP, PSA, or both. On the other hand, staining for vimentin, which is an intermediate filament and a major component of the cytoskeleton of all mesenchymal cells and derived tumors, is not helpful since it is also expressed in a large number of sarcomatoid carcinomas, not only of the prostate, but also of the urinary bladder.[71]

SMALL CELL CARCINOMA

Small cell carcinoma of the prostate is a rare neoplasm characterized by aggressive clinical behavior. Morphologically, it is similar to the lung counterpart, but in some cases it may appear in association with microacinar carcinoma. Ultrastructural and immunocytochemical evidence indicates that a significant number of these cases display neuroendocrine differentiation. Since prostatic tumors with endocrine features may not respond to hormone therapy, they should be differentiated from poorly differentiated prostatic adenocarcinoma.[72] In contrast to

poorly differentiated adenocarcinoma, immunostaining for PAP and PSA are almost invariably negative in small cell carcinoma of the prostate. These tumors, however, usually react with antibodies to endocrine markers, especially neuron-specific enolase (NSE), chromogranin, and synaptophysin, which are expressed independently from the hormone or neurotransmitter produced by the tumor (Fig. 9-5).

NSE is an isoenzyme of the glycolytic enzyme enolase, first localized in neurons and, subsequently found in central and peripheral neuroendocrine cells. Antibodies to NSE have been widely used in the diagnosis of endocrine tumors.[73-75] Because NSE is present in the cytosol, the intensity of the immunostaining for NSE does not correlate with the number of secretory granules. In two recent series, NSE immunostaining was reported in 55.5 and 85.7 percent of cases of small cell carcinoma of the prostate.[72, 76] Recently, however, it has become apparent that NSE is not a specific marker for neuroendocrine cells, as was previously believed. NSE reactivity has been found in a variety of non-neuroendocrine neoplasms, including carcinoma of the kidney, breast and ovary, seminoma, chordoma, and some sarcomas and lymphomas.[77-80]

Fig. 9-5. Small cell carcinoma of the prostate showing numerous NSE immunoreactive cells.

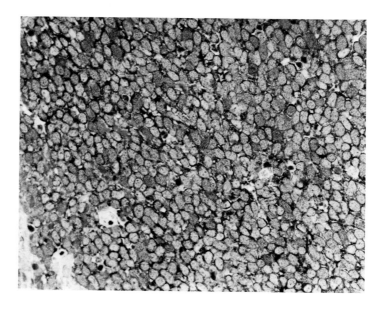

Chromogranins are a group of acidic monomeric proteins of various sizes that form a major part of the soluble protein of the secretory granules of the adrenal medulla. The largest polypeptide is chromogranin A (molecular weight 75 kDa), which is the most abundant.[81] Antibodies to chromogranin A have been used in the diagnosis of a variety of endocrine and neuroendocrine tumors, including tumors derived from the adrenal medulla, C cell of the thyroid, parathyroid gland, anterior pituitary, and islets of the pancreas.[82-84] Since immunostaining for chromogranin A closely parallels the reaction obtained with some argyrophilic stains (Grimelius), endocrine tumors that contain small, sparse endocrine granules stain weakly or not at all with antibodies to chromogranin A. Weakly staining neoplasms include Merkel cell tumor of the skin, neuroblastoma, and small cell carcinoma of the lung and prostate. In spite of this limitation of the staining, Turbat-Herrera and colleagues[72] were able to demonstrate immunoreactivity in all seven small cell carcinomas of the prostate studied, although staining was limited to scant cells in some of the cases.

Synaptophysin is a major transmembrane protein isolated from presynaptic vesicles of bovine neurons.[85] It is not only a highly specific neuroendocrine marker that can be detected in routinely fixed tissues, but it has an advantage over other neuroendocrine markers such as NSE in that it does not react with melanomas.[86] Synaptophysin reactivity has been demonstrated in some small cell carcinomas of the prostate, confirming the endocrine differentiation of some of these tumors.[72]

The monoclonal antibody HNK-1, also known as anti-Leu-7, was raised against a human T-lymphomatoid cell line.[87] This antibody, originally characterized as specific for human cells with natural killer activity, has also been used in the diagnosis of primary and metastatic adenocarcinoma of the prostate,[88-90] as well as normal and neoplastic neuroendocrine cells.[91,92] Because of the broad reactivity of Leu-7 with prostatic tumors, positive staining with this antibody cannot be used as unequivocal evidence of neuroendocrine differentiation of a tumor involving this organ.

Mammalian neurofilaments (NF) are protein triplets composed of three distinct subunits with respective molecular weights of 68, 150, and 200 kDa.[93] Immunocytochemical studies have shown NF in tumors displaying neural features, such as ganglioneuromas, medulloblastomas, and pinealomas.[94-96] In addition, NF reactivity has also been found in carcinoid tumors, pheochromocytomas, and small cell carcinomas of the skin (Merkel cell tumor) and lung.[97, 98] At present, there are no studies investigating the presence of NF in prostatic tumors with endocrine differentiation.

Hormone polypeptides, such as calcitonin, adrenocorticotropic hormone, and bombesin, have been reported in small cell carcinomas of the prostate.[72, 99-101] However, these substances are not consistently expressed in all tumors with endocrine differentiation, so that their value in surgical pathology is limited compared to the previously described markers.

APPLICATION OF KERATIN IMMUNOSTAINING IN THE DIAGNOSIS OF ATYPICAL HYPERPLASIAS OF THE PROSTATE

Keratins are a complex multigenic family of polypeptides that, by double-diffusion gel electrophoresis, can be subdivided according to their molecular weight and isoelectric point into at least 19 subclasses, ranging from 40 to 68 kDa. In human tissues, eight type II keratins (Moll's catalog numbers 1 to 8)[102] and 11 type I keratins (numbers 9 to 19) have been identified. They are expressed in pairs of one larger basic and a smaller acidic member of a similar molecular size rank.[103] Different normal epithelia express different keratins. This differentiation-dependent expression permits subdivision of keratin polypeptides into two groups: those keratins (numbers 7 and 8 of type II, and 18 and 19 of type I) typical of simple, one-layer epithelia of the small intestine and colon, and those characteristic of, but not exclusive to, stratified squamous epithelia (keratins numbers 1 to 6 of type II, and 9 to 17 of type I).[102, 103] The normal prostatic epithelium contains keratins 5, 8, 18, and 19.[104]

Many monoclonal antibodies against keratin proteins have been generated. These can be divided into two principal groups: a broadly reactive group, which recognizes epitopes produced by many keratin proteins, and a selective group, which recognizes epitopes restricted to fewer proteins or even to a single keratin. Broadspectrum antibodies reactive to several keratin proteins can be used to establish the epithelial nature of poorly differentiated carcinoma, and selective antibodies that react with a restricted number of keratins can be used in the study of specific pathological conditions.

Since paraformaldehyde fixation tends to inactivate the antigenic determinants recognized by these antibodies, some antibodies require frozen sections or special fixation (i.e., ethanol or methacarn). Although some antibodies can be applied to formalin-fixed tissues, in order to obtain optimal results, tissue specimens must be treated with proteolytic enzymes during the immunostaining procedure.[105]

BASAL CELL HYPERPLASIA

The glandular acini of the prostate are lined by two distinct cell types. The inner layer consists of columnar secretory cells. The outer layer is formed by flattened, polygonal, triangular-shaped basal cells that are adjacent to the basal lamina. Basal cell hyperplasia is a benign lesion of the prostate that can be confused with carcinoma. Typically, it consists of a proliferation of hyperchromatic cells resembling basal cells that fills and expands the acini (Fig. 9-6). This proliferation may be diffuse, but usually involves one or several lobules. A rare variant of basal cell hyperplasia exhibits lumina in the majority of the affected acini; in these cases, the pattern closely simulates microacinar carcinoma of the prostate. By the use of the 34βE11 antikeratin monoclonal antibody (EAB-903, Enzo Biochem), which recognizes 49-, 57-, 59-, and 66-kDa keratin proteins, it is possible to selectively stain basal cells of normal and hyperplastic prostate.[106, 107] Immunohistochemical studies using this antikeratin antibody, together with PAP and PSA immunostaining, can be helpful in the differentiation of basal cell hyperplasia from adenocarcinoma. Basal cell hyper-

Fig. 9-6. Basal cell hyperplasia. This photomicrograph illustrates basaloid cells forming solid nests. A few nests show central lumens (right upper corner).

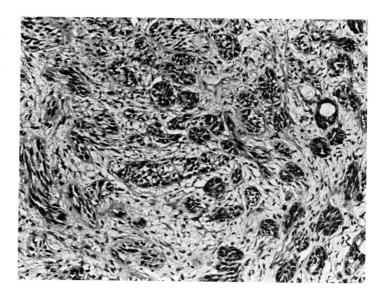

plasia stains strongly with 34βE11 antibody, but reactivity is weak or absent for PAP or PSA[107] (Fig. 9-7A). The latter immunostaining, however, may be seen in the cells lining the inner lumina (Fig. 9-7B). In contrast, adenocarcinoma stains strongly for the prostate-specific markers but not with the 34βE11 antikeratin antibody. Adenoid cystic carcinoma of the prostate and adenoid basal tumor typically react with 34βE11 antikeratin antibody. Based on this keratin immunoreactive staining pattern, it has been suggested that these tumors, as well as basal cell hyperplasia, are derived from true basal cells of the normal prostate.[107]

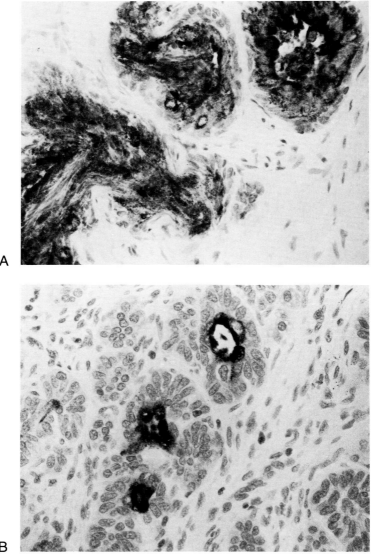

Fig. 9-7. (A) High-molecular-weight keratin (903) immunostaining of basal cell hyperplasia. There is diffuse, intense staining of basaloid cells. **(B)** Immunoperoxidase preparation showing PAP immunostaining of luminal lining cells.

CLEAR CELL CRIBRIFORM HYPERPLASIA OF
PROSTATE

This is a rare proliferative process that may be confused with carcinoma of the prostate owing to its cribriform pattern.[108, 109] It consists of a complex intra-acinar papillary-cribriform proliferation of clear cells that show no nuclear atypia. Nucleoli are not present in the majority of the cases, but when present, are small and inconspicuous (Fig. 9-8A). The cytoplasmic borders are well delineated, and immunostaining with the 34βE11 antikeratin antibody demonstrates the presence of the basal cell layer, supporting the benign nature of this lesion (Fig. 9-8B).

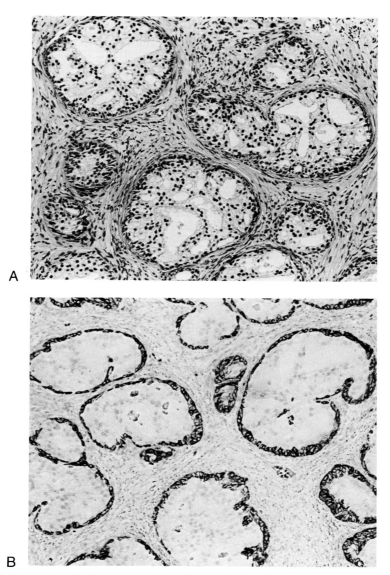

Fig. 9-8. **(A)** Clear cell cribriform hyperplasia. The acini are involved by complex papillary-cribriform proliferation. **(B)** The intact basal cell layer is demonstrated with 903 antikeratin antibody.

SCLEROSING ADENOSIS

Sclerosing adenosis of the prostate is a recently described lesion that has some morphologic similarities to sclerosing adenosis of the breast.[110, 111] It simulates carcinoma of the prostate and adenomatoid tumor.[112, 113] Histologically, the lesion is characterized by numerous, small, irregular, and distorted glandular structures embedded in a cellular stroma. The acini are generally round to oval, and some are elongated with a branching configuration. Because of the small glandular proliferation, this lesion may be confused with well-differentiated adenocarcinoma. Although sclerosing adenosis is a small glandular proliferation, the presence of irregular sized and shaped acini with a basal cell layer and the lack of prominent nucleoli and pleomorphism indicate the benign nature of the lesion. Additionally, the fibromuscular stroma surrounding the glands is more cellular than that seen in cases of well-differentiated adenocarcinoma. Immunostaining with 34βE11 antikeratin antibody demonstrates the presence of the basal cell layer. The stromal cells are also positive for keratin, S-100 protein, and smooth muscle actin, indicating myoepithelial differentiation.

PROSTATIC INTRAEPITHELIAL NEOPLASIA

Prostatic intraepithelial neoplasia (PIN), or intraductal dysplasia, is considered a precursor for invasive carcinoma. The highest grade of PIN is considered carcinoma in situ.[114-116] Immunocytochemical studies using 34βE11 antikeratin antibody demonstrated that PIN with early invasion is characterized by disruption of the normal basal layer of the prostatic acini.

ATYPICAL ADENOMATOUS HYPERPLASIA

Atypical adenomatous hyperplasia (AAH) is another premalignant lesion that, although less frequent than PIN, has also been associated with carcinoma of the prostate. AAH and carcinoma of the prostate are both characterized by a microglandular proliferation with loss of the basal cell layer[114, 115] (Fig. 9-9). Because of these similarities in the immunostaining patterns, the differential diagnosis of these two lesions is based on cytologic criteria.

PROSTATIC SARCOMAS

Sarcoma of the prostate is an unusual condition comprising less than 0.1 percent of prostatic malignant diseases.[117] Most of the sarcomas in the prostate are leiomyosarcomas or rhabdomyosarcomas.[118-122]

A large number of markers have been used for the diagnosis of rhabdomyosarcoma, including myoglobin, β-enolase, titin, creatinine phosphokinase-MM, creatinine phosphokinase-BB, protein-Z, desmin, fast and slow myosins, and fetal heavy-chain myosin; only a few of these markers have proved to be specific for skeletal muscle differentiation.[123-125] Antibodies to muscle antigens that are most commonly used in the diagnosis of rhabdomyosarcoma include myoglobin, desmin, muscle actins, and sarcomeric myosins.[124, 126, 127]

Antibodies to myoglobin, although skeletal muscle specific, are not very helpful because they are reactive only with well-differentiated tumors, which usually do not pose much diagnostic difficulty. Even in such cases, staining is limited to only scattered cells.

Desmin is an intermediate filament having a molecular weight of 50 to 55 kDa that is found in smooth, cardiac, and skeletal muscle cells. In spite of its lack of specificity for skeletal muscle cells, antibodies to desmin are extremely helpful in the diagnosis of rhabdomyosarcoma, particularly in those cases in which smooth muscle tumors are not in the differential diagnosis. In our experience, as well as that of others,[128, 129] almost all rhabdomyosarcomas, regardless of their degree of differentiation, react for desmin.

Actin is a contractile cytoskeletal protein that is widely distributed in all tissue cells. To date, six different actin isotypes, based on differences

Fig. 9-9. Keratin immunostaining shows complete absence of basal cell layer in invasive adenocarcinoma, while surrounding dysplastic acini still retain the basal layer.

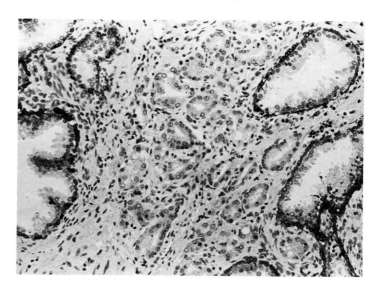

in isoelectric point and amino acid sequence, have been described in vertebrates.[130] Among these isoforms, skeletal muscle α-, smooth muscle α-, cardiac α-, and smooth muscle γ-actin are known to be expressed exclusively in muscle cells. We have found that the recently developed monoclonal antibody to muscle-specific actin (HHF35) stains most leiomyosarcomas, regardless of their location or degree of differentiation. HHF35 monoclonal antibody recognizes α-actin from skeletal and cardiac muscle tissues, as well as α- and γ-actin from smooth muscle tissue, but not the nonmuscle β-actin.[131, 132] Because of its strong reaction in formalin-fixed, paraffin-embedded tissue, this antibody can be extremely helpful in the diagnosis of all types of muscle-derived neoplasms, especially leiomyosarcomas, which react more often with HHF35 monoclonal antibody than with those directed against desmin.

Adult sarcomeric myosins are specific constituents of skeletal and cardiac muscle that are chemically and antigenically different from myosins of smooth muscle origin. These proteins are not always present in rhabdomyosarcomas and, as a result, they are infrequently observed in poorly differentiated tumor cells.[124, 126] Fetal heavy-chain myosin, a contractile skeletal protein absent in adult skeletal muscle fiber, is specific for rhabdomyosarcoma. Also, antibodies to this oncofetal antigen stain rhabdomyoblasts as well as morphologically immature myosarcoma cells.[124] Although antibodies to sarcomeric myosins react in formalin-fixed, paraffin-embedded tissues, they may require frozen or specially fixed tissue specimens to produce optimal results.

Vascular tumors of the prostate are rare; however, cases of angiosarcomas have been reported.[133] Actin, myosin, vimentin, and blood group antigens have been demonstrated in vascular tumors, but they are not specific for endothelial cells. Factor VIII-related antigen (FVIII:RAg) is elaborated exclusively by megakaryocytes and endothelial cells, but is not always present in angiosarcoma.[134, 135] *Ulex europaeus* agglutinin I (UEAI) is a lectin that can be used to evaluate the H antigen that corresponds to the blood group O. It has proved to be a powerful marker for all types of endothelial cells, regardless of the patient's blood group, and will stain angiosarcomas that do not display immunoreactivity for FVIII:RAg.[135]

In addition to aiding in the diagnosis of vascular tumors, immunocytochemical markers for endothelial cells and components of the basement membrane have also been reported to be helpful in establishing the diagnosis of lymphovascular invasion.[136] In our experience, the use of basement membrane markers such as laminin and collagen IV is limited by the need for frozen sections and special fixation procedures in order to obtain optimal results. Although some investigators have indicated that FVIII:RAg can be a useful marker for lymphovascular invasion, the value of antibodies to this substance is limited by the fact that not all endothelial cells appear to express this marker.[135] In our experience, UEAI is the only marker with practical value in the diagnosis of lymphovascular invasion.

Primary and secondary involvement of the prostate by lymphomas is uncommon.[137-140] Recently, a variety of antibodies that can mark lymphocytes on routinely processed specimens have been developed. These include various murine monoclonal antibodies that react broadly with leukocyte-common antigen (LCA). LCA constitutes a group of four related glycoproteins (molecular weights of 185-, 200-, 215-, and 230 kDa) that are present on the cell membrane of a variety of bone marrow-derived cells, such as granulocytes, thymocytes, macrophages/monocytes, and immature erythroid cells. Since the molecular weight of the glycoproteins that define LCA closely average 200 kDa, the generic term *anti-T200* is frequently used to refer to these antibodies.[141, 142]

MISCELLANEOUS RARE NEOPLASMS

Primary melanomas of the prostate have rarely been reported.[143] Since amelanotic melanomas can be confused with other poorly differentiated neoplasms, immunohistochemical studies can be very helpful in establishing the differential diagnosis. S-100 protein, an acidic protein of unknown function that was first detected in nervous tissue, has proven to be useful in the diagnosis of melanoma.[144, 145] Unfortunately, because it is not a melanocyte-specific marker, positive immunostaining cannot be considered as unequivocally diagnostic of melanoma. A variety of other nonmelanocytic neoplasms, such as neural tumors, certain types of histiocyte-derived neoplasms, and a variety of carcinomas and sarcomas, may contain this substance.[146-148] The recently developed HMB-45 monoclonal antibody has been reported to immunoreact with melanomas in formalin-fixed, paraffin-embedded tissues.[146, 149, 150] In our experience, HMB-45, although less sensitive for melanoma than S-100, is a highly specific marker for this tumor and, when used in conjunction with S-100 or incorporated into a panel of cell markers such as keratin and LCA, makes the diagnosis of melanoma much more accurate.

Rare cases of endodermal sinus (yolk sac) tumor originating in the prostate have been reported.[151-153] Demonstration of α-fetoprotein within tumor cells can be helpful in establishing the diagnosis.

METASTATIC NEOPLASMS

Metastatic neoplasms to the prostate are uncommon and, when they occur, are usually due to direct invasion from carcinoma originating in the bladder or rectum. Clinical information, together with negative staining for PSA and PAP, allows separation of prostatic adenocarcinoma and carcinoma originating in the bladder. Immunoreactivity for CEA, together with negative immunostaining for PSA and PAP, permits differentiation of tumors originating in the rectum and mucin producing or signet ring cell prostatic adenocarcinoma. The prostate can also be involved by metastases from a distant organ. The most commonly recorded tumors metastatic to the prostate are malignant melanoma and carcinoma of the lung.[154] Immunohistochemical studies using antibodies against PSA, PAP, CEA and melanoma markers can be helpful in establishing the diagnosis.

ONCOGENES

New techniques in molecular biology, particularly in the area of recombinant DNA, have created a revolution in the way cancer can be studied. Refined resolution of genetic structure, organization, and expression has led to the identification of specific molecular changes in cells that resulted in cancer development. Some of these alterations may be secondary, but others may be the basis for the evolution of a normal cell to a malignant one. The typical examples are the oncogenes, which are often found in normal cells and are associated with normal cellular functions. On the other hand, oncogenes that are homologous to transforming genes of RNA tumor viruses are also known to play critical roles in cancer cells.

By definition, oncogenes are genes that cause cancer. They represent altered versions of a group of normal genes that exist in every cell. The normal genes are known as *proto-onco-genes,* of which there are approximately 30 in the cellular genome and an additional 10 or more in the genome of tumor viruses, and that are encoding proteins required for the assembly of normal cellular structural framework and for normal growth and development. When these proto-oncogenes are altered by mutation, site-specific translocation, or faulty initiation-transcription, new homologous proteins may be produced at a suboptimal concentration or at an inappropriate time in the cell cycle. These changes have been shown to confer transforming properties leading to neoplasia; these genes are then referred to as *oncogenes.*

The proto-oncogenes can be grouped according to their function or location in the cell: growth factors, growth factor receptors, nuclear proteins, and membrane proteins. Changes activating normal proto-oncogenes to transforming oncogenes could occur at the DNA, RNA, or protein level. Theoretically, these changes should be easily amenable to molecular, biochemical, and immunologic manipulations. For example, when cellular proteins are structurally altered during oncogenesis, the modified proteins in cancer cells can be detected by immunologic techniques utilizing monoclonal antibody generated against the modified cellular proteins. Experiments are in progress in many laboratories to investigate further uses of DNA and antibody probes for detection of these differences between

normal and neoplastic tissue. Qualitative and quantitative alterations in oncogene-related sequences and their translational protein products in normal and neoplastic cells may provide diagnostically useful information. Oncogenes and their products may serve as useful tumor markers and improve our capabilities for diagnosing cancer.

Although studies are in progress to determine how frequently oncogenes are activated in prostatic cancer and whether activation is related to tumor progression, thus far, few oncogene studies have been reported in the field of prostatic cancer. Rijnders et al.[155] studied oncogene expression in human prostatic carcinoma cell lines and reported that transcripts of H-*ras* and *myc* were consistently found in all cell lines. Further experiments showed that *fos* and H-*ras* were decreased, but *myc* expression was not changed, by withdrawal of androgen. Therefore, the expressions of these oncogenes may be related to prostatic tumor cell growth, and some oncogenes appeared to be androgen regulated in vitro. Further studies indicated high expression of c-*myc* proto-oncogene in patients with adenocarcinoma, especially those with poorly differentiated adenocarcinoma.[156] A study by Viola et al.[157] with *ras* oncogene revealed that the *ras* p21 product was not found in benign or hyperplastic prostates, but only in prostatic carcinoma, especially in high-grade carcinoma (grade III/III).

They suggested that *ras* p21 antigen in prostate adenocarcinoma correlated strongly with nuclear anaplasia, and suggested that oncogene p21 may represent a biologically relevant tumor marker. However, this finding has not been supported by other experiments,[158, 159] in which the expression of p21 was unchanged from normal in hyperplastic prostates and in prostatic carcinoma. The different results between Viola et al.[157] and others[158, 159] could be due to different experimental procedures employed. Furthermore, this discrepancy may be due to different human tissue specimens used. It is conceivable that the human specimens employed in these studies may differ in the expression of other oncogenes, which can be detected by accompanying RNA in situ hybridization studies. Thompson and Land[160] have recently induced hyperplastic and cancerous prostatic growth in mouse prostates by transfection of the fetal urogenital sinuses with *ras* and *myc* oncogenes.

A number of growth factors have also been implicated in the pathogenesis of benign prostatic hyperplasia and prostatic cancer.[161] Immunohistochemistry of oncogene-associated growth factors has been underutilized. If used appropriately, it potentially can provide insight into the biology of prostate cells and be an adjunct to conventional histology.[161] The number of antibodies available against oncogene protein products is far less than the molecular probes that are available. Preliminary studies using antibodies for the characterizations of oncogene protein expression on human tissues have, nevertheless, been initiated. Antibodies specific for *ras* p21 proteins have been the most extensively used thus far. Hand et al.,[162] using monoclonal antibodies that they developed, found that *ras* protein expression was high in human mammary and colon carcinomas, and that the extent of antibody labeling could be used to distinguish benign from malignant colonic disease.[162, 163]

The definitive role of oncogenes in human cancer development remains uncertain. It is unlikely that any single oncogene is capable of complete cellular transformation. Rather, combinations of oncogene activations are probably responsible for neoplastic development, in accord with the well-known initiation-promotion concept of carcinogenesis. Future clinical applications of oncogenes include tumor diagnosis, tumor prognosis, and responsiveness to therapy. Our understanding of oncogene expression is still in its infancy. It is important to standardize tissue processing, methodology, and reagent usage with cross-validation of technology for exploring oncogenes.

REFERENCES

1. Mackay, B, Ordóñez NG: Role of the pathologist in the evaluation of poorly differentiated tumors and metastatic tumors of unknown origin. p. 3. In Greco FA, Oldham PK (eds): Tumors of Unknown Origin and Poorly Differentiated Neoplasms. Grune & Stratton, Orlando, FL, 1986

2. Gittes RF: Serum acid phosphatase and screening for carcinoma of the prostate. New Engl J Med 309:852, 1983

3. Stamey TA, Yang N, Hay AR, et al: Prostate specific antigen as a serum marker for adenocarcinoma of the prostate. New Engl J Med 317:909, 1987

4. Friedman NW, Steffen SJ, Lobeck H, et al: Immunohistochemical demonstration of tumor-associated antigens in prostatic carcinoma of various histologic differentiation. Eur Urol 11:52, 1985

5. Ford TF, Butchner DN, Masters JRW, Parkinson MC: Immunohistochemical localization of prostatic specific antigen: specificity and application to clinical practice. Br J Urol 57:50, 1985

6. Tell DT, Khoury JM, Taylor G: Atypical metastasis from prostate cancer. JAMA 253:3574, 1985

7. Baker WC, Mayers FJ, Melrite RWD: Prostatic-specific antigen: clinical experience using immunoperoxidase staining techniques in patients with metastatic prostate cancer. J Surg Oncol 37:165, 1988

8. Katz RL, Raval P, Brooks TE, Ordóñez NG: Role of immunocytochemistry in diagnosis of prostatic neoplasia by fine needle aspiration biopsy. Diagn Cytopathol 1:28, 1985

9. Travis WD, Wold LE: Immunoperoxidase staining of fine needle aspiration specimens previously stained by the Papanicolaou technique. Acta Cytol 31:517, 1987

10. Flisch CW, Toccanier M-F, Kapanci Y: Immunohistochemical detection of prostatic acid phosphatase in 110 cases of bone metastases. p. 169. In Fenoglio-Preiser CM, Wolff M, Rilke F (eds): Progress In Surgical Pathology. Volume VIII. MacMillan, New York, 1988

11. Nadji M, Tabei SZ, Castro A, et al: Prostatic specific antigen: an immunohistologic marker for prostatic neoplasms. Cancer 48:1299, 1981

12. Bentz MS, Cohen C, Demers LM, Budgeon LR: Immunohistochemical demonstration of prostatic origin of metastases. Urology 19:584, 1982

13. Mukai M, Yoshimura S, Anzai M: Effect of decalcification on immunoperoxidase staining. Am J Surg Pathol 10:413, 1986

14. Choe BK, Pontes JE, McDonald J, Rose NR: Purification and characterization of human prostatic acid phosphatase. Preparative Biochem 8:73, 1973
15. Liu MF, Lee CL, Wojcieszyn FW, et al: Fundamental biochemical and immunological aspects of prostatic acid phosphatase. Prostate 1:415, 1980
16. Lange PH, Winfield HN: Biological markers in urologic cancer. Cancer 60:464, 1987
17. Chu TM, Wang MC, Scott WW, et al: Immunochemical detection of serum prostatic acid phosphatase. Methodology and clinical evaluation. Invest Urol 15:319, 1978
18. Foti G, Fennimore-Cooper JF, Hershman H, Malvaez RR: Detection of prostatic cancer by solid phase radioimmunoassay of serum prostatic acid phosphatase. New Engl J Med 279:1357, 1977
19. Vihko P, Lukkarinen O, Konturri M, Vihko RR: Effectiveness of radioimmunoassay of human prostate-specific phosphatase in the diagnosis and follow-up of therapy in prostatic carcinoma. Cancer Res 41:1180, 1981
20. Loor R, Wang MC, Valenzuela L, Chu TM: Expression of prostatic acid phosphatase in human prostate cancer. Cancer Lett 14:63, 1981
21. Li CY, Lam WK, Yam LT: Immunohistochemical diagnosis of prostatic cancer with metastasis. Cancer 46:706, 1980
22. Keshgegian AA, Kline TS: Immunoperoxidase demonstration of prostate acid phosphatase in aspiration biopsy cytology (ABC). Am J Clin Pathol 82:586, 1984
23. Jobsis AC, deVries GP, Meijer AEFM, Ploem JS: The immunohistochemical detection of prostate acid phosphatase, its possibilities and limitations in tumor histochemistry. Histochem J 13:961, 1981
24. Limas C: Monoclonal and polyclonal antibodies to prostatic acid phosphatase and prostatic-specific antigen. p. 383. In Wick MR, Siegal GP (eds): Monoclonal Antibodies in Diagnostic Immunohistochemistry. Marcel Dekker, New York, 1988
25. Yam LT, Lackila AJ, Lam WKW, Li CY: Immunohistochemistry of prostatic acid phosphatase. Prostate 2:97, 1981
26. Cohen C, Bentz MS, Budgeon LR: Prostatic acid phosphatase in carcinoid and islet cell tumors. Arch Pathol Lab Med 107:277, 1983
27. Epstein JI, Kuhajda FP, Lieberman PH: Prostate-specific acid phosphatase immunoreactivity in adenocarcinomas of the urinary bladder. Hum Pathol 17:939, 1986
28. Schevchuk MM, Romas NA, Ng PY, et al: Acid phosphatase localization in prostatic carcinoma. Cancer 52:1642, 1983
29. Wang MC, Valenzuela LA, Murphy GP, Chu TM: Purification of human prostate specific antigen. Invest Urol 17:159, 1979
30. Graves HCB, Sensabaugh GF, Blacke ET: Postcoital detection of a male-specific serum protein: application to the investigation of rape. New Engl J Med 312:338, 1985
31. Warhol MJ, Longtine JA: The ultrastructural localization of prostatic specific antigen and prostatic acid phosphatase in hyperplastic and neoplastic prostates. J Urol 134:607, 1985
32. Sinha AA, Wilson MJ, Gleason DF: Immunoelectron microscopic localization of prostatic-specific antigen in human prostate by the protein A-gold complex. Cancer 60:1288, 1987
33. Killian CS, Emrich LJ, Vargas FP, et al: Relative reliability of five serially measured markers for prognosis of progression in prostate cancer. J Natl Cancer Inst 76:179, 1986
34. Seamonds B, Yang N, Anderson K, et al: Evaluation of prostate-specific and prostatic acid phosphatase in prostate carcinomas. Urology 28:472, 1986
35. Svanholm H: Evaluation of commercial immunoperoxidase kits for prostatic specific antigen and prostatic specific acid phosphatase. Acta Pathol Microbiol Immunol Scand [A] 94:7, 1986
36. Stein BS, Peterson RO, Vangore S, Kendall AR: Immunoperoxidase localization of prostatic specific antigen. Am J Surg Pathol 2:553, 1982
37. Epstein JI, Eggleston TC: Immunohistochemical localization of prostatic specific acid phosphatase and prostate-specific antigen in stage A$_2$ adenocarcinoma of the prostate. Human Pathol 15:853, 1984
38. Ellis DW, Leffers S, Davies JS, Ng ABP: Multiple immunoperoxidase markers in benign hyperplasia and adenocarcinoma of the prostate. Am J Clin Pathol 81:279, 1984
39. Allhoff EF, Proppe KH, Chapman CM, et al: Evaluation of prostatic acid phosphatase and prostatic specific antigen in identification of prostate cancer. J Urol 129:315, 1983
40. Feiner HD, Gonzalez R: Carcinoma of the prostate with atypical immunohistological features: clinical and histologic correlates. Am J Surg Pathol 10:765, 1986

41. Melicow MM, Pachter MR: Endometrial carcinoma of prostatic utricle (uterus masculinus). Cancer 20:1715, 1967

42. Melicow MM, Tannenbaum M: Endometrial carcinoma of uterus masculinus (prostatic utricle): report of 6 cases. J Urol 106:892, 1971

43. Langman J: Medical Embryology. 4th ed. Williams & Wilkins, Baltimore, 1981, p. 251

44. McNeal JE: The prostate and prostatic urethra: a morphologic synthesis. J Urol 107:1008, 1972

45. Arey LB: Developmental Anatomy: A Textbook and Laboratory Manual of Embryology. 7th ed. WB Saunders, Philadelphia, 1974, p. 328

46. Glenister TW: The development of the utricle and of the so-called middle or median lobe of the human prostate. J Anat 96:443, 1962

47. Hamilton WJ, Mossman HW: Hamilton, Boyd and Mossman's Human Embryology. 4th ed. Williams & Wilkins, London, 1972, p. 411

48. Ro JY, Ayala AG, Wishnow KI, Ordóñez NG: Prostatic duct adenocarcinoma with endometrioid features: immunohistochemical and electron microscopic study. Semin Diagn Pathol 5:301, 1988

49. Bostwick DG, Kindrachuk RW, Rouse RV: Prostatic adenocarcinoma with endometrioid features: clinical, pathologic, and ultrastructural findings. Am J Surg Pathol 9:595, 1985

50. Epstein JI, Woodruff JM: Adenocarcinoma of the prostate with endometrioid features: a light microscopic and immunohistochemical study of ten cases. Cancer 57:111, 1986

51. Mendelsohn G: Signet-cell simulating microfollicular adenoma of the thyroid. Am J Surg Pathol 8:705, 1984

52. Schroder S, Bocker W: Signet-ring-cell thyroid tumors. Follicle cell tumors with arrest of folliculogenesis. Am J Surg Pathol 9:619, 1985

53. Kim H, Dorfman RF, Rappaport H: Signet-ring-cell lymphoma: a rare morphologic and functional expression of nodular (follicular) lymphoma. Am J Surg Pathol 2:119, 1978

54. Weiss LM, Wood GS, Dorfman RF: T-cell signet-ring-cell lymphoma: A histologic, ultrastructural, and immunohistochemical study of two cases. Am J Surg Pathol 9:273, 1985

55. Shebani K, Battifora H: Signet-ring cell melanoma. A rare morphologic variant of malignant melanoma. Am J Surg Pathol 12:28, 1988

56. Rubinstein LJ: Tumors of the central nervous system. p. 85. In Atlas of Tumor Pathology.

2nd series, Fascicle 6. Armed Forces Institute of Pathology, Bethesda, 1972

57. Enzinger FM, Weiss SW: Epithelioid smooth muscle tumors. p. 316. In Enzinger FM, Weiss SW (eds): Soft Tissue Tumors. CV Mosby, St. Louis, 1983

58. Remmele W, Weber A, Harding P: Primary signet-ring carcinoma of the prostate. Hum Pathol 19:478, 1988

59. Ro JY, el-Naggar A, Ayala AG, et al: Signet ring cell carcinoma of the prostate: electron microscopy and immunohistochemical studies of eight cases. Am J Surg Pathol 12:453, 1988

60. Ro JY, Grignon DJ, Troncoso P, Ayala AG: Mucin in prostatic adenocarcinoma. Semin Diag Pathol 5:273, 1988

61. Alguail-Garcia A: Artifactural changes mimicking signet-ring-cell carcinoma of transurethral prostatectomy specimens. Am J Surg Pathol 10:795, 1986

62. Schned AR: Artifactural signet-ring cells. Am J Surg Pathol 11:736, 1987

63. Patel RC, Dias R, Fernandes M, Lavengood RW: Adenocarcinoma of the prostate. Mucin secreting. NY State J Med 81:936, 1981

64. Franks LM, O'Shea JD, Thomson AER: Mucin in the prostate: a histochemical study in normal glands, latent, clinical, and colloid cancers. Cancer 17:983, 1964

65. Cricco RP, Kassis J: Mucinous adenocarcinoma of prostate. Urology 14:276, 1979

66. Sika JV, Buckley JJ: Mucus-forming adenocarcinoma of prostate. Cancer 17:949, 1964

67. Odom DG, Donatucci CF, Deshon GE: Mucinous adenocarcinoma of the prostate. Human Pathol 17:863, 1986

68. Hsueh Y, Tsung SH: Prostatic mucinous adenocarcinoma. Urology 24:626, 1984

69. Ordóñez NG, Ayala AG, von Eschenback AC, et al: Immunoperoxidase localization of prostatic acid phosphatase in carcinoma of the prostate with sarcomatoid changes. Urology 19:210, 1982

70. Shannon RL, Grignon DJ, Ro JY, et al: Sarcomatoid carcinoma of the prostate. Lab Invest 60:87A, 1989

71. Ro JY, Ayala AG, Wishnow KI, Ordóñez NG: Sarcomatoid bladder carcinomas: clinicopathologic and immunohistochemical study of 44 cases. Surg Pathol 1:359, 1988

72. Turbat-Herrera EA, Herrera GA, Gore I, et al: Neuroendocrine differentiation in prostatic

carcinomas. A retrospective autopsy study. Arch Pathol Lab Med 112:1100, 1988

73. Vinores SA, Bonnin JM, Rubinstein LJ, Marangos PJ: Immunohistochemical demonstration of neuron-specific enolase in neoplasms of the CNS and other tumors. Arch Pathol Lab Med 108:536, 1984

74. Battifora H, Silva EG: The use of antikeratin antibodies in the immunohistochemical distinction between neuroendocrine (Merkel cell) carcinoma of the skin, lymphoma, and oat cell carcinoma. Cancer 58:1040, 1986

75. Tsokis M, Linnoila RI, Chandra RS, Triche TJ: Neuron-specific enolase in the diagnosis of neuroblastoma and other small round-cell tumors in children. Hum Pathol 15:575, 1984

76. Ro JY, Tetu B, Ayala Ag, Ordóñez NG: Small cell carcinomas of the prostate. Part II. Immunohistochemical and electron microscopic studies of 18 cases. Cancer 59:977, 1987

77. Haimoto H, Takashi M, Koshikawa T, et al: Enolase enzymes in renal tubules and renal cell carcinoma. Am J Pathol 124:488, 1986

78. Leader M, Collins M, Patel J, Henry K: Anti-neuron specific enolase staining reactions in sarcomas and carcinomas: Its lack of neuroendocrine specificity. J Clin Pathol 39:1186, 1986

79. Kizmits R, Schernthaner G, Krisch K: Serum neuron-specific enolase: a marker for response to therapy in seminoma. Cancer 60:1017, 1987

80. Nemeth J, Galian A, Mikol J, et al: Neuron-specific enolase and malignant lymphomas (23 cases). Virchows Arch [A] 412:89, 1987

81. Hagan C, Schmidt KW, Fischer-Colbrie R, Winkley H: Chromogranin A, B, and C in human adrenal medulla and endocrine tissues. Lab Invest 55:405, 1986

82. Wilson BS, Lloyd RV: Detection of chromogranin in neuroendocrine cells with a monoclonal antibody. Am J Pathol 115:458, 1984

83. Lloyd RV, Mervak T, Schmidt K, et al: Immunohistochemical detection of chromogranin and neuron-specific enolase in pancreatic endocrine neoplasms. Am J Surg Pathol 8:607, 1984

84. Lloyd RV, Shapira B, Sisson JC, et al: Immunohistochemical study of pheochromocytomas. Arch Pathol Lab Med 108:541, 1984

85. Wiedenmann B, Franke WW, Kuhn C, et al: Synaptophysin: a marker protein for neuroendocrine cells and neoplasms. Proc Natl Acad Sci USA 83:3500, 1986

86. Gould VE, Wiedenmann B, Lee I, et al: Synaptophysin expression in neuroendocrine neoplasms as determined by immunocytochemistry. Am J Pathol 126:243, 1987

87. Abo T, Balch CM: A differentiation antigen of human NK and K cells identified by a monoclonal antibody (HNK-1). J Immunol 127:1024, 1981

88. Wahab ZA, Wright GL Jr: Monoclonal antibody (anti-Leu 7) directed against natural killer cells reacts with normal, benign and malignant prostate tissues. Int J Cancer 36:677, 1985

89. Rusthoven JJ, Robinson JB, Kolin A, Pinkerton PH: The natural-killer-cell-associated HNK-1 (Leu-7) antibody reacts with hypertrophic and malignant prostatic epithelium. Cancer 56:289, 1985

90. May EE, Perentes E: Anti-Leu 7 immunoreactivity with human tumours: its value in the diagnosis of prostatic adenocarcinoma. Histopathology 11:295, 1987

91. Bunn PA, Linnoila I, Minna JD, et al: Small cell lung cancer, endocrine cells of the fetal bronchus and other neuroendocrine cells express leu-7 antigenic determinant present in natural killer cells. Blood 65:764, 1985

92. Tischler AS, Mobtaker H, Mann K, et al: Anti-lymphocytes antibody leu-7 (HNK-1) recognizes a constituent of neuroendocrine granule matrix. J Histochem Cytochem 34:1213, 1986

93. Osborne M, Weber K: Tumor diagnosis by intermediate filament typing: a novel tool for surgical pathology. Lab Invest 48:372, 1983

94. Tischler AS, Mobtaker H, Mann K, et al: Anti-lymphocyte antibody Leu-7 (HNK-1) recognizes a constitutent of neuroendocrine granule matrix. J Histochem Cytochem 34:1213, 1986

95. Lee V, Wu HL, Schlaepfer WW: Monoclonal antibodies recognize individual neurofilament triplet proteins. Proc Natl Acad Sci USA 79:6089, 1982

96. Mukai M, Torikata C, Iri H, et al: Expression of neurofilament triplet proteins in human neural tumors: an immunohistochemical study of paraganglioma, ganglioneuroma, ganglioneuroblastoma, and neuroblastoma. Am J Pathol 122:28, 1986

97. Sibley RK, Dahl D: Primary neuroendocrine (Merkel cell?) carcinoma of the skin. II. An immunocytochemical study of 21 cases. Am J Surg Pathol 9:109, 1985

98. Gould VE, Lee I, Moll R, et al: Synaptophysin

expression in neuroendocrine neoplasms determined by immunocytochemistry. Lab Invest 54:23A, 1986

99. di Sant'Agnese PA, de Mesy Jensen KL: Neuroendocrine differentiation in prostatic carcinoma. Hum Pathol 18:849, 1987

100. Wenk RE, Bhagavan BW, Levy R, et al: Ectopic ACTH, prostatic oat cell carcinoma and marked hypernatremia. Cancer 40:773, 1977

101. Vuitch MF, Mendelsohn G: Relationship of ectopic ACTH production to tumor differentiation: a morphologic and immunohistochemical study of prostatic carcinoma with Cushing's syndrome. Cancer 47:396, 1981

102. Moll R, Franke WW, Schiller DL, et al: The catalog of human cytokeratins: patterns of expression in normal epithelia, tumors, and culture cells. Cell 31:11, 1982

103. Cooper D, Schermer A, Tung-Tien S: Classification of human epithelia and their neoplasms using monoclonal antibodies to keratins: strategies, applications, and limitations. Lab Invest 52:243, 1985

104. Achtstatter T, Moll R, Moore B, Franke WW: Gel electrophoresis studies of prostate cytokeratins. J Histochem Cytochem 33:415, 1985

105. Ordóñez NG, Manning JT, Brooks T: Effect of pre-trypsinization on the immunostaining of formalin-fixed, paraffin-embedded tissues. Am J Surg Pathol 12:121, 1988

106. Brawer MK, Peehl DM, Stamey TA, Bostwick DG: Keratin immunoreactivity in the benign and neoplastic human prostate. Cancer Res 45:3663, 1985

107. Grignon DJ, Ro JY, Ordóñez NG, et al: Basal cell hyperplasia, adenoid basal cell tumor, and adenoid cystic carcinoma of the prostate gland: an immunohistochemical study. Human Pathol 19:1425, 1988

108. Ayala AG, Srigley JR, Ro JY, et al: Clear cell cribriform hyperplasia of prostate: report of 10 cases. Am J Surg Pathol 10:665, 1986

109. Gleason DF: Atypical hyperplasia, benign hyperplasia and well-differentiated adenocarcinoma of the prostate. Am J Surg Pathol 9(Suppl):53, 1985

110. Young RH, Clement PB: Sclerosing adenosis of the prostate. Arch Pathol Lab Med 111:363, 1987

111. Srigley JR: Small-acinar patterns in the prostate gland with emphasis on atypical adenomatous hyperplasia and small-acinar carcinoma. Semin Diagn Pathol 5:254, 1988

112. Sesterhenn IA, Mostofi FK, Davis CJ: Fibroepithelial nodules of the prostate simulating carcinoma. Lab Invest 58:83A, 1988

113. Chen KTK, Schiff JJ: Adenomatoid prostatic tumor. Urology 21:88, 1983

114. Bostwick DG, Brawer MK: Prostatic intra-epithelial neoplasia and early invasion in prostate cancer. Cancer 59:788, 1987

115. Bostwick DG: Premalignant lesions of the prostate. Semin Diagn Pathol 5:240, 1988

116. McNeal JE, Bostwick DG: Intraductal dysplasia: a premalignant lesion of the prostate. Hum Pathol 17:64, 1986

117. Mostofi FK, Price EB: Tumors of the male genital system. In Atlas of Tumor Pathology. 2nd series, Fascicle 8. Armed Forces Institute of Pathology, Washington, DC, 1973

118. Tannenbaum M: Sarcomas of the prostate gland. Urol 5:810, 1975

119. Narayana AS, Loening S, Weimar GW, Culp DA: Sarcoma of the bladder and prostate. J Urol 119:72, 1978

120. Rogers PCJ, Howard SS, Komp DM: Urogenital rhabdomyosarcomas in childhood. J Urol 115:738, 1976

121. Schmidt JD, Welch MJ: Sarcoma of the prostate. Cancer 37:1908, 1976

122. Tungekar MF, Al Adnani MS: Sarcomas of the bladder and prostate: the role of immunohistochemistry and ultrastructure in diagnosis. Eur Urol 12:180, 1986

123. Tsokos M: The role of immunocytochemistry in the diagnosis of rhabdomyosarcoma. Arch Pathol Lab Med 110:776, 1986

124. Ceccarelli C, Eusebi V, Bussolati G: Desmin and sarcomeric myosins in the diagnosis of rhabdomyosarcomas. p. 223. In DeLellis RA (ed): Advances in Immunohistochemistry. Raven Press, New York, 1988

125. Osborn M, Hill C, Altmannsberger M, Weber K: Monoclonal antibodies to titin in conjunction with antibodies to desmin separate rhabdomyosarcomas from other tumor types. Lab Invest 55:101, 1986

126. De Jong ASH, Van Raamsdonk W, Van Vark M, Voute PA, Albus-Lutter CE: Myosin and myoglobin as tumor markers in the diagnosis of rhabdomyosarcoma: a comparative study. Am J Surg Pathol 8:521, 1984

127. Schmidt RA, Cone R, Haas JE, Gown AM: Diagnosis of rhabdomyosarcomas with HHF35, a monoclonal antibody directed against muscle actins. Am J Pathol 131:19, 1988

128. Azumi N, Ben-Ezra J, Battifora H: Immuno-phenotypic diagnosis of leiomyosarcomas and rhabdomyosarcomas with monoclonal antibodies to muscle-specific actin and desmin in formalin-fixed tissue. Mod Pathol 1:469, 1988

129. Altmannsberger M, Weber K, Droste R, Osborn M: Desmin is a specific marker for rhabdomyosarcoma of human and rat origin. Am J Pathol 118:85, 1985

130. Vandekerckhove J, Weber K: At least six different actins are expressed in a higher mammal: an analysis based on the amino acid sequence of the amino-terminal tryptic peptide. J Mol Biol 126:783, 1978

131. Tsukada T, Tippens D, Gordon D, et al: HHF35, a muscle-actin-specific monoclonal antibody. I. Immunohistochemical and biochemical characterization. Am J Pathol 126:51, 1987

132. Tsukada T, McNutt MA, Ross R, Gown AM: HHF35, a muscle actin-specific monoclonal antibody. II. Reactivity in normal, reactive, and neoplastic human tissues. Am J Pathol 127:389, 1987

133. Tannenbaum M: Urologic Pathology: The Prostate. Lea & Febiger, Philadelphia, 1977

134. Guarda LA, Ordóñez NG, Smith JL, Hanssen G: Immunoperoxidase localization of factor VIII in angiosarcomas. Arch Pathol Lab Med 106:515, 1982

135. Ordóñez NG, Batsakis JG: Comparison of Ulex europaeus I lectin and factor VIII-related antigen in vascular lesions. Arch Pathol Lab Med 108:129, 1984

136. Ordóñez NG, Brooks T, Thompson S, Batsakis JG: Use of Ulex europaeus agglutinin I in the identification of blood vessel invasion in previously stained microscopic slides. Am J Surg Pathol 11:543, 1987

137. West WO: Primary lymphosarcoma of prostate bland. Arch Intern Med 109:469, 1962

138. Heaney JA, DeLellis RA, Rudders RA: Non-Hodgkin lymphoma arising in lower urinary tract. Urology 25:479, 1985

139. Fell P, O'Connor M, Smith JM: Primary lymphoma of the prostate presenting a bladder outflow obstruction. Urology 29:555, 1987

140. Ben-Ezra J, Sheibani K, Kendrick FE, et al: Angiotropic large cell lymphoma of the prostate gland: an immunohistochemical study. Hum Pathol 17:964, 1986

141. Pinkus GS: Leukocyte common antigen. p. 261. In DeLellis RA (ed): Advances in Immunohistochemistry. Raven Press, New York, 1988

142. Salter DM, Krajewski AS, Dewar AE: Immunohistochemical staining of non-Hodgkin's lymphoma with monoclonal antibodies specific for the leukocyte common antigen. J Pathol 146:345, 1985

143. Berry NE, Reese L: Malignant melanoma which had its first clinical manifestations in the prostate gland. J Urol 69:286, 1953

144. Nakajima T, Watanabe S, Sato Y, et al: Immunohistochemical demonstration of S100 protein in human malignant melanoma and pigmented nevi. Gann 72:335, 1981

145. Nakajima T, Watanabe S, Sato Y, et al: Immunohistochemical demonstration of S100 protein in malignant melanoma and pigmented nevus, and its diagnostic application. Cancer 50:912, 1982

146. Ordóñez NG, Xiaolong J, Hickey RC: Comparison of HMB-45 monoclonal antibody and S-100 protein in the immunohistochemical diagnosis of melanoma. Am J Clin Pathol 90:385, 1988

147. Têtu B, Ordóñez NG, Ayala AG, Mackay B: Chondrosarcoma with additional mesenchymal component (dedifferentiated chondrosarcoma). II. An immunohistochemical and electron microscopic study. Cancer 58:287, 1986

148. Drier JK, Swanson PE, Cherwitz DC, Wick MR: S-100 protein immunoreactivity in poorly differentiated carcinomas. Immunohistochemical comparison with malignant melanoma. Arch Pathol Lab Med 111:447, 1987

149. Gown AM, Vogel AM, Hoak D, et al: Monoclonal antibodies specific for melanocytic tumors distinguish subpopulation of melanocytes. Am J Pathol 123:195, 1986

150. Ordóñez NG, Sneige N, Hickey RC, Brooks TE: Use of monoclonal antibody HMB-45 in the cytologic diagnosis of melanomas. Acta Cytol 32:684, 1988

151. Benson RC, Segne JW, Cornay JA: Primary yolk sac (endodermal sinus) tumor of the prostate. Cancer 41:1395, 1978

152. Michel F, Gattengo B, Roland J, et al: Primary nonseminomatous germ cell tumor of the prostate. J Urol 135:595, 1986

153. Palma PD, Dante S, Guazzieri S, Sperandio P: Primary endodermal sinus tumor of the prostate. Report of a case. Prostate 12:255, 1988

154. Johnson DE, Chalbaud R, Ayala AG: Secondary tumors of the prostate. J Urol 112:507, 1974

155. Rijnders AWM, van der Korput JAGM, van

Steenbrugger GJ, et al: Expression of cellular oncogenes in human prostatic carcinoma cell lines. Biochem Biophys Res Comm 132:548, 1985

156. Heming WH, Hamel A, MacDonald R, et al: Expression of the *c-myc* protooncogene in human prostatic carcinoma and benign prostatic hyperplasia. Cancer Res 46:1535, 1986

157. Viola MV, Fromowitz F, Oravez S, et al: Expression of *ras* oncogenes p21 in prostate cancer. New Engl J Med 314:133, 1986

158. Varma VA, Austin GE, O'Connell AC: Antibodies to *ras* oncogenes p212 proteins lack immunohistochemical specificity for neoplastic epithelium in human prostate tissue. Arch Pathol Lab Med 113:16, 1989

159. Peehl DM, Wehner N, Stamey TA: Activated *Ki-ras* oncogene in human prostate adenocarcinoma. Prostate 10:281, 1987

160. Thompson TC, Land H, Southgate J, Kitchener G: Multi-stage carcinogenesis induced by *ras* and *myc* oncogenes in a reconstituted organ. Cell 56:917, 1989

161. Fowler JE, Lau JLT, Ghosh L, et al: Epidermal growth factor and prostatic carcinoma: an immunohistochemical study. J Urol 139:857, 1988

162. Hand PH, Thor A, Wunderlich D, et al: Monoclonal antibodies of predefined specificity detected activated *ras* gene expression in human mammary and colon carcinomas. Proc Natl Acad Sci USA 81:5227, 1984

163. Thor A, Hand PH, Wunderlich D, et al: Monoclonal antibodies define different *ras* gene expression in malignant and benign colonic disease. Nature 311:562, 1984

10

Aspiration Biopsy Cytology of the Prostate

John A. Maksem, Cirilo F. Galang, Paul W. Johenning,
Chanho H. Park, and Myron Tannenbaum

The prostate is commonly biopsied to diagnose carcinoma and to determine optimal treatment.[1] Transrectal aspiration biopsy is a useful method for examining prostate glands with (1) palpable discrete nodules; (2) induration; (3) fixation; (4) benign enlargement, especially prior to transurethral or suprapubic prostatectomy; (5) sonographic abnormalities suggestive of carcinoma; (6) elevated serum levels of prostate tumor markers such as prostatic acid phosphatase and prostate-specific antigen (PSA); (7) metastatic adenocarcinoma of unknown primary outside of the prostate in male patients; and (8) nonoperable prostatic carcinoma, in which an objective and reproducible method is desired to determine the effect of treatment on the primary tumor.[2] In this chapter, the diagnostic criteria for interpretation of aspiration biopsy of the prostate are presented.

COMPLICATIONS

Aspiration biopsy of the prostate gland is a relatively safe procedure. Infections are the most frequent complication, occurring in less than 2 percent of cases. Esposti et al.[3] related the experience at the Karolinska Institute with approximately 14,000 transrectal aspiration biopsies. In the first report of this series, appearing in 1966, these investigators noted no noteworthy complications in 1,430 biopsies. By 1968, over 3,000 cases had been reported, with a 0.4 percent incidence of complications, including epididymitis (two cases) transient hematuria (two

cases), hemospermia (three cases), and febrile reactions (five cases). Of 14,000 biopsies reported in 1975, there were four cases of *Escherichia coli* sepsis, one of which was fatal.

Patients at the Karolinska Institute referred from the Department of Rheumatology had the highest incidence of complications: of 42 biopsies from 32 patients with chronic polyarthritis, 7.2 percent had complications, significantly higher than the 1 percent complication rate observed in 508 biopsies from patients in the Department of Urology. Most of the patients from Rheumatology had been referred for aspiration biopsy to establish prostatitis as the cause of polyarthritis, and not with suspicion of carcinoma; similarly, four of five patients with complications from Urology had prostatitis.

Because of these complications associated with prostatitis, Esposti et al. ''. . . ceased to perform TAB (transrectal aspiration biopsy) of the prostate in order to reveal inflammatory reactions,'' although they noted that ''. . . a history of prostatitis is not in itself a contraindication to TAB of the prostate.'' Ten percent of their patients with a clinical diagnosis of prostatitis also had carcinoma on aspiration biopsy, similar to the 14.1 percent and 17.5 percent frequency reported by us in previous series.[2, 4, 5]

Several other reports have confirmed the low complication rate of aspiration biopsy.[1, 6, 7] Also, transrectal aspiration biopsy has been suggested as an alternative to transperineal core biopsy in the prevention of tumor seeding.[8] Furthermore, there have been no fistulae to adjacent organs or pulmonary emboli reported following aspiration biopsy, in contrast with large-bore cutting needle biopsies.

THE PRODUCTS OF ASPIRATION BIOPSY

Aspiration biopsy produces small sheets and clusters of cells, similar to core biopsy, but without the stromal component.[3] In aspirations, the epithelial component is amplified because all of the epithelium that is harvested is available for examination, not just a representative cross section. Aspiration biopsy cytology permits evaluation of cell-to-cell associations within epithelial cell aggregates (similar to tissue pattern) in addition to the evaluation of single-cell morphology. Sampling error is decreased by performing more than one collection from the prostate, and the greatest quantity of material is obtained by a sustained back-and-forth sawing motion of the aspiration needle during the biopsy. There may be difficulty in targeting small lesions or in extracting a satisfactory sample from an area of fibrosis or desmoplasia, even with an adequate sawing motion. Low suc-

tion pressure minimizes the amount of contamination by blood and tissue juices. Poor collections should be repeated, and multiple samples from a suspicious site should be collected to decrease the probability of inadequate sampling.

BENIGN EPITHELIUM

Cytologic preparations display the epithelial cells en face. In this arrangement, the cells of the prostatic epithelium lie in an orderly sheet-like pattern. Cell borders have a distinct honeycomb or chicken-wire configuration, especially at the apical intercellular zone[1, 2, 6, 7] (Fig. 10-1).

In hyperplastic epithelium, clusters of epithelial cells rise out of the plane of the epithelial sheet, forming "hills and valleys" and club-like aggregates on low-power examination (Figs. 10-2 and 10-3). In atrophy, epithelial cells are more cuboidal and cell boundaries are distinct, but without prominent apical scalloping of cytoplasm on the luminal surface. Hyperplasia and atrophy may both be present in the same microscopic field, a remarkable characteristic of the prostate.[9]

Nuclei are similar in all types of benign pros-

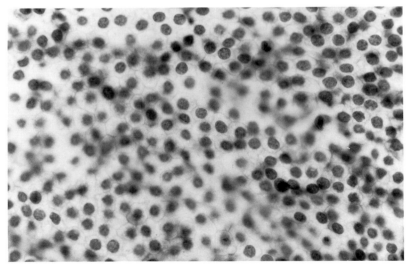

Fig. 10-1. The apicalmost portion of a benign epithelial sheet, in which the apical intercellular junction assumes a distinct honeycomb or chicken-wire configuration in the en face preparation.

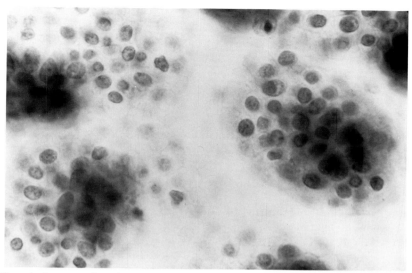

Fig. 10-2. The apicalmost portion of a hyperplastic epithelial sheet, in which only the hillock-like arrangement of epithelial cells are seen in the en face preparation.

tatic epithelium. Benign nuclei are evenly distributed, rather monotonous, unilayered, and round to oval (Fig. 10-4). The chromatin pattern is finely granular, and the nuclear size is comparable to that of an erythrocyte (approximately 7 μm in diameter). Nucleoli of benign epithelial cells are usually indistinct, except in occasional cases of epithelial hyperplasia, in which chromocenters or micronucleoli may be seen.[1, 2, 6, 7]

Basal cells are present in normal, atrophic, and hyperplastic epithelium, lying immediately below the epithelial cell layer (Fig. 10-5). Basal

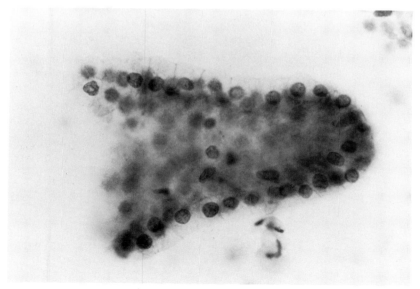

Fig. 10-3. A lateral view of a hyperplastic epithelial papilla presenting as a club-like structure. Note that the apical cell cytoplasm is well delineated along the external surface of the structure.

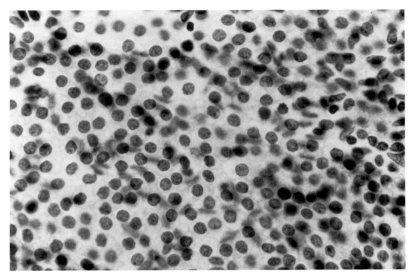

Fig. 10-4. The same benign epithelial sheet shown in Figure 10-1, but focused at the plane of the epithelial cell nuclei. The nuclei are regularly distributed, rather monotonous, unilayered, and round to oval in this en face preparation.

cells form a discontinuous dendritic network of cells whose nuclear polarity appears haphazard (Fig. 10-6). The density of the basal cells varies from less dense in atrophic epithelium to more dense in hyperplastic epithelium.

The number of basal cells is increased in cases of hyperplasia and reactive atypia, and their nuclear contours may appear enlarged and rounded (Fig. 10-7). In dysplasia, the density of the basal cells may decrease as the severity of dysplasia increases (crude inverse proportionality) (see below).[2, 10]

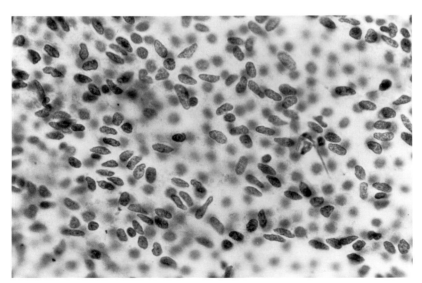

Fig. 10-5. The same benign epithelial sheet shown in Figures 10-1 and 10-4, but focused at the plane of the basal cell nuclei. Basal cell nuclei lie immediately below the epithelial cell layer in this en face preparation.

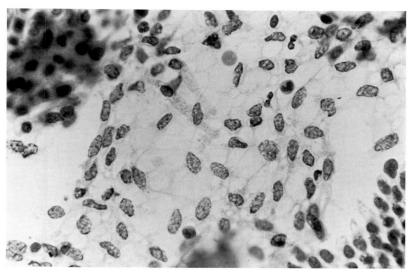

Fig. 10-6. Basal cells that have been isolated from their epithelial layer in the course of biopsy. They form a dendritic, discontinuous network of cells whose nuclear polarity seems haphazard.

PROSTATITIS

Prostatitis is a common urologic condition whose diagnosis is not always based on standardized criteria. Clinically, the term is often applied randomly to any condition associated with prostatic inflammation or various prostatic syndromes.[4, 5, 11, 12]

The histologic patterns of prostatic inflammation are varied and confusing, and often over-

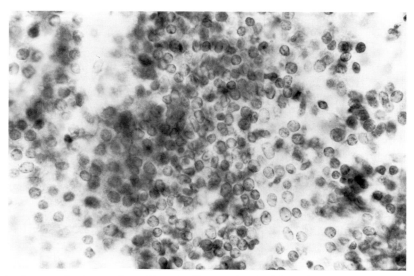

Fig. 10-7. An increase in the number of basal cells associated with benign prostatic enlargement. In this case the basal cell nuclei are enlarged, more rounded, vesicular, and more densely crowded than in normal prostatic epithelium.

looked. The most frequent finding in chronic prostatitis is a lymphoplasmacytic infiltrate, appearing diffusely, scattered in a patchy distribution, or as discrete foci. Prostatitis may involve ducts, acini, periductal and periacinar stroma, and the fibromuscular stroma. The cytologic features of prostatitis have been defined precisely, and standardization of the diagnosis and classification of the prostatitides is feasible.[2, 4, 5]

Drach et al.[13] proposed a clinical and etiologic classification of prostatitis with four major categories: acute bacterial prostatitis, chronic (more often subacute) bacterial prostatitis, nonbacterial prostatitis or prostatosis, and prostatodynia. A histologic classification of prostatitis has also been proposed: acute, chronic, and granulomatous prostatitis[14] (see Ch. 2). Leistenschneider and Nagel[7] have proposed a similar but more complex classification to be applied to aspiration biopsy cytology: purulent, abscessing, chronic, chronic recurrent, granulomatous, and tuberculous prostatitis. The most frequent type of inflammation they observed was chronic recurrent (i.e., subacute), and tuberculous was the rarest.[7]

ACUTE PROSTATITIS

Acute (bacterial) prostatitis is a contraindication to fine-needle aspiration biopsy because of the risk of sepsis; one case of fatal sepsis attributable to acute prostatitis was recorded in Esposti's[3] series of 14,000 transrectal aspiration biopsies.

Cytologically, virtually all of the inflammation consists of polymorphonuclear leukocytes. Scattered necrotic epithelial cell aggregates may also be found, admixed with histiocytes, eosinophils, and sometimes bacteria (Fig. 10-8). Frequently, the preparation appears quite cellular, but the epithelial cells appear as small aggregates in a sea of neutrophils. Other specimens contain sheets of epithelial cells with morphologic abnormalities, including loss of distinct cell borders, slight to moderate anisonucleosis, crowding, overlapping and indentation of nuclei, and small- to intermediate-size nucleoli[2, 4, 5] (Fig. 10-9).

CHRONIC PROSTATITIS

Chronic prostatitis may be due to bacterial infection of the urinary tract, but is usually idiopathic. It is difficult to diagnose and treat; consequently, the identification of florid chronic inflammation by aspiration biopsy warrants culture of aspiration material. Urine culture and culture of secretions obtained by prostatic massage may also be useful.

Histiocytes are the hallmark of chronic prostatitis (Fig. 10-10). These cells are round and plump, with finely granular cytoplasm, frequently containing coarse pigmented or irregular phagocytized material. Neutrophils, eosinophils, lymphocytes, and plasma cells may also be seen, but are not as prominent in aspirations as in tissue sections. Epithelial atypia is usually not severe, but other reactive epithelial changes may be seen, including incomplete squamous or transitional cell metaplasia (Fig. 10-11), basal cell hyperplasia (see Fig. 10-7), and epithelial cells containing refractile golden brown pigment (coarse basophilic material in tetrachrome stains), probably derived from "constipated" tertiary lysosomes[2, 4, 5] (Fig. 10-12).

GRANULOMATOUS PROSTATITIS

Epithelial atypia is often associated with granulomatous prostatitis. The epithelial cells exhibit slight to moderate nuclear pleomorphism, small- to medium-size nucleoli, and finely granular chromatin (Fig. 10-13). Metaplasia, basal cell hyperplasia, and epithelial cell pigmentation may also be seen. Special stains for bacteria and fungi are frequently useful in determining etiology, but should not substitute for a careful clinical history.[14-19]

Inflammation in granulomatous prostatitis is similar to chronic prostatitis, but also includes multinucleated giant cells and granulomas. Multinucleated giants cells are not specific for granulomatous prostatitis, occasionally appearing as an isolated finding within prostatic lumens in the absence of significant inflammation, unrelated to a specific disease (Fig. 10-14). We consider the presence of ill-defined cellular aggre-

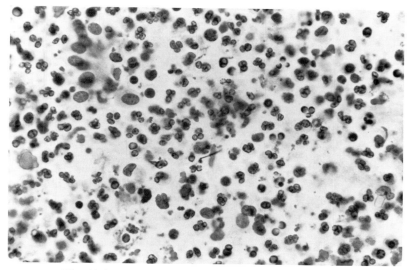

Fig. 10-8. Purulent exudate in a case of acute prostatitis.

gates of immobilized macrophages in aspiration biopsy specimens pathognomonic of granulomatous disease (Fig. 10-15). We refer to these aggregates of apparent intact granulomata as "fibrohistiocytic aggregates." Cytoplasmic fu-sion among adjacent cells in such aggregates probably leads to formation of giant cells with prominent dendritic processes (Fig. 10-16). Occasionally, there is an admixture of amorphous and granular necrotic debris.[2, 4, 5]

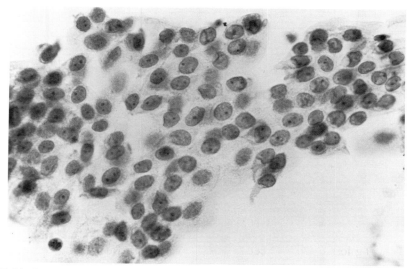

Fig. 10-9. Epithelial atypia in a case of prostatitis. In response to inflammation, sheets of epithelial cells may show disruption of their usual morphology, with loss of distinct cell borders, slight to moderate anisonucleosis, crowding, overlapping and indentaton of adjacent nuclei, and the acquisition of small nucleoli.

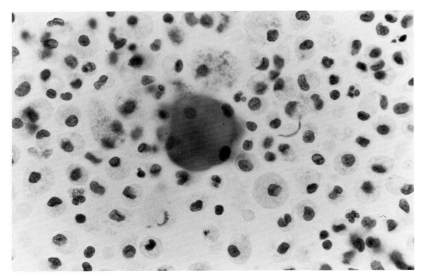

Fig. 10-10. Exudate in a case of chronic prostatitis; the predominant inflammatory cell is the histiocyte.

DYSPLASIA

Dysplasia of the prostate gland is considered a potential diagnostic pitfall in histologic sections and in cytologic preparations. These lesions have a variety of names: primary atypical epithelial hyperplasia, doubtful carcinoma, hyperplasia, small and large acinar carcinoma, marked atypia, atypical glandular hyperplasia, dysplastic lesions, adenosis, and atypical hyperplasia, among others.[9, 20]

Reactive atypia is a non-neoplastic response

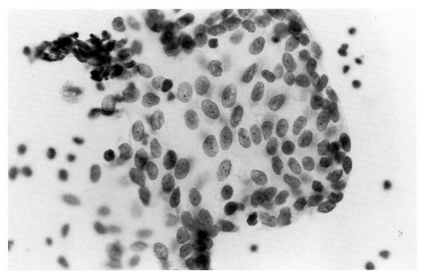

Fig. 10-11. Metaplasia in a case of prostatitis. The type of metaplasia, whether transitional or squamous, is indeterminate; therefore, we prefer to call this *incomplete metaplasia*.

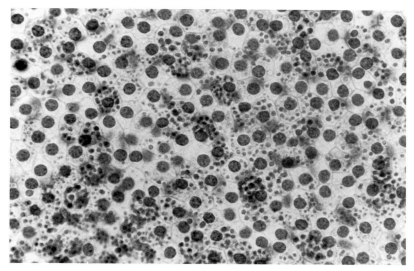

Fig. 10-12. Course pigmentation, probably derived from ''constipated'' tertiary lysosomes in an otherwise normal appearing prostatic epithelial sheet.

to inflammation, radiation, or other idiopathic injury that can mimic dysplasia. We reserve the term *dysplasia* for primary proliferations of abnormal epithelium, excluding reactive changes owing to transient injury-repair phenomena and metaplasia. Bostwick and Brawer[10] coined the term *prostatic intraepithelial neoplasia* (PIN) for these lesions, considering them to be precancerous. Kovi et al.[20] step sectioned 429 whole prostate glands, and concluded that dysplasia poses a significant cancer risk, especially when found in younger patients. Helpap[21]

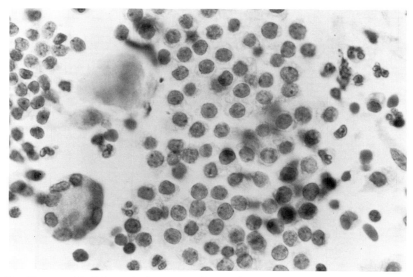

Fig. 10-13. Significant epithelial atypia in a case of granulomatous prostatitis. Note the giant cell in the lower left-hand corner.

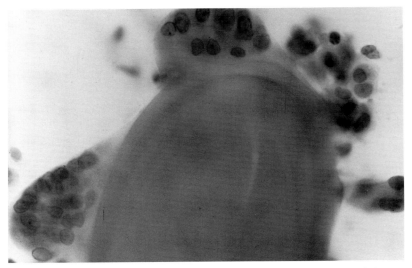

Fig. 10-14. Multinucleated giant cells derived from the intraluminal compartment of the prostatic glands may be seen in the absence of any significant stromal inflammation, and these cannot be correlated with a specific disease process such as granulomatous prostatitis.

showed that the labeling index of ''primary atypical epithelial hyperplasia'' was similar to that of poorly differentiated adenocarcinoma and cribriform carcinoma. Also, he reported the development of adenocarcinoma in about 25 percent of patients with dysplasia.[21]

In prostates without carcinoma, we have found that the frequency of dysplasia in aspiration biopsy specimens is no higher than in core biopsies or transurethral resection specimens; that is, the diagnosis of dysplasia does not appear to be a hedge against the diagnosis of well-

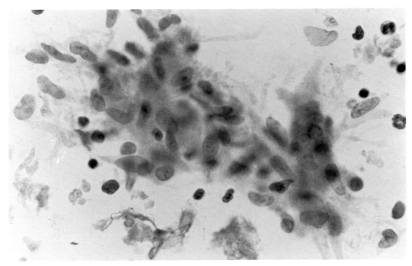

Fig. 10-15. A fibrohistiocytic aggregate, composed of immobilized macrophages resembling both epithelioid and fibrositic cells. We believe that such structures are pathognomonic for stromal granulomatous disease.

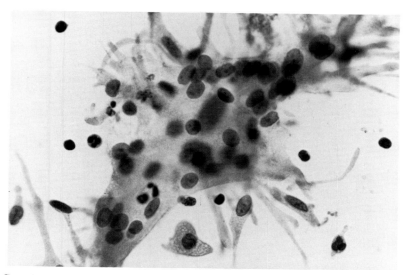

Fig. 10-16. Cytoplasmic fusion among adjacent cells in fibrohistiocytic aggregates may give rise to giant cells with prominent dendritic processes, which we believe are indicative of stromal granulomatous disease.

differentiated carcinoma in cytologic material. However, in prostates with carcinoma, we have seen significant dysplasia about twice as often in aspiration biopsy specimens when compared with matched core biopsies. This difference probably reflects the geographically wider sampling of aspiration biopsy. McNeal and Bostwick[22] observed that the highest grades of dysplasia were found more often in specimens that also contain carcinoma. Furthermore, the extent of dysplasia was greater in glands harboring carcinoma; when dysplasia was multifocal, the prostate more often contained multifocal carcinoma.

We identify dysplasia more easily in aspiration biopsies than in histologic specimens. In the aspiration specimen, several hundred nuclei are laid side to side en face, allowing detection of small aberrations among groups of adjacent nuclei. In our aspiration biopsy laboratory, dysplasia is present without carcinoma in about 10 to 15 percent of cases; dysplasia is associated with low-volume carcinoma (see below) in more than 98 percent of cases, representing about 8 percent of all diagnoses; and dysplasia is associated with outright carcinoma in about 52 percent of cases, representing about 13 percent of all

diagnoses.[2] Well-differentiated and moderately differentiated carcinoma are commonly associated with dysplasia. In contrast, poorly differentiated carcinoma is infrequently associated with dysplasia. Similar findings have been reported in histologic studies.[23]

Dysplasia is classified by aspiration biopsy cytology according to Tannenbaum and Droller[23]: (1) small- (adenomatous) to intermediate-size (tubular) gland pattern with mild to moderate nuclear anaplasia, but without a well-defined basal cell investment (Figs. 10-17 to 10-20); (2) cribriform pattern (Fig. 10-21); and (3) papillary pattern, characterized by ill-defined fibrovascular stalks protruding from sheets of atypical cells with an intact (although often reduced) basal cell investment (Fig. 10-22). The observations of Bostwick and Brawer[10] suggest an additional pattern of dysplasia: nuclear anaplasia in otherwise morphologically preserved epithelial sheets with retained basal cells (Figs. 10-23 and 10-24). This additional pattern, in our experience, is frequently seen in the papillary and cribriform patterns, suggesting a continuum of morphologic patterns.[2] Prostatic crystalloids are also seen with increased frequency in dysplasia and adenocarcinoma, and are con-

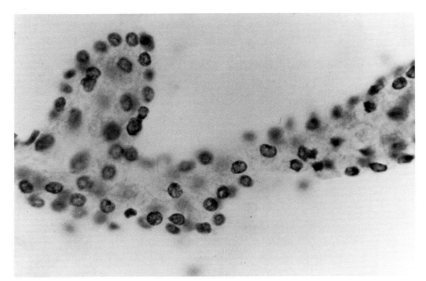

Fig. 10-17. "Roof view" of an irregular small gland without nuclear abnormalities, but lacking a well-defined basal cell investment and showing occasional rosettes of nuclei. This was interpreted as dysplasia, small gland (adenomatous) type, with minimal to moderate nuclear atypia.

sidered an epiphenomenon (Fig. 10-25; also see Fig. 10-10). Ro et al.[24] recently reviewed the significance of crystalloids, and concluded that their presence in benign and atypical prostate glands warranted study of additional material (repeat biopsy) owing to the frequent association with adenocarcinoma.

The morphologic criteria of dysplasia are cytologic atypia, irregular glandular architecture, and disorganization of epithelial-stromal

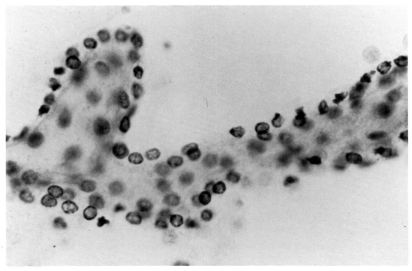

Fig. 10-18. Same case as depicted in Figure 10-17, "wall level," with a clear view of the gland lumen.

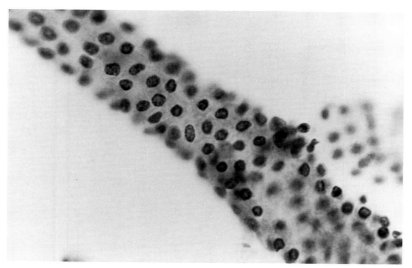

Fig. 10-19. A case similar to that illustrated in Figures 10-17 and 10-18, interpreted as dysplasia, small gland (adenomatous) type, with minimal to moderate nuclear atypia.

integrity.[23] Two of these criteria (atypia and irregular architecture) are recognizable in aspiration biopsy specimens.

Dysplasia signifies an increased incidence of coexisting carcinoma elsewhere in the prostate, or of carcinoma developing in the future. Stil-

mant et al.[18] group atypical hyperplasia with biopsy specimens showing malignancy, because of the 90 percent risk of concomitant carcinoma. At present, there is no evidence that dysplasia is an immediate hazard to the patient, and, in the absence of outright carcinoma, frequent clin-

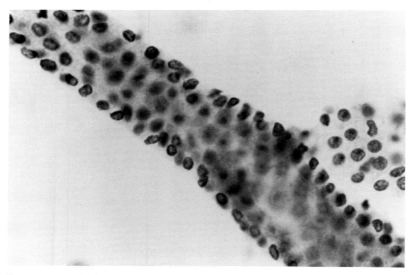

Fig. 10-20. Same case as depicted in Figure 10-19, "wall level," with a clear view of the gland lumen. Note the lack of basal cells in all of these illustrations (see Figs. 10-29 to 10-32).

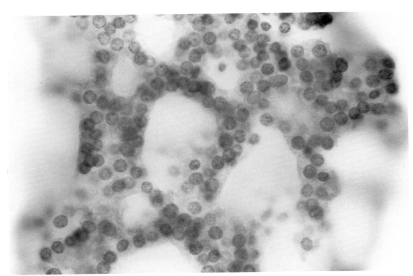

Fig. 10-21. A large cell aggregate arranged in a cribriform pattern, but lacking significant nuclear atypia, interpreted as dysplasia, cribriform type, with minimal nuclear atypia. Regardless of the nature of the nuclei, it has been our experience that this pattern alteration is very frequently associated with overt carcinoma within the prostate gland. The presence of cribriform dyplasia in the absence of carcinoma should be an indicator for close clinical follow-up and re-evaluation.

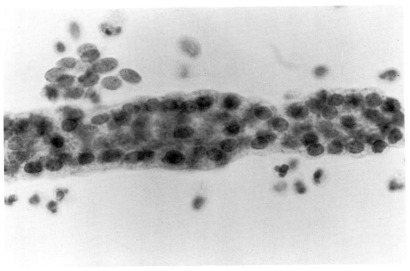

Fig. 10-22. A long pseudopapillary structure with minimal nuclear atypia, interpreted as dysplasia, pseudopapillary type, with minimal nuclear atypia. Similar structures may occasionally be seen with florid hyperplasia.

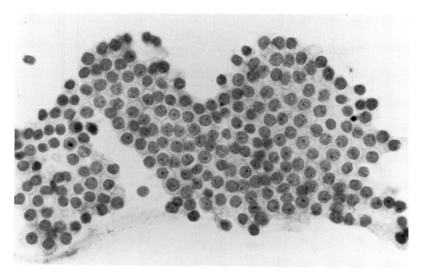

Fig. 10-23. A flat sheet of epithelial cells with moderate nuclear atypia, characterized by mild crowding, enlargement, and nucleolar prominence, interpreted as dysplasia, large acinar type, with moderate nuclear atypia. Basal cells are generally seen in markedly reduced numbers under such situations.

ical follow-up or repeat biopsy is considered adequate management.[10] Those patients with dysplasia on aspiration biopsy, core needle biopsy, or subtotal sampling of the prostate gland should be carefully followed and periodi-cally examined for the development of cancer.[2, 22, 23] If aspiration biopsy is used to follow the patient, it should be performed every 3 to 6 months, and should include complete digital rectal examination.

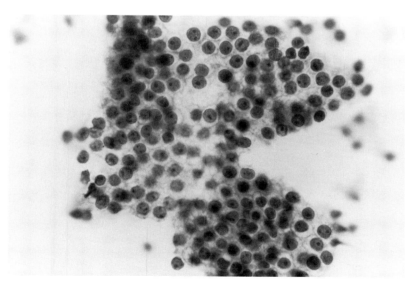

Fig. 10-24. Another example of dysplasia, large acinar type, with moderate nuclear atypia.

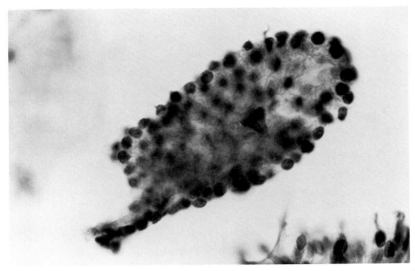

Fig. 10-25. A normal-size gland with a poorly defined basal cell investment containing a prostatic crystalloid. When crystalloids are detected in prostatic glands that appear histologically benign or merely atypical, study of additional material or repeat biopsy should be undertaken because of their more frequent association with adenocarcinoma.

Imaging studies may also be useful in identifying nonpalpable prostatic abnormalities. There have been no reported studies on the utility of tumor markers in the follow-up of dysplasia, but it would be reasonable to expect that a serial rise in serum prostate-specific tumor markers in a patient with dysplasia would indicate concomitant carcinoma; in such instances, rebiopsy would be appropriate.[2]

CYTOLOGIC FEATURES OF CARCINOMA

We rely on three major criteria for the diagnosis of cancer by aspiration biopsy: cellularity, anaplasia, and dysdifferentiation.[2]

CELLULARITY

In a biopsy of good technical quality containing cell clusters diagnostic of well- or moderately differentiated carcinoma, we modify the diagnosis based on the quantity of tumor[2]:

1. *Highly suspicious for carcinoma*: for cases in which there are fewer than three cancer cell aggregates per slide present on two slides; the morphologic criteria for the diagnosis of carcinoma are met, but the cellular criteria are not.

2. *Small amount of carcinoma*: for cases in which there are three or more cancer cell aggregates per slide on two slides, but when such cell aggregates represent less than 10 percent of the total epithelial cell component.

3. *Outright carcinoma*: same as 2, but when the cancer cell aggregates represent more than 10 percent of the total epithelial cell component on the slides, or when poorly differentiated carcinoma is present.

The first two categories (''highly suspicious for carcinoma'' and ''small amount of carcinoma'') suggest the presence of either a small carcinoma that has been adequately sampled, or a large carcinoma that has been inadequately sampled. When only rare malignant cell aggregates are observed, other studies, including imaging studies, tumor markers, and rebiopsy, may help in determining the extent of carcinoma and appropriate therapy.

ANAPLASIA AND DYSDIFFERENTIATION

Carcinoma is distinguished from benign epithelium by the same criteria used in most malignancies: dyshesion, variation in nuclear size (anisonucleosis) and shape (poikilonucleosis), and nucleolar prominence. The cytomorphology of prostate cancer is dependent upon the degree of differentiation (the extent of the tumor's resemblance to benign epithelium) and the degree of nuclear anaplasia.[2, 25] Prominent nucleoli, when present, are characteristic of malignancy. However, nucleoli may occasionally be inconspicuous in the cells of prostatic carcinoma. Another hallmark of malignancy, numerous abnormal mitotic figures, is infrequently present in prostatic carcinoma, and then only in poorly differentiated tumors.

Decreasing differentiation is usually accompanied by increasing anaplasia. However, differentiation and anaplasia should be considered separately in prostatic aspiration biopsy specimens.[2]

GRADING OF CARCINOMA

Cytologic grading of prostate carcinoma relies on the degree of nuclear anaplasia, with two possible exceptions: the recognition of microadenomatous complexes in well-differentiated carcinoma, and cellular dissociation and dyshesion in poorly differentiated carcinoma.

The microadenomatous complex (microglandular complex, microadenoma, or microacinus) is of diagnostic importance for well-differentiated adenocarcinoma in aspiration biopsy specimens prepared by the usual smear techniques.[1, 3, 6, 7] The microacinus is a rosette of 5 to 10 tumor cell nuclei arranged about a central space. These nuclei vary from slightly abnormal, with only minimal anisopoikilonucleosis and small nucleoli, to frankly anaplastic. Kline[6] reported microacini in about 60 percent of cases of well-differentiated adenocarcinoma. Leistenschneidier and Nagel[7] warned that the giant cells of granulomatous prostatitis may simulate the microadenomatous complex of carcinoma. In aspiration biopsies that have been fixed in suspension and subsequently prepared by filtration or cytocentrifuge techniques, microacini may be seen. Nuclear rosettes may also be found within solid cell aggregates displaying minimal nuclear atypia, features characteristic of cribriform adenocarcinoma of low nuclear grade (moderately to poorly differentiated carcinoma).

The Uropathological Study Group on Prostatic Carcinoma[2, 26, 27] has identified six malignant cytologic criteria: (1) average nuclear size; (2) nuclear variability (size); (3) average nucleolar size; (4) nucleolar variability (size, shape, and number); (5) disturbance of nuclear arrangement; and (6) cellular and nuclear dissociation. Each of these six criteria is graded as slight, moderate, or severe, and assessed 1, 2, or 3 points, respectively. The criteria are totaled, with scores ranging from 6 to 18. Scores of 6 to 10 are considered grade I (well-differentiated carcinoma); 11 to 14, grade II (moderately differentiated); and 15 to 18, grade III (poorly differentiated). In reporting cytologic findings in prostatic carcinoma, tumor grade and score are both given (e.g., grade II, score 13). According to the Uropathological Study Group on Prostatic Carcinoma,[27] the classification of carcinoma is based on the least-differentiated component. However, it is recognized that prostatic carcinoma is usually heterogeneous.[9]

We feel that tissue patterns of prostate carcinoma can be accurately predicted by aspiration biopsy, with estimates made of Gleason's scores.[2, 26, 27]

Well-differentiated carcinoma, with normal- or intermediate-size glands, appears as sheets of cells in a single layer, similar to the single-cell-layer sheet morphology of benign and hyperplastic gland preparations (Fig. 10-26). This appearance results from the aspiration needle slicing portions of glands free from the prostatic stroma. Some intact glands may also be observed. At low magnification, it may be difficult to distinguish well-differentiated carcinoma from normal prostatic epithelium. Consequently, higher magnification is necessary in evaluating seemingly benign specimens to avoid a missed diagnosis of carcinoma.[7] As the size

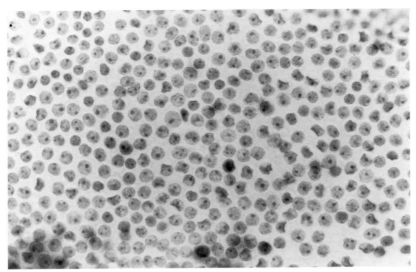

Fig. 10-26. Well-differentiated adenocarcinoma of the prostate gland by pattern criteria. This sheet of anaplastic nuclei could only be derived from a gland whose size and morphology would recapitulate that of a gland giving rise to benign epithelial aggregates, as illustrated in Figures 10-1, 10-3, and 10-4. Such glands are lined by a single layer of anaplastic epithelial cells without adherent basal cells.

of the glands decreases, the probability of harvesting intact gland structures increases. Normal- or intermediate-size glands are related to Gleason's pattern 1 or 2 carcinoma (Figs. 10-27 to 10-30) with one exception: so-called large acinar adenocarcinoma with pseudopapillary structures (Gleason's pattern 3 carcinoma) (Figs. 10-31 and 10-32). The distinction between Gleason's patterns 1 and 2 is not possible in cytology specimens because the gland-to-

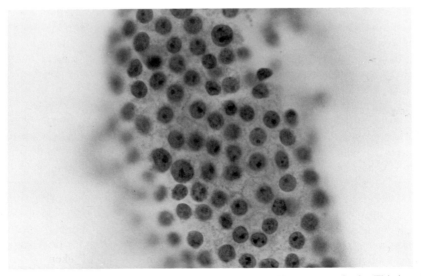

Fig. 10-27. Well-differentiated adenocarcinoma of the prostate gland by pattern criteria. This is an intermediate-size gland structure viewed from the "roof portion" of an intact neoplastic gland laid on its side. The nuclei are anaplastic and no basal cells are seen.

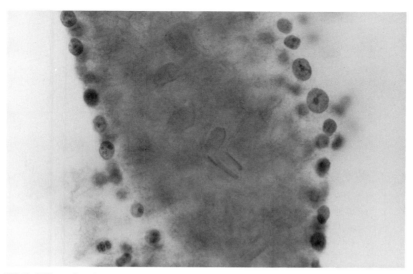

Fig. 10-28. Well-differentiated adenocarcinoma of the prostate gland by pattern criteria. This is the same gland illustrated in Figure 10-25 viewed at the "wall level" of an intact neoplastic gland. Within the gland lumen are various secretions as well as a somewhat refractile body interpreted as a prostatic crystalloid. Prostatic crystalloids are not infrequently seen in association with well- and moderately differentiated adenocarcinomas of tubular pattern.

gland tissue arrangement cannot be assessed. Small glands, whether straight or irregular, correspond to Gleason's pattern 3 carcinoma (Figs. 10-33 and 10-34). Irregular small glands that are also branched or fused correspond to Gleason's pattern 4 carcinoma (Figs. 10-35 to 10-38).

Cribriform carcinoma (Fig. 10-39) appears as either regular cribriform structures (smooth, uniform arborization of lumens punctuating a solid core of epithelial cells, with an even, smooth external surface) or irregular cribriform structures, indistinguishable from small fused glands (irregular, angulated arborization of variably sized lumens punctuating an epithelial cell core with an irregular external surface). These cribriform patterns are associated with pseudopapillary structures (Fig. 10-40), composed of clubbed aggregates of tumor cells whose cytoplasm is scalloped over the outer surface. Apocrine snouts may occasionally be seen on the surface of such aggregates. Regular cribriform structures and pseudopapillary aggregates usually correspond to Gleason's pattern 3 carcinoma, and irregular cribriform structures with or without hypernephroid clear cells correspond to Gleason's pattern 4 carcinoma (Fig. 10-41). Sheets of neoplastic cells with papillary or pseudopapillary fronds and a cribriform pattern may originate in the primary or secondary ducts of the prostate gland.[9] Tumors with signet ring cells (Fig. 10-42) have been observed with cribriform carcinoma, associated with broad sheets of anaplastic cells (assumed to have been derived from large prostatic acini or ducts) (Fig. 10-43). Rarely, signet ring cells are associated with small acinar tumors.

Undifferentiated carcinoma appears as either solid clusters of tumor cells or dissociated single tumor cells with infrequent or missing glands. Such tumors probably represent terminal dysdifferentiation, and invariably correspond to Gleason's pattern 5 carcinoma (Figs. 10-44 and 10-45). Poorly differentiated invasive transitional cell carcinoma, arising from prostatic ducts or secondarily invading the prostate by contiguous extension, may be mistaken for undifferentiated carcinoma (Fig. 10-46). Immunohistochemistry may be helpful in resolving this diagnostic dilemma (see Ch. 9).

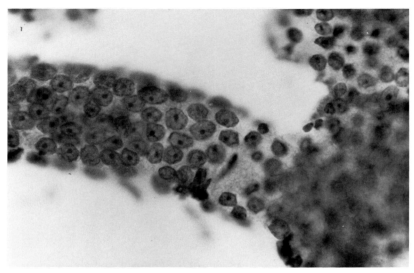

Fig. 10-29. Well-differentiated adenocarcinoma of the prostate gland by pattern criteria. This is a relatively normal-size gland viewed at the "roof level." It has a tubular structure and obviously neoplastic nuclei.

FALSE-POSITIVE BIOPSIES (ERRONEOUS
CARCINOMA)

False-positive cytologic diagnosis is of greater clinical concern than failure to demonstrate carcinoma on the first attempt.[7] Sunder-

land and Lederer[28] obtained optimal quality-assured aspiration biopsy specimens from 100 fresh autopsy specimens and 100 unfixed prostates removed surgically, and in their study, no incorrect diagnosis of carcinoma was made (no false-positive results). Trott et al.[29] de-

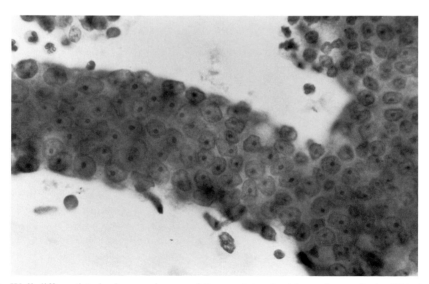

Fig. 10-30. Well-differentiated adenocarcinoma of the prostate gland by pattern criteria. This is the same gland as that illustrated in Figure 10-29. Note how the "walls" and the "floor" of this somewhat smaller gland structure are in nearly the same plane of focus, attesting to the smaller gland size.

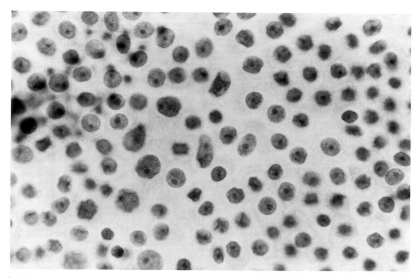

Fig. 10-31. Moderately differentiated adenocarcinoma of the prostate gland with both large flat sheets and pseudopapillary structures (see Fig. 10-32).

scribed 165 positive aspiration biopsies obtained at the Institute of Urology Laboratory of St. Paul's Hospital between 1965 and 1973. Their single false-positive cytologic diagnosis was from a patient who, at autopsy, was found not to have prostatic carcinoma; review of the pre-mortem slides showed slight cellular abnormalities attributable to prostatic abscess that were misinterpreted as carcinoma. Such diagnostic difficulties underscore the need for caution in interpretation in the presence of fulminant prostatitis.[18, 29]

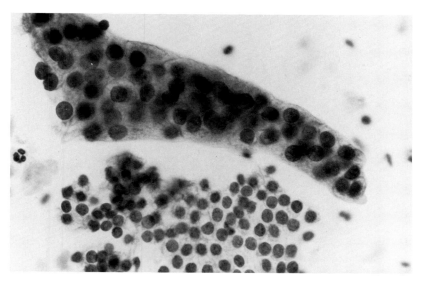

Fig. 10-32. Moderately differentiated adenocarcinoma of the prostate: pseudopapillary structures (same case as in Figure 10-31).

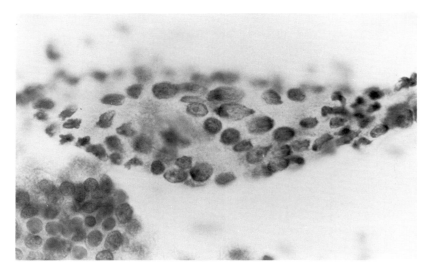

Fig. 10-33. Moderately differentiated adenocarcinoma of the prostate by pattern criteria. Viewed from the "roof level," this small neoplastic gland is somewhat irregular in comparison to the neoplastic glands illustrated in earlier figures. Also note that there is a suggestion of rosetting of the nuclei within the wall of the gland, interpreted as microadenomatous structures. No basal cells are seen on the outer shell of this three-dimensional glandular structure.

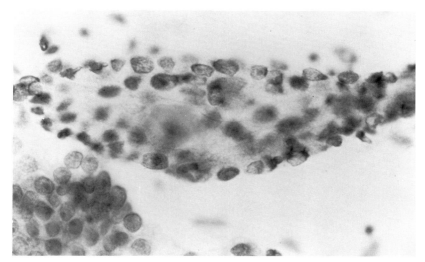

Fig. 10-34. Moderately differentiated adenocarcinoma of the prostate by pattern criteria. Viewed from the "wall level," the lumen of this gland is well defined.

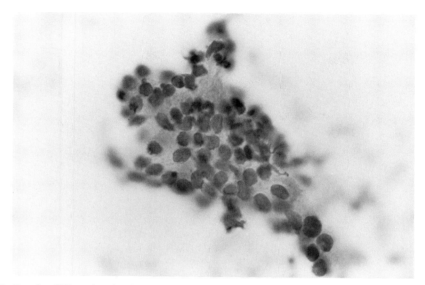

Fig. 10-35. Poorly differentiated adenocarcinoma of the prostate by pattern criteria. Viewed from the ''roof level,'' irregular gland branching or fusing is noted. The nuclei are hyperchromatic, condensed, angulated, and irregular, but appear less overtly neoplastic than some cases illustrated earlier—such is the nature of the nucleus in prostate cancer. The next three figures are derived from the same case and demonstrate a real problem with prostate cancer cytology which is practiced in a solely nuclear-dependent fashion: anisopoikilonucleosis and hyperchromatism may at times outweigh or supplant nucleolar prominence in prostate cancer diagnosis and grading.

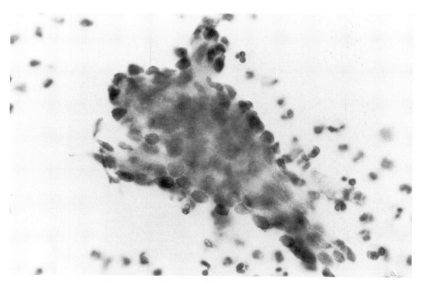

Fig. 10-36. Poorly differentiated adenocarcinoma of the prostate gland by pattern criteria. Same gland as that illustrated in Figure 10-35. A definite lumen is identified in this irregularly branched small gland.

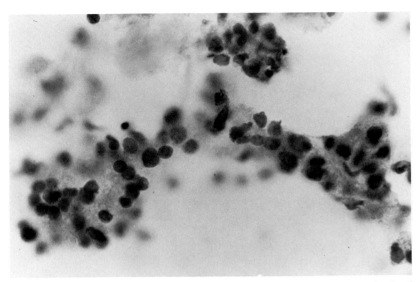

Fig. 10-37. Poorly differentiated adenocarcinoma of the prostate gland by pattern criteria. Same case as that illustrated in Figures 10-35 and 10-36. Irregularly branched small gland fragments viewed from the "roof level."

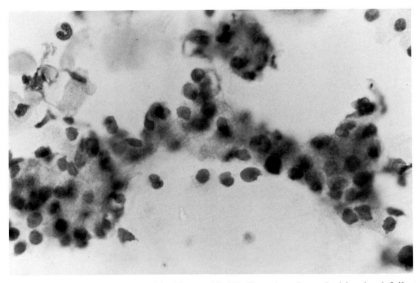

Fig. 10-38. Same gland as that illustrated in Figure 10-37. Focusing through this gland fails to identify a well-formed central lumen. Such groups may be properly described as "cords of cells," but most likely represent highly attenuated small gland structures.

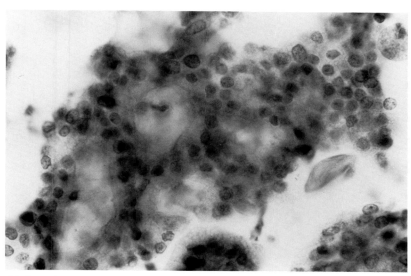

Fig. 10-39. Moderately to poorly differentiated adenocarcinoma with a cribriform pattern. In this case, the neoplastic cell aggregate is composed of what seems to be a repetitive gland within gland structure; however, arborizing lumens may also be thought of as interrupting a solid core of tumor cells, allowing one to mentally construct a continuum between the cribriform pattern and the comedo pattern, where the solid cell plug is not otherwise interrupted.

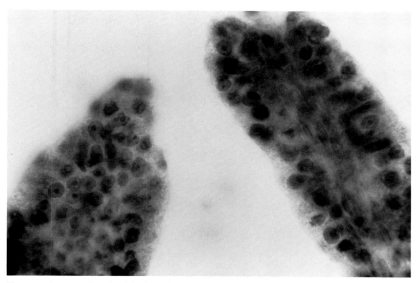

Fig. 10-40. Frequently associated with the cribriform pattern are papillary (with vascular core) and pseudo-papillary (without vascular core) structures. These suggest a continuum between the large-acinar-with-papillae type of neoplasm with the cribriform pattern of adenocarcinoma of the prostate gland.

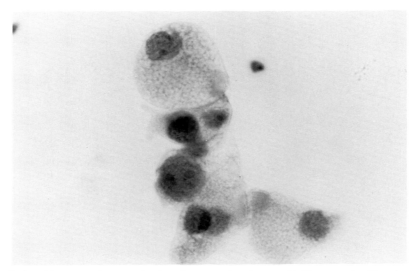

Fig. 10-41. Isolated foamy to clear neoplastic cells suggesting the so-called hypernephroid variant of adenocarcinoma of the prostate gland.

Anandan et al.[30] reported that most patients with malignant aspiration biopsies who had contradictory benign core biopsies were found to have early well-differentiated tumors. If an aspirate was correctly obtained, processed, and evaluated by persons experienced in cytodiagnosis of the prostate, then the diagnosis of outright carcinoma in a patient without prostatitis should not be dismissed as false positive even when the histologic diagnosis was contradictory.[7]

In order to avoid false-positive results, carcinoma should be diagnosed only when all criteria are met. For example, when small numbers of atypical cells suspicious for malignancy are present, repeat biopsy is recommended. Also, otherwise normal sheets of prostatic epithelium

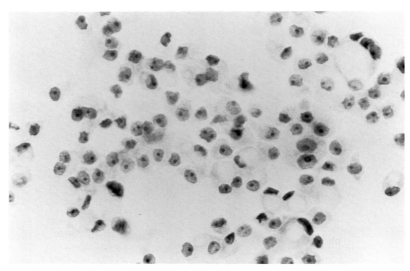

Fig. 10-42. Signet ring cells in an adenocarcinoma of the prostate gland.

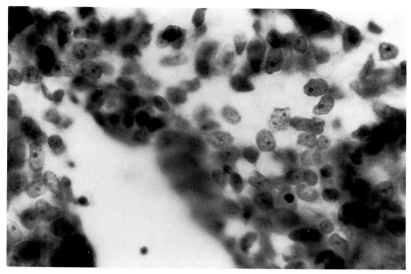

Fig. 10-43. Large gland variant of prostate adenocarcinoma with numerous signet ring cells. The PSA positivity of this tumor indicated prostatic origin of this neoplasm.

containing cellular foci with prominent nucleoli, variable nuclear size, and nuclear hyperchromasia should not be considered sufficient for the diagnosis of carcinoma.[7] The simplicity of aspiration biopsy of the prostate allows acquisition of additional specimens to resolve diagnostic difficulties.

FALSE-NEGATIVE BIOPSIES (MISSED CARCINOMA)

Missed carcinoma (false-negative biopsy) may be due to the following: (1) inadequate specimen; (2) tumor missed in the course of the biopsy; (3) the lesion is histologically border-

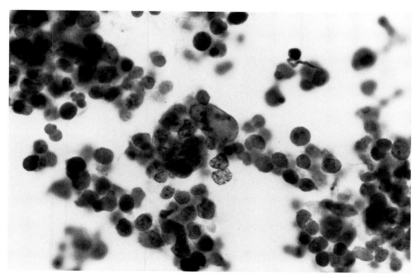

Fig. 10-44. Undifferentiated adenocarcinoma of the prostate gland.

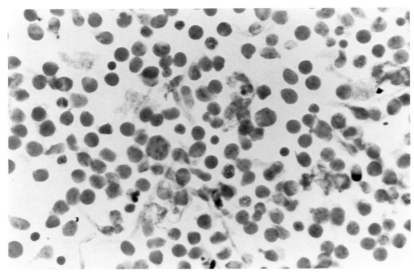

Fig. 10-45. Undifferentiated adenocarcinoma of the prostate gland. This neoplasm was positive for both PSA and neuron-specific enolase. Leukocyte-common antigen testing was negative in this case, which was interpreted as a small-cell anaplastic carcinoma of prostatic origin.

line, and thus difficult to interpret as outright carcinoma; or (4) the tumor has occurred in association with fulminant prostatitis. In our experience, when carcinoma is missed on aspira-tion biopsy, the cellularity of the preparation is inadequate or the carcinoma is well to moder-ately differentiated, with sampling error owing to small tumor size.[2]

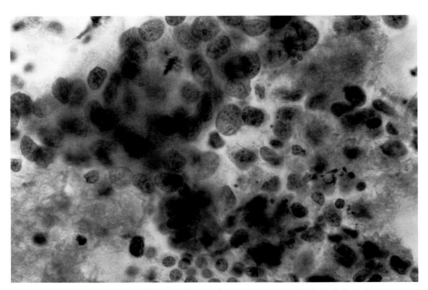

Fig. 10-46. Poorly differentiated transitional cell carcinoma secondarily involving the prostate gland. This patient had a prior nephrectomy for transitional cell carcinoma of the renal pelvis, with the subsequent development of a pelvic mass. PSA was negative but keratin was positive.

DISTINGUISHING PROSTATITIS AND CARCINOMA

Prostatic inflammation can produce palpable abnormalities on digital rectal examination, and may mimic the physical findings of carcinoma. However, the effect of inflammation on the cytologic diagnosis of carcinoma may be overstated. Koss et al.[1] warned that prostatic carcinoma must be diagnosed with extreme care in the presence of inflammation; however, "extreme care" must not be confused with "over-caution," especially in dealing with such a ubiquitous problem as prostatitis.[18] Our studies have demonstrated carcinoma in about 15 percent of cases of prostatitis.[2, 4, 5] In cases of diagnostic difficulty, it is appropriate to report suspicious abnormal epithelial changes as "atypical beyond the degree and stage of inflammation." This approach will avoid overdiagnosis of epithelial dysplasia and avoid an erroneous diagnosis of carcinoma. Since aspiration biopsy of the prostate gland is easily performed and well tolerated, rebiopsy should be attempted 6 to 12 weeks after appropriate treatment for prostatitis, especially if clinical suspicion of carcinoma remains.

COMPLEMENTARY ROLES OF ASPIRATION AND CORE BIOPSY

In comparing the relative benefits of core and aspiration biopsy, many investigators have implied that one method will supersede the other in the diagnosis of prostatic carcinoma.[31-42] However, we and others have observed that these techniques are complementary.[31-42] When used together at a single operative sitting, there is a significant increase in the diagnostic sensitivity of the examination for the detection of carcinoma.

Among 228 ultrasound-guided matched core and aspiration biopsy specimens that we gathered from the files of the Aspiration Biopsy Laboratory, Inc. (Cleveland, OH), there were 90 cases (40 percent) of carcinoma, with agreement between core and aspiration biopsy in 80 of these 90 cases (89 percent). Eighty-four carci-

nomas (93 percent) were detected by core biopsy. Six carcinomas missed by core biopsy were detected by aspiration biopsy. Among these six cases, two had a predicted Gleason's score of 6, three had a predicted score of 5, and one had a predicted score of 3. Two of the six false-negative core biopsies were technically poor. Interestingly, four of the six false-negative core biopsies showed moderate to severe dysplasia. Eighty-six cases of carcinoma (96 percent) were detected by aspiration biopsy. Four carcinomas missed by aspiration biopsy were detected by core biopsy. Among these four cases, one had a Gleason's score of 7, two had a score of 6 and one had a score of 5. Two of the four false-negative aspiration biopsies were technically poor. Moderate to severe dysplasia was present on two of the four false-negative aspiration biopsies.

False-negative results adversely affect both core biopsy and aspiration biopsy. Zincke et al.[43] showed that digitally directed needle biopsies of the prostate gland had a 12 percent false-negative rate, based on patient follow-up of 4 years. The cumulative data that we have cited[31-42] suggest a problem of similar magnitude; among 1,522 digitally guided matched core and aspiration biopsies, there were 743 cases (49 percent) of carcinoma. Core biopsy identified 663 cases (85 percent), and aspiration biopsy identified 625 (81 percent) cases. Core and aspiration biopsies agreed on the diagnosis of carcinoma in 546 cases (74 percent). Our limited sample of 228 cases (enhanced by ultrasound guidance) showed a greater degree of agreement between core and aspiration biopsies (89 percent compared to 74 percent): nonetheless, the cumulative data indicate that 5 percent of carcinomas are missed by either method alone.

Our data and the indexed literature indicate that core and aspiration biopsies have statistically equivalent sensitivity in the diagnosis of prostate carcinoma. Both techniques have the inherent limitation of small sample size from a relatively large organ. Use of both of these sampling modalities appears to minimize sampling error. Each biopsy method offsets the potential shortcomings of the other; core biopsy is specific, and aspiration biopsy can sample more widely, allowing the recognition of multifocal disease. Aspiration biopsy allows wider blind screening of sonographically normal prostates that may harbor isoechoic tumor foci, a useful feature with the increasing use of ultrasound-guided biopsy.

CONCLUSION

Aspiration biopsy is a rapid and relatively painless technique for evaluating the abnormal prostate. It can be performed as an outpatient procedure without anesthesia, and is easily tolerated. The sensitivity of aspiration biopsy to detect cancer appears to be equivalent to that of core biopsy, and the use of both techniques at a single operative sitting may amplify cancer detection. Few complications are encountered by this method.

We feel that aspiration biopsy is a valuable diagnostic tool for the practicing urologist, and should be widely applied for initial evaluation. In our experience, four-quadrant aspiration biopsy appears to be a valuable adjunct to digitally-directed core biopsies. Aspiration biopsy allows widespread blind screening of sonographically occult neoplasms in those instances when ultrasonography is either unrevealing, as with isoechoic lesions, or when sonographic abnormalities prove to be inconsequential. It is expected that aspiration biopsy will contribute to the early diagnosis of prostate cancer.

REFERENCES

1. Koss LG, Woyke S, Schreiber K, et al: Thin needle aspiration biopsy of the prostate. Urol Clin North Am 11:237, 1984
2. Maksem JA, Park CH, Johenning PW, Galang CF, Tannenbaum M: Aspiration biopsy of the prostate gland. Urol Clin North Am Nov, 15(4):555 1988
3. Esposti PL: Aspiration Biopsy Cytology in the Diagnosis and Management of Prostatic Carcinoma. Stahl and Accidenstryck, Stockholm, 1974
4. Maksem JA, Johenning PW: Prostatitis and aspiration biopsy cytology of the prostate. Urology 32:263, 1988
5. Maksem JA, Johenning PW, Park CH, Galang CF: Prostatitis and aspiration biopsy of the prostate gland. ASCP check sample. Cytopathology 16(1), 1988
6. Kline TS: Guides to Clinical Aspiration Biopsy: Prostate. Igaku-Shoin, New York, 1984
7. Leistenschneider W, Nagel R: Atlas of Prostatic Cytology. Springer-Verlag, New York, 1984
8. Haddad FS, Somsin AA: Seeding and perineal implantation of prostatic cancer in the tract of the biopsy needle: 3 cases and literature review. J Surg Oncol 35:184, 1987
9. Miller GJ: An atlas of prostatic biopsies: dilemmas of morphologic variance. Prog Surg Pathol 8:81, 1988
10. Bostwick DG, Brawer MK: Prostatic intraepithelial neoplasia and early invasion in prostate cancer. Cancer 59:788, 1987
11. Madsen PO, Gasser TC: Prostatitis. Infection 14:253, 1986
12. Stamey TA: Pathogenesis and Treatment of Urinary Tract Infections. Williams & Wilkins, Baltimore, 1980
13. Drach GW, Mears EM, Fair WR, et al: Classification of benign diseases associated with prostatic pain: prostatitis or prostatodynia? J Urol 120:266, 1978
14. Peterson RO: Urological Pathology. JB Lippincott, Philadelphia, 1986
15. Stillwell TJ, DeRemee RA, McDonald TJ, et al: Prostatic involvement in Wegener's granulomatosis. J Urol 138:1251, 1987
16. Schned AR: Prostatic granulomas. Am J Surg Pathol 8:797, 1984
17. Stilmant M, Siroky MB, Johnson KB: Fine needle aspiration cytology of granulomatous prostatitis induced by BCG immunotherapy of bladder cancer. Acta Cytol 29:961, 1985
18. Stilmant MM, Freedlund MC, De Las Morenas A, et al: Expanded role for fine needle aspiration of the prostate. A study of 335 specimens. Cancer 63:583, 1989
19. Oates RD, Stilmant MM, Freedlund MC, Siroky MB: Granulomatous prostatitis following Bacillus Calmette-Guérin immunotherapy of bladder cancer. J Urol 140:751, 1988

20. Kovi J, Mostofi FK, Heshmat MY, et al: Large acinar atypical hyperplasia and carcinoma of the prostate. Cancer 61:555, 1988
21. Helpap B: The biological significance of atypical hyperplasia of the prostate. Virchows Arch [A] 387:307, 1980
22. McNeal JE, Bostwick DG: Intraductal dysplasia: a premalignant lesion of the prostate. Hum Pathol 17:64, 1986
23. Tannenbaum M, Droller M: Primary atypical hyperplasia of the prostate gland: a premalignant lesion. World J Urol 5:92, 1987
24. Ro JY, Ayala AG, Ordonez NG, et al: Intraluminal crystalloids in prostatic adenocarcinoma. Immunochemical, electron microscopic and x-ray microanalytical studies. Cancer 57:2397, 1986
25. Mostofi FK: Problems of grading carcinoma of prostate. Semin Oncol 3:161, 1976
26. Maksem JA, Resnik MI, Johenning PW: Can a cytological grading system be predictive of Gleason's scores in aspiration biopsy cytology specimens of prostate carcinoma? World J Urol 5:99, 1987
27. Maksem JA, Johenning PW: Is cytology capable of adequately grading prostate carcinoma? Matched series of 50 cases comparing cytologic and histologic pattern diagnosis. Urol 31:437, 1988
28. Sunderland H, Lederer H: Prostatic aspiration biopsy. Br J Urol 43:603, 1971
29. Trott PA, Hendry WF, Pugh RBC, et al: Franzen-needle transrectal prostatic biopsy. Lancet (Sept. 15):620, 1973
30. Anandan N, Mackenzie E, Gingell JC, et al: Role of Franzen needle aspiration biopsy in carcinoma of the prostate. J R Med Soc 76:828, 1983
31. Ekman H, Hedberg K, Persson PS: Cytological versus histological examination of needle biopsy specimens in the diagnosis of prostatic cancer. Br J Urol 39:544, 1967
32. Epstein NA: Prostatic biopsy. A morphologic correlation of aspiration cytology with needle biopsy histology. Cancer 38:2078, 1976
33. Kline TS, Kelsey DM, Kohler FP: Prostatic carcinoma and needle aspiration biopsy. Am J Clin Pathol 67:131, 1977
34. Zattoni F, Pagano F, Rebuffi A, Constantin G: Transrectal thin needle aspiration biopsy of prostate: four years' experience. Urology 22:69, 1983
35. Hosking DH, Paraskevas M, Hellsten OR, Ramsey EW: The cytological diagnosis of prostatic carcinoma by transrectal fine needle aspiration. J Urol 129:998, 1983
36. Chodak GW, Bibbo M, Strauss FH, Wied GL: Transrectal aspiration biopsy versus transperineal core biopsy for the diagnosis of carcinoma of the prostate. J Urol 132:480, 1984
37. Maier U, Czerwenka K, Neuhold N: The accuracy of transrectal aspiration biopsy of the prostate: an analysis of 452 cases. Prostate 5:147, 1984
38. Whelan JP, Chin JL, Shapre JR, Davis IR: Transrectal needle aspiration versus transperineal needle biopsy in diagnosis of carcinoma of prostate. Urology 27:410, 1986
39. Carter HB, Riehle RA, Koizumi JH, et al: Fine needle aspiration of the abnormal prostate: a cytohistological correlation. J Urol 294, 1986
40. Bodner DR, Hampel N, Maksem JA, et al: Aspiration biopsy of the prostate. World J Urol 5:62, 1987
41. Alfthan O, Klintrup H-E, Koivuniemi A, Taskinen E: Cytological aspiration biopsy and Vim-Silverman biopsy in the diagnosis of prostatic carcinoma. Chir Gynaecol Fenn 59:226, 1970
42. Chodak GW, Steinberg GD, Bibbo M, et al: The role of transrectal aspiration biopsy in the diagnosis of prostate cancer. J Urol 135:299, 1986
43. Zincke U, Campbell JT, Utz D, et al: Confidence in the negative transrectal needle biopsy. Surg Gynecol Obstet 136:78, 1973

11

Interpretation of Postradiation Prostate Biopsies

Michael K. Brawer and David G. Bostwick

Radiation therapy is commonly employed as an alternative to radical prostatectomy for treatment of localized prostatic adenocarcinoma. This chapter discusses the efficacy of radiation therapy and the importance of local tumor control, with emphasis on the interpretation of postradiation biopsies.

EFFICACY OF RADIATION THERAPY

Ionizing radiation may be delivered to the prostate by a variety of modalities. In their pioneering work in 1910, Paschkis and Pittinger[1] employed an intraurethral radium source. Subsequently, Young[2] described successful results with radium placement intravesically, intraurethrally, and transrectally. External beam radiation therapy was first used in the 1920s, but the introduction of the linear accelerator by Bagshaw and associates[3, 4] in the 1950s heralded the beginning of the modern age of radiation therapy for prostate cancer. Refinements in interstitial radiation therapy, including retropubic and perineal implants, have also emerged as useful methods. Several centers employ a combination of external beam and interstitial radiotherapy. These methods have proven effective in treating prostate cancer, with local tumor control and improved patient survival.

Survival and Disease-Free Survival

Survival of patients treated with radiation therapy is similar to that following radical prostatectomy. With cancer confined to the prostate,

Bagshaw[4] noted actuarial survival at 5, 10, and 15 years of 81, 59, and 36 percent, respectively; for cancers with extracapsular extension, the corresponding survivals were 62, 36, and 18 percent. Although one prospective randomized study demonstrated a slight advantage of surgery in halting tumor progression, that report has been criticized on numerous points, including experimental study design.

Patients with prostatic carcinoma tend to be elderly, so survival statistics that do not control for intercurrent illness are biased. Disease-free survival, utilized by numerous investigators to assess efficacy of therapy, is also problematic owing to significant understaging at the time of diagnosis. Staging pelvic lymph node dissections have not been performed in the majority of these studies, and the use of noninvasive imaging studies in assessing pelvic lymph node status is controversial (see Ch. 13).

Importance of Local Tumor Control

The best indicator of treatment efficacy is the ability to achieve local tumor control by eradicating tumor from the site of origin. Clinical assessment of tumor eradication may be difficult, however, particularly in visceral organs like the prostate. Digital rectal examination is unreliable after irradiation because of fibrosis and anterior displacement of the gland.[5-9] Scardino and associates[10] demonstrated a significant decrease in prostatic volume following combined interstitial and external beam irradiation. Transrectal ultrasound is unproven as a method of imaging the irradiated prostate.

Needle biopsy appears to be the best method available for objective assessment of local tumor control after irradiation.[10-31] Needle biopsy has a low level of sampling error, which is minimized by taking serial specimens.

Residual carcinoma was identified in 87 percent of serial prostatic needle biopsies in patients irradiated with curative intent, according to Rhamy and associations.[24] Other studies confirmed these results, identifying residual tumor in 50 percent or more of irradiated prostates.[11, 13, 14] Scardino[10] recently reviewed 10 published studies, and, of 506 aggregate patients, 228 (45 percent) had positive postradiation biopsies; 54 percent of these also had clinical evidence of tumor recurrence. Of the 278 patients with negative postradiation biopsies, only 21 percent had tumor recurrence. He concluded that a positive biopsy after irradiation indicated probable tumor progression. Other studies have also shown a statistically significant correlation between positive postradiation biopsy and subsequent treatment failure and tumor progression.[29-31]

Histopathologic evaluation should only be made after the full therapeutic impact of irradiation, including delayed effects.[12, 15] Cox and Stoffel[15] observed positive biopsies postradiation in 63 percent of samples taken within 12 months, decreasing to 46 percent of samples after 12 months, a finding confirmed by others.[12] The interval required before procurement of prognostic tissue cannot be precisely defined, although certain trends are apparent. Kagan and colleagues[5] identified four patients with positive biopsies at 6 months who continued to show gradual decrease of tumor on rectal palpation, and had subsequent negative biopsies at 1 and 2 years. Biopsy conversion from positive to negative 1 to 2 years after irradiation occurred in 7 of 53 patients reported by Kurth et al.[23] From experience with 34 biopsies, Carlton et al.[7] suggested that biopsy prior to 6 months may be misleading.

Accurate interpretation of postradiation biopsies is also important because of the potential for salvage therapy following radiation failure.[32-37] According to Rainwater and Zincke,[32] salvage prostatectomy is feasible following radiation failure, and the associated mor-

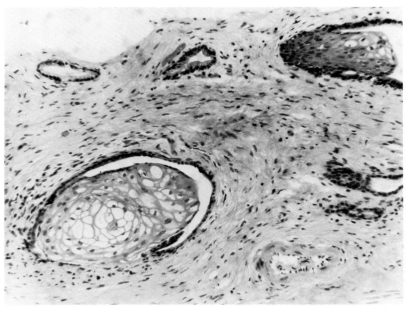

Fig. 11-1. Radiation-induced squamous metaplasia of prostatic ductules. The patient had not received hormonal therapy. (H&E, ×64.)

bidity is acceptable. Although they identified no significant correlation between local recurrence and systemic progression or cause-specific survival, they attributed this to the small number of patients in their series.

TUMOR VIABILITY AFTER IRRADIATION

No definitive method exists for assessment of tumor viability after irradiation. Musselman and associates[38] demonstrated monolayer growth from explants of prostatic carcinoma 2 years or more after definitive radiation. Conversely, Mollenkamp et al.[39] were unable to culture any of 19 irradiated tumors, and they concluded that radiation suppressed mitotic activity and growth potential; however, their success rate for in vitro cultivation of untreated carcinoma was also poor (less than 7 percent). Mahan et al.[40] identified intense cytoplasmic immunoreactivity for prostatic acid phosphatase in 23 of 27 irradiated adenocarcinomas, leading them to suggest that tumor cells capable of protein production probably retain the potential for

cell division and consequent metastatic spread. Other reports have claimed that if prostatic carcinoma is not histologically ablated by radiotherapy after a reasonable time interval, it is probably wise to consider the cancer biologically active.[12, 41] Bostwick et al.[12] studied pre- and postirradiation samples from 40 patients, and concluded that malignant glands identified 12 to 18 months or more following radiation therapy should be considered viable; the consequences of denying viability of such foci of apparent residual neoplasm outweighed the side effects incurred by additional therapeutic intervention.

POSTRADIATION BIOPSY

RADIATION CHANGES IN THE NON-NEOPLASTIC PROSTATE

A variety of morphologic changes occur in the non-neoplastic prostate following radiation[12, 42] (Figs. 11-1 to 11-3). The number of glands per unit of stromal area is unaffected

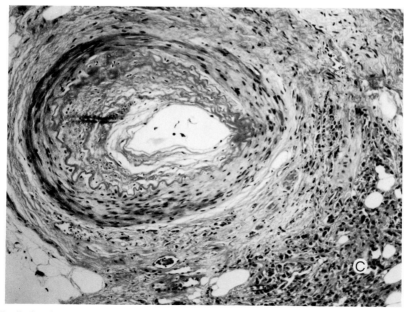

Fig. 11-2. Radiation-induced myointimal proliferation of vessel. Extensive residual carcinoma is present in the adjacent stroma. *C*, carcinoma. (H&E, ×135.)

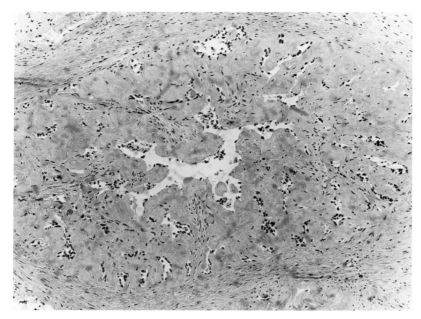

Fig. 11-3. Marked atrophy and fibrosis of the seminal vesicle following radiation therapy. (H&E, ×40.)

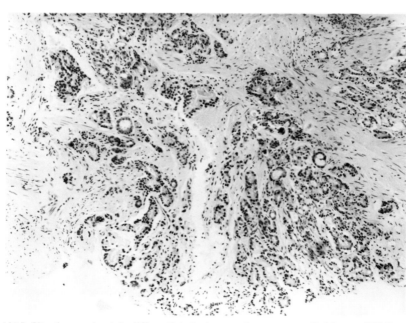

A

Fig. 11-4. (A) Infiltrating moderately differentiated adenocarcinoma on needle biopsy. (H&E, ×40.) Compare with Figures B and C, obtained 14 years after definitive external beam radiation therapy. (*Figure continues.*)

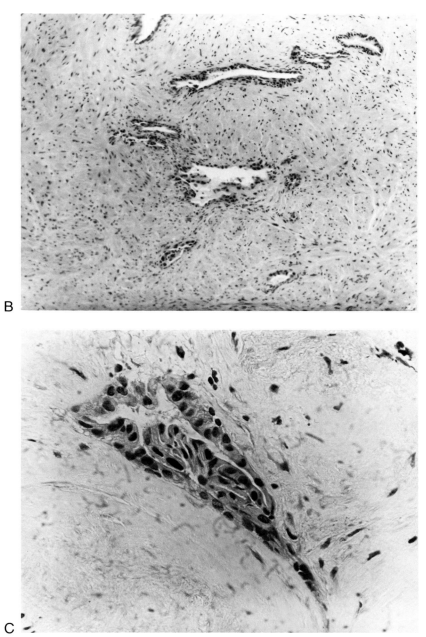

Fig. 11-4 (*Continued*). In (**B**), the glands are shrunken and atrophic, with no evidence of residual or recurrent tumor. (H&E, ×40.) At higher magnification (**C**), the glands display nuclear and cytologic atypia. (H&E, ×160.)

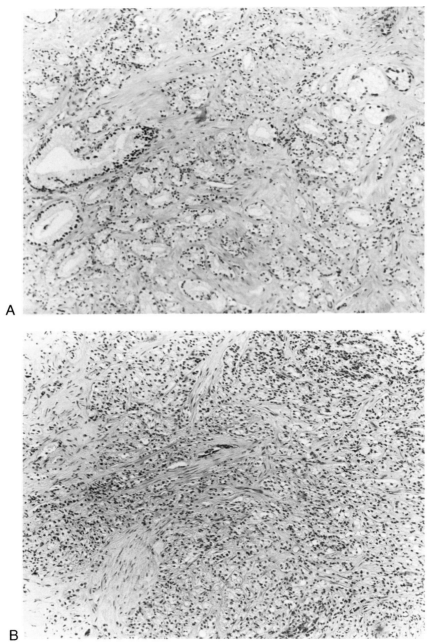

Fig. 11-5. Prostatic adenocarcinoma before and after radiation therapy. No significant differences were observed in tumor grade following irradiation. (**A**) Original diagnostic biopsy from a 62-year-old man. Compare with (**B**), obtained 3 years after administration of 6,500 rads. (*Figure continues.*)

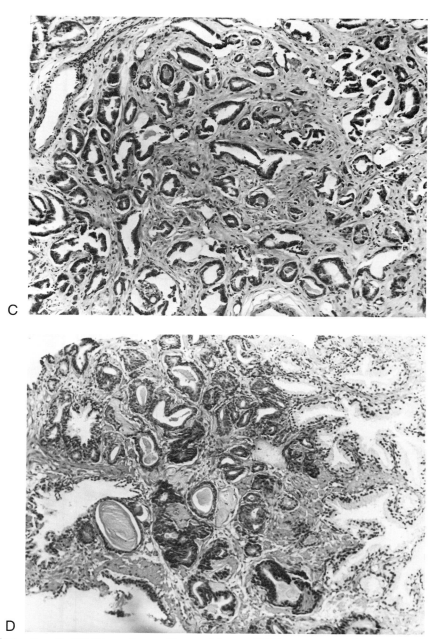

Fig. 11-5 (*Continued*). (**C**) Biopsy from a 57-year-old man. (**D**) Tumor recurred 6 years after administration of 7,000 rads. (H&E, ×40.)

by radiation therapy, although the proportion of atrophic glands increases from 5 to 27 percent.[12] Squamous metaplasia and squamous-like metaplasia are significant findings after radiation therapy, present in 63 percent of irradiated prostates (Fig. 11-1) and only rarely prior to radiation. The incidence of cytologic atypia of epithelial cells increases from 11 to 78 percent following radiation therapy, with variation in nuclear size and shape, nuclear hyperchromasia, and a high nuclear cytoplasmic ratio.[12] Secretory activity of luminal cells is markedly decreased.

The prostatic stroma reveals prominent fibrosis after radiation, with occasional foci of smooth muscle atrophy. Acute inflammation is observed within 4 months of surgical intervention, and is interpreted as postsurgical prostatitis. Only 6 of 56 postradiation samples studied by Bostwick et al.[12] displayed atypical fibroblasts. Myointimal proliferation of vessels was observed in 67 percent of cases, with lipid-laden macrophages within the intima of arteries in 21 percent of specimens (Fig. 11-2). Phlebothrombosis was identified rarely.

The seminal vesicles showed atrophy and fibrosis in 89 percent of cases, but retained the characteristic golden-brown epithelial pigment (Fig. 11-3). Squamous metaplasia and cytologic atypia were observed in the transitional epithelium of large prostatic ducts and the prostatic urethra.

RADIATION CHANGES IN PROSTATIC CARCINOMA

According to Bostwick et al.,[12] the only finding indicative of radiation injury in the neoplastic prostate was a decrease in the number of tumor glands; in 43 percent of samples, the tumor was absent (Fig. 11-4). Most specimens harboring residual carcinoma had decreased tumor mass. In cases exhibiting an abundance of tumor postradiation, tumor regrowth from incompletely ablated neoplasm was assumed.

The grade of the tumor did not appear to change following radiation therapy (Fig. 11-5).

There was no evidence of tumor dedifferentiation, and the response to irradiation appeared to be equal in well-, moderately, and poorly differentiated neoplasms. Cytologic abnormalities, including variations in nuclear size and shape, abnormal chromatin staining pattern, and prominent nucleoli, were observed after radiation in both neoplastic and non-neoplastic glands. Mitotic figures were scarce before and after radiation therapy, without an increase in the number of atypical forms.

In the majority of postradiation specimens, there was no difficulty in determining the presence or absence of neoplasm. The few cases in which there were suspicious cells or glands were resolved by examining multiple levels or employing acid mucin stains. Perineural and lymphatic invasion was identified in 6 of 40 pretreatment biopsies (15 percent), with a similar incidence in biopsies displaying residual tumor following irradiation.[12]

Keisling et al.[41] noted that the ultrastructural features of prostatic adenocarcinoma postradiation were indistinguishable from those of untreated carcinoma, and they concluded that residual tumor is viable.

A grading system for assessing tumor aggressiveness following radiation or hormonal treatment has recently been described.[19,42]

IMMUNOHISTOCHEMISTRY AS A DIAGNOSTIC AID

Basal cell-specific antikeratin monoclonal antibodies have been shown to be useful in distinguishing benign glands from prostatic carcinoma, with only the former displaying immunoreactivity (Figs. 11-6 and 11-7).[43-45] Recently, Brawer et al.[46] employed antibodies directly against cytokeratin number 5 (basal cell-specific)[47] to stain biopsy specimens of 37 patients who had undergone definitive external beam radiation therapy. Positive immunoreactivity was observed in all benign acini and ductules, but there was no staining of malignant glands (Figs. 11-8 and 11-9). In four cases, the diagnosis of carcinoma was believed to be

Fig. 11-6. Preirradiation prostatic biopsy showing normal glands stained with basal cell-specific antikeratin monoclonal antibody KA1. Note staining restricted to the basal cell layer, with nonreactivity of lumenal cells. (PAP, ×190.) (From Brawer et al,[46] with permission.)

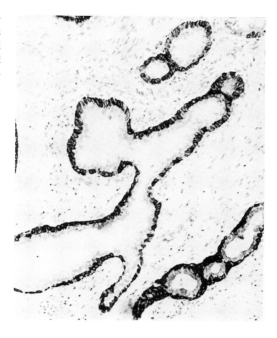

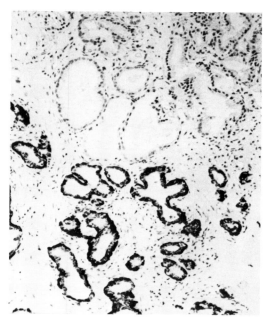

Fig. 11-7. Preirradiation prostatic biopsy showing normal glands (lower field) and low-grade carcinoma (upper field) reacted with KA1. Note the loss of basal cell reactivity in the carcinomatous glands. (PAP, ×190.) (From Brawer et al,[46] with permission.)

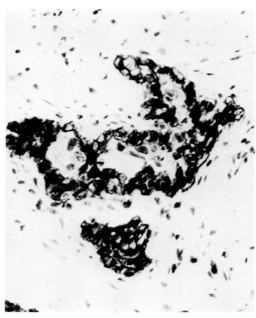

Fig. 11-8. Postradiation prostatic biopsy showing atypical proliferation within a benign gland. Note the lack of normal basal cell/lumenal cell polarity, cellular atypia, and increased proportion of cells reacting with KA1. (PAP, ×480.) (From Brawer et al,[46] with permission.)

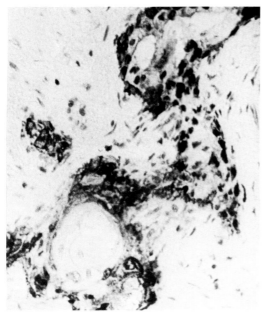

Fig. 11-9. Postradiation prostatic biopsy showing an area of squamous metaplasia. Note the large squamoid cells are only focally reactive with KA1. (PAP, ×480.) (From Brawer et al,[46] with permission.)

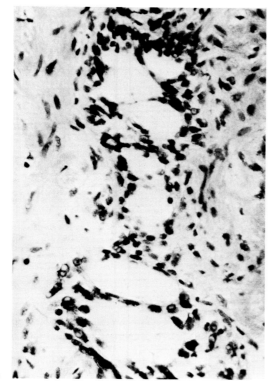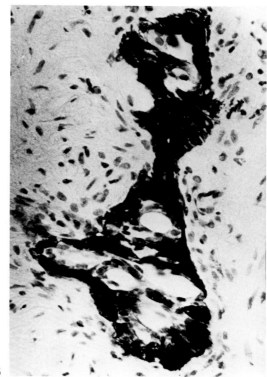

A   B

Fig. 11-10. Serial sections of a postradiation prostatic biopsy stained with hematoxylin and eosin (**A**) and reacted with KA1 (**B**). Note cellular atypia and cribriform patterns seen in the hematoxylin and eosin-stained section in Figure A. Staining with KA1 (Figure B) reveals basal cell reaction pattern typical of irradiated glands. (PAP, ×480.) (From Brawer et al,[46] with permission.)

equivocal based on hematoxylin and eosin-stained slides; in these cases, the glands displayed disordered proliferation of atypical cells (Fig. 11-10). These proliferations displayed basal cell-specific antikeratin immunoreactivity with extension of staining throughout the cell layers; the pattern was different from that seen in basal cell hyperplasia, in which the normal lumenal (secretory cell layer) was devoid of basal cell-specific immunoreactivity. This unique pattern was observed only in irradiated specimens, and they concluded that the lesion was benign. The authors noted that basal cell-specific keratin staining was a useful adjunct to surgical pathologic diagnosis postradiation, allowing differentiation of benign atypical lesions from carcinoma.[46]

REFERENCES

1. Paschkis R, Pittinger W: Radiumbehandlung eines Prostatasarkoms. Wein Klin Wochensch 48, 1910
2. Young HH: Technique of radium treatment of cancer of prostate and seminal vesicles. Surg Gynecol Obstet 34:93, 1922
3. Bagshaw MA, Kaplan HS, Sagerman RH: Linear accelerator supervoltage radiotherapy. VII. Carcinoma of the prostate. Radiology 85:121, 1965
4. Bagshaw MA: Radiation therapy for cancer of the prostate. p. 345. In Skinner DG, Lieskovsky G (eds): Diagnosis and Management of Genitourinary Cancer. WB Saunders, Philadelphia, 1988
5. Kagan AR, Gordon J, Cooper JF, et al: A clinical appraisal of post-irradiation biopsy in prostatic cancer. Cancer 39:637, 1977

6. Schellhammer PF, Lagada LE, El-Mahdi A: Histological characteristics of prostatic biopsies after iodine-125 implantation. J Urol 123:700, 1980

7. Carlton CE Jr, Dawoud F, Hudgins P, Scott R Jr: Irradiation treatment of carcinoma of the prostate: a preliminary report based on eight years of experience. J Urol 108:924, 1972

8. Pistenma DA, Bagshaw MA, Freiha FS: Extended-field radiation therapy for prostatic adenocarcinoma: status report of a limited prospective trial. p. 229. In Johnson DE, Samuels ML (eds): Cancer of the Genitourinary Tract. Raven Press, New York, 1979

9. Fujino A, Scardino PT: Transrectal ultrasonography for prostatic cancer II. The response of the prostate to definitive radiotherapy. Cancer 5:935, 1986

10. Scardino PT, Frankel JM, Wheeler TM, et al: The prognostic significance of post-irradiation biopsy results in patients with prostatic cancer. J Urol 135:510, 1986

11. Freiha FS, Bagshaw MA: Carcinoma of the prostate: results of post-irradiation biopsy. Prostate 5:19, 1984

12. Bostwick DG, Egbert BM, Fajardo LF: Radiation injury of the normal and neoplastic prostate. Am J Surg Pathol 6:541, 1982

13. Scardino PT: The prognostic significance of biopsies after radiotherapy for prostatic cancer. Semin Urol 1:243, 1983

14. Kiesling VJ, McAninch JW, Goebel JL, Agee RE: External beam radiotherapy for adenocarcinoma of the prostate: a clinical followup. J Urol 124:851, 1980

15. Cox DJ, Stoffel TJ: The significance of needle biopsy after irradiation for stage C adenocarcinoma of the prostate. Cancer 40:156, 1977

16. Leach GE, Cooper JF, Kagan AR: Radiotherapy for prostatic carcinoma: post-irradiation prostatic biopsy and recurrence patterns with long-term followup. J Urol 128:505, 1982

17. Herr HW, Whitmore WF Jr: Significance of prostatic biopsies after radiation therapy for carcinoma of the prostate. Prostate 3:339, 1982

18. Cosgrove MD, George FW, Terry T: The effects of treatment on the local lesion of carcinoma of the prostate. J Urol 109:861, 1973

19. Dhom G, Degro S: Therapy of prostatic cancer and histopathologic followup. Prostate 3:531, 1982

20. Bagshaw MA: Radiation therapy of prostatic carcinoma. p. 405. In Crawford ED, Borden TA (eds): Genitourinary Cancer Surgery, Lea & Fibeger, Philadelphia, 1982

21. Whitmore WF Jr: Interstitial radiation therapy for carcinoma of the prostate. Prostate 1:157, 1980

22. Neglia WJ, Hussey DH, Johnson DE: Megavoltage radiation therapy of carcinoma of the prostate. Int J Radiat Oncol Biol Phys 2:873, 1977

23. Kurth KH, Altwein JE, Skoluda D, Hohenfellner R: Followup of irradiated prostatic carcinoma by aspiration biopsy. J Urol 117:615, 1977

24. Rhamy RK, Wilson SK, Caldwell WL: Biopsy-proved tumor following definitive radiation for resectable carcinoma of the prostate. J Urol 107:627, 1972

25. Cupps RE, Utz DC, Fleming TR, et al: Definitive radiation therapy for prostatic carcinoma: Mayo Clinic experience. J Urol 124:855, 1980

26. Nachtshein DA, McAninch JW, Stutzman RE, Goubel JL: Latent residual tumor following external radiotherapy for prostate adenocarcinoma. J Urol 120:312, 1978

27. Jacobi GH, Hohenfellner R: Staging management and post-treatment reevaluation of prostate cancer: dogma questioned. p. 31. In Jacobi GH, Hohenfellner R (eds): Prostate Cancer. Williams & Wilkins, Baltimore, 1982

28. Lytton B, Collins JT, Weiss RM, et al: Results of biopsy after early stage prostatic cancer treatment by implantation of I-125 seeds. J Urol 121:306, 1979

29. Leibel SA, Pino Y, Torres JL: Improved quality of life following radical radiation therapy for early stage carcinoma of the prostate. Urol Clin North Am 7:593, 1980

30. Perez CA, Walz BH, Zivnuska FR, et al: Irradiation of carcinoma of the prostate localized to the pelvis: analysis of tumor response and prognosis. Int J Radiat Oncol Biol Phys 6:555, 1980

31. Gibbons RP, Mason JT, Correa RJ Jr, et al: Carcinoma of the prostate: local control with external beam radiation therapy. J Urol 121:310, 1979

32. Rainwater LM, Zincke H: Radical prostatectomy after radiation therapy for cancer of the prostate: feasibility and prognosis. J Urol 140:1455, 1988

33. Cumes DM, Gofinnet DR, Martinez A, Stamey

TA: Complications of Iodine-125 implantation in pelvic lymphadenectomy for prostatic cancer with special reference to patients who have failed external beam therapy as their initial mode of therapy. J Urol 126:620, 1981

34. Goffinet DR, Martinez A, Freiha F, et al: Iodine-125 prostate implants for recurrent carcinoma after external beam irradiation: preliminary results. Cancer 45:2717, 1980

35. Mador DR, Huben RP, Wajsman Z, Pontes JE: Salvage surgery following radical radiotherapy for adenocarcinoma of the prostate. J Urol 133:58, 1985

36. Carson CC, Zincke H, Utz DC, Radical prostatectomy after radiotherapy for prostatic cancer. J Urol 124:237, 1980

37. Ahlering TE, Lieskovsky G, Skinner DG: Salvage options following radiotherapy failures. p. 454. In Skinner DG, Lieskovsky G: Diagnosis and Management of Genitourinary Cancer. WB Saunders, Philadelphia, 1988

38. Musselman PW, Tubbs R, Connelly RW, et al: Biological significance of prostatic carcinoma after definitive radiation therapy. J Urol 137: 114A, 1987

39. Mollenkamp JS, Cooper JF, Kagan AR: Clinical experience with supervoltage radiotherapy in carcinoma of the prostate: a preliminary report. J Urol 113:374, 1975

40. Mahan DE, Bruce AW, Manley PN, Franchi

L: Immunohistochemical evaluation of prostatic carcinoma before and after radiotherapy. J Urol 124:488, 1980

41. Kiesling VJ, Friedman HI, McAninch JW, et al: The ultrastructural changes of prostatic adenocarcinoma following external beam radiation therapy. J Urol 122:633, 1979

42. Helpap B: Treated prostatic carcinoma: histological, immunohistochemical, and cell kinetic studies. Appl Pathol 3:230, 1985

43. Brawer MK, Bostwick DG, Peehl DM, Stamey TA: Keratin protein in human prostatic tissue and cell culture. Ann NY Acad Sci 455:729, 1986

44. Brawer MK, Peehl DM, Stamey TA, Bostwick DG: Keratin immunoreactivity in the benign and neoplastic human prostate. Cancer Res 45:3663, 1985

45. Bostwick DG, Brawer MK: Prostatic intraepithelial neoplasia (PIN) and early invasion in prostatic cancer. Cancer 59:788, 1987

46. Brawer MK, Nagle RB, Pitts W, et al: Keratin immunoreactivity as an aid to the diagnosis of persistent adenocarcinoma in irradiated human prostates. Cancer 63:454, 1989

47. Nagle RFB, Ahmann FR, McDaniel KM, et al: Cytokeratin characterization of human prostatic carcinoma and its derived cell lines. Cancer Res 47:281, 1987

12

Surgical Pathology of the Male Urethra and Seminal Vesicles

John R. Srigley and R. Warren J. Hartwick

THE MALE URETHRA

SURGICAL ANATOMY AND HISTOLOGY

The male urethra can be anatomically divided into prostatic, bulbomembranous, and penile regions (Fig. 12-1). The prostatic and membranous portions have been referred to as the proximal (posterior) urethra, and the bulbous and penile as the distal (anterior) urethra.[1] The prostatic urethra begins at the bladder neck in the region of the internal urethral orifice and continues to the level of the urogenital diaphragm. The prostatic urethra usually measures about 4 cm in length, and can be further subdivided into proximal and distal segments with the verumontanum as the dividing point. The prostatic urethra at the base of the verumontanum angles anteriorly at about 35 degrees.[2] The prostatic utricle and ejaculatory ducts pass through the verumontanum to open into the prostatic urethra. The ostia of the prostatic ducts are situated in a double row on either side of the verumontanum continuing proximally and distally along the prostatic urethra. The membranous urethra, which measures about 2 to 2.5 cm in length, traverses the urogenital diaphragm and is surrounded by muscle fibers serving a sphincteric function. The bulbous urethra is a capacious segment located immediately distal to the urogenital diaphragm at the root of the penis. It is about 3 to 4 cm in length, and usually is considered together with the membranous portion when discussing neoplastic disease. The penile or pendulous urethra continues from the bulbous portion for about 12 to 14 cm. The penile segment ends in the region of the fossa navicularis, which is immediately proximal to the external urethral meatus.

The proximal prostatic urethra is lined by transitional epithelium similar to that seen in the bladder. Superficial (umbrella) cells are readily identified. This typical transitional mucosa blends imperceptibly into pseudostratified or stratified columnar epithelium typifying the distal prostatic, bulbomembranous, and most of the penile urethra (Fig. 12-2). In the distal portion of the penile urethra and fossa navicularis, a stratified nonkeratinizing squamous epithelium is seen that is continuous with the mucosa of the external meatus. The subepithelial connective tissue of the urethra is variable in amount and nearly always contains a slight infiltrate of lymphocytes.

Shallow periurethral prostatic glands composed of short ducts and acini are identified along the proximal segment of the prostatic urethra. The bulbourethral or Cowper's glands are paired tubuloalveolar glands that reside in the fibromuscular tissue of the urogenital diaphragm. Their paired excretory ducts enter the posterior aspect of the bulbous urethra. The secretory acini of Cowper's glands are composed of cuboidal to columnar cells with dark, basally located nuclei and abundant mucinous cytoplasm. These glands may be occasionally encountered in transurethral resectates and needle biopsies. A number of shallow mucus-secreting glands (Littre's glands) are situated in the lateral walls of the anterior urethra.

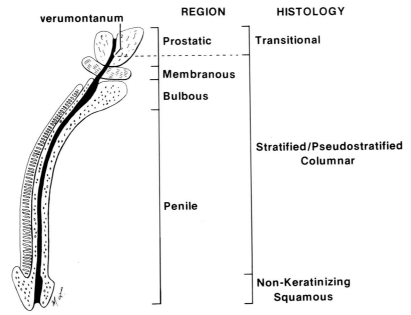

REGION   **HISTOLOGY**

verumontanum

Prostatic — Transitional

Membranous

Bulbous

Penile — Stratified/Pseudostratified Columnar

Non-Keratinizing Squamous

Fig. 12-1. Line drawing showing anatomic regions of male urethra with histologic correlates.

Surgical specimens representing urethral disease are usually incisional or excisional biopsies of ulcers, nodules, polyps, or strictures. Transurethral resectates are commonly obtained from the prostatic urethra. Formal urethrectomy specimens may be seen either alone or in combination with cystoprostatectomies. Super-radical excisions, including portions of pubic bone, penis, scrotum, and anorectal canal, may be encountered in cases of advanced urethral cancer.

CONGENITAL ANOMALIES

A number of congenital abnormalities may affect the urethra, including hypospadias, epispadias, urethral duplication, congenital cysts, and megalourethra.[3, 4] Additionally, both posterior and anterior urethral valves may occur, resulting in complete or incomplete outflow obstruction with or without urinary tract infection.[4] These congenital diseases are usually encountered in the pediatric population and are rarely, if ever, seen by practicing surgical pathologists.

DIVERTICULUM

Urethral diverticula are usually seen in women, and are thought to be secondary to trauma and/or obstruction of periurethral ducts. Malignancy, usually in the form of adenocarcinoma, may complicate urethral diverticula in women.[5] Diverticula of the male urethra are exceedingly uncommon, but have been associated with prior surgery or infection such as tuberculosis. Carcinoma arising in a diverticulum in a male has only rarely been described.[6]

URETHRITIS

A variety of specific and nonspecific infections may affect the urethra. Acute urethritis may be subdivided into gonorrheal and nongonorrheal varieties. Gonorrhea is caused by *Neisseria gonorrhoeae*, a gram-negative diplococcus. Patients with gonorrhea usually present with a yellow urethral discharge often accompanied by irritative voiding symptoms. The diagnosis is usually made on clinical grounds. Bi-

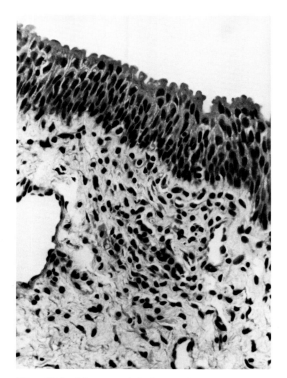

Fig. 12-2. Mucosa of bulbomembranous urethra. Note the pseudostratified columnar epithelium with mild chronic inflammation in lamina propria. (H&E, ×250.)

opsies from acute gonorrheal urethritis are exceedingly uncommon, but may show florid suppurative inflammation along with the typical diplococci. Progression to chronic urethritis with or without stricture formation may be seen. Biopsy from a gonorrhea-associated stricture usually shows only nonspecific chronic inflammation. Definitive diagnosis is usually made on clinical and microbiologic grounds rather than with histopathology.

A host of other groups of organisms, including staphylococci, *Escherichia coli, Mycoplasma,* and *Chlamydia,* have been implicated in nongonorrheal (nonspecific) urethritis. *Chlamydia* is most often implicated as causative in nonspecific urethritis.[7] However, biopsies are rarely performed, and if done usually show only nonspecific chronic inflammation.

Granulomatous inflammation of the urethra is relatively uncommon. Urethral tuberculosis is well described and usually thought to be secondary to upper urinary tract foci.[8] Tuberculosis may present as a stricture, urethral dilatation, or fistulization. The histologic specimen shows typical caseous granulomas in which acid-fast organisms may be identified. Other fungal or parasitic causes of granulomatous urethritis are exceptionally rare. With the increasing usage of Calmette-Guerin bacillus (BCG) to treat superficial bladder cancer, BCG-associated granulomas may occasionally be encountered in prostatic urethral biopsies (Fig. 12-3).

Uncommon forms of urethritis include follicular urethritis and polypoid urethritis. These lesions are identical to their counterparts in the bladder.[9, 10] Polypoid urethritis can endoscopically simulate papillary neoplasms of the

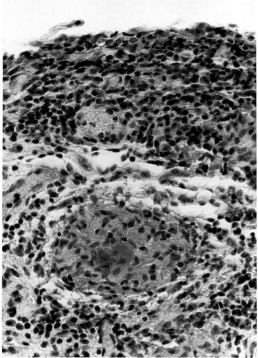

Fig. 12-3. Biopsy of prostatic urethra from patient receiving intravesical BCG therapy. Note denuded mucosa (top) with underlying chronic inflammation and noncaseating granuloma. (H&E, ×250.)

urethra.[11] Histologically, these polyps are covered with a urethral mucosa and the cores are markedly edematous, often with a sprinkling of acute and chronic inflammatory cells (Fig. 12-4). In many cases, this process is thought to be secondary to catheterization or instrumentation.

CONDYLOMA

Condyloma acuminatum of the male urethra is relatively common and usually occurs in young men. Most cases are confined to the distal urethra, but involvement of the proximal urethra and bladder may be seen. Most cases have a typical exophytic appearance, although papular variants of flat condyloma may be seen.

The histologic appearance is typical of condyloma at other sites. Mucosal acanthosis, papillomatosis with hyper- and parakeratosis, and focal koilocytotic atypia are seen. The differential diagnosis includes nonspecific fibroepithelial polyps and squamous papilloma. Condylomata are strongly associated with human papillomaviruses, especially types 6 and 11 (Fig. 12-5). Interestingly, in patients with clinical or subclinical human papillomavirus infection of the penis, the distal urethra is thought to be a reservoir for virus even in the absence of a clinical urethral lesion.[12]

MALAKOPLAKIA

Rare examples of malakoplakia of the urethra are noted in the literature.[13, 14] It may involve the urethra alone or be associated with bladder lesions. The histology is typical of malakoplakia at other sites. Sheets of histiocytes with granular eosinophilic cytoplasm admixed with neutrophils, lymphocytes, and plasma cells are noted. Typical Michaelis-Gutmann bodies must be present in order to make a diagnosis (Fig. 12-6). Malakoplakia is believed to be an unusual manifestation of bacterial infection in which there is an incomplete metabolism of bacteria.[15]

LOCALIZED AMYLOIDOSIS

Occasional examples of localized amyloidosis of the male urethra have been reported.[16, 17] The patients usually have hematuria, and a thickened urethral segment may be palpable. These lesions often present as indurated tumor-like

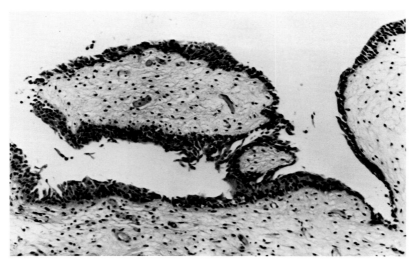

Fig. 12-4. Polypoid urethritis. Note the edematous polyp covered by focally attenuated urothelium. This patient had a history of urethral instrumentation. (H&E, ×100.)

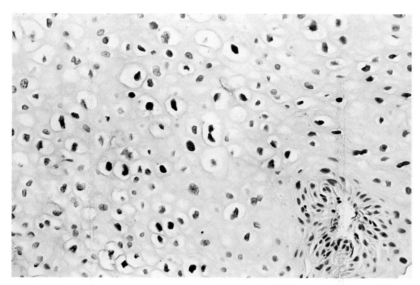

Fig. 12-5. Photomicrograph of urethral condyloma showing positivity for human papillomavirus types 6 and 11. Note the intense staining of koilocyte nuclei. (In situ hybridization using HPV 6/11 probe with the avidin-biotin detection system.) (Case courtesy of Dr. Rita Kandel, Mount Sinai Hospital, Toronto, Ontario, Canada.) (×450.)

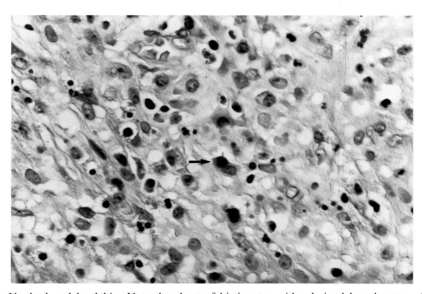

Fig. 12-6. Urethral malakoplakia. Note the sheet of histiocytes with admixed lymphocytes. Centrally, a laminated Michaelis-Guttman body is seen (arrow). (H&E, ×400.)

masses that are suspicious for carcinoma. At the microscopic level, typical amorphous sheets of eosinophilic material are seen, frequently with nonspecific chronic inflammation and foreign-body giant cells. The amyloid nature of the process can be confirmed by histochemistry or ultrastructural analysis.

PROLIFERATIVE (METAPLASTIC) URETHRITIS INCLUDING NEPHROGENIC ADENOMA

The urethra, as part of the "urothelial field," can undergo metaplastic changes similar to counterparts seen in the bladder and upper urinary tract. Not uncommonly, Von Brunn's nests of minor foci of squamous metaplasia may be noted. Squamous metaplasia is more frequently encountered in patients with chronic indwelling catheters, and may also be seen after urethral infection such as gonorrhea.[18] Urethritis cystica and glandularis may also be noted in the urethra. Frequently, these metaplastic changes are associated with a mild nonspecific chronic inflammatory infiltrate that may or may not be pathogenetically related. A causal relationship between these forms of metaplasia and urethral carcinoma is at best speculative.

Nephrogenic adenoma (metaplasia) may also be encountered in the urethra, especially the prostatic segment.[19] Patients may present with hematuria or hemospermia and have a papillary or nodular lesion detected by urethroscopy. Histologically, a papillary lesion is often seen in which transitional epithelium is replaced by a

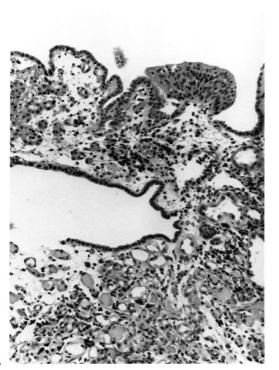
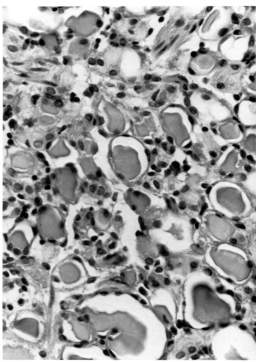

A   B

Fig. 12-7. Nephrogenic adenoma of the urethra. **(A)** Note the papillary surface configuration. An island of transitional epithelium (upper right) alternates with cuboidal surface epithelium. In the underlying stroma, a proliferation of tubules is seen. (H&E, ×100.) **(B)** Nephrogenic tubules containing hyalinized luminal material. (H&E, ×400.)

single layer of cuboidal to columnar cells. This glandular epithelium may dip into the underlying connective tissue and be associated with a proliferation of small tightly packed tubules containing eosinophilic luminal secretions. The appearance is similar to the "thyroidization" of chronic pyelonephritis. The small tubules in the lamina propria bear a striking resemblance to renal tubules (Fig. 12-7). This lesion enters the differential diagnosis of a urethral polyp, and, when encountered in the prostatic urethra, may simulate prostatic acinar carcinoma. Nephrogenic adenoma is generally considered benign, although some investigators have noted the rare association of nephrogenic adenoma and urethral carcinoma, suggesting a relationship between these two conditions.[20, 21]

URETHRAL POLYPS

The differential diagnosis of urethral polyps is shown in Table 12-1. A variety of developmental, inflammatory, metaplastic, and neoplastic processes may appear as urethral polyps to the endoscopist. Polypoid (papillary) urethritis, condyloma, and nephrogenic adenoma have been previously discussed, and papillary neopla-

sia is addressed in the subsequent section. The discussion in this section will be confined to nonspecific fibroepithelial polyps and adenomatous polyps of prostatic origin.

Fibroepithelial Polyps

Fibroepithelial polyps are uncommon urethral lesions usually seen in young boys, with about 70 percent of cases occurring in boys under the age of 10. The usual fibroepithelial polyp consists of a fibrovascular core covered by transitional and/or squamous epithelium. These polyps bear a striking resemblance to the well-described fibroepithelial polyps of the upper urinary tract. Patients usually present with bladder outlet obstruction, with or without urinary tract infection. Some investigators regard these lesions are congenital anomalies, although their occurrence in older patients would argue against this hypothesis.[22] Some investigators have identified nerve fibers and smooth muscle in the stroma of pediatric cases, raising the possibility of a hamartoma.[22] Alternatively, fibroepithelial polyps may arise from pre-existing polypoid urethritis, in which the edematous stroma undergoes fibrosis.[23]

Table 12-1. Differential Diagnosis of Urethral Polyps in Males

Type	Usual Age Range (yrs)	Usual Location[a]	Proposed Pathogenesis
Fibroepithelial polyp	< 10	P	Developmental (? postinflammatory)
Polypoid urethritis	Wide range	P	Inflammatory
Nephrogenic adenoma	Wide range	P	Metaplastic
Condyloma accuminatum	20-40	D	Virus-associated proliferation
Urethral polyp of prostatic origin	20-40	P	Developmental ectopia +/− hyperplasia
Squamous papilloma	20-40	D	Hyperplastic/neoplastic
Transitional cell papilloma	> 40	P	Neoplastic
Papillary carcinoma	> 40	T (P>D)	Neoplastic

[a] P, proximal urethra; D, distal urethra; T, total urethra.

Urethral Polyps of Prostatic Origin

Exophytic lesions containing prostatic tissue are occasionally encountered in the prostatic urethra, especially in the region of the verumontanum.[24] A variety of terms have been applied to these lesions, including *adenomatous polyp of prostatic urethra, prostatic urethral polyp, papillary adenoma of prostatic urethra,* and *prostatic caruncle,* to name a few.[25-28] Their etiology is not well established, although they probably represent ectopia secondary to developmental anomalies. A recent paper, which discussed prostatic-type polyps involving bladder, ureteric orifices, and urethra suggested that the pathogenesis at each site may be different.[29] The bladder lesions were thought to possibly be variants of cystitis cystica glandularis and the ureteric orifice polyps, developmental abnormalities. The urethral prostatic polyps were thought to represent a hyperplastic process.

The typical patient is a young male in the third or fourth decade of life presenting with hemospermia or hematuria. The endoscopist identifies a posterior urethral polyp and takes a biopsy. Histologically, these lesions are polypoid nodules covered in part by a papillary/glandular prostatic epithelium or by a mixture of prostatic and transitional epithelium (Fig. 12-8A). The core of the polyp frequently contains prostatic glands, often surrounded by typical fibromuscular stroma. Corpora amylacea may be identified. Using immunohistochemical markers for prostate-specific antigen and pros-

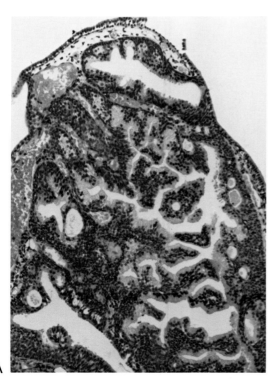
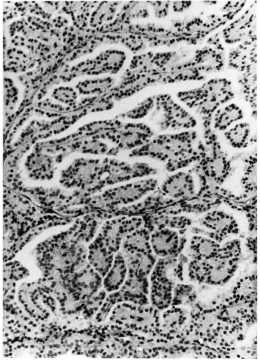

A   B

Fig. 12-8. Two examples of prostatic polyps in the posterior urethra. Both cases were positive for prostate-specific markers. **(A)** Note the relatively normal-appearing prostate epithelium within the polyp. (H&E, ×80.) **(B)** Note the micropapillary proliferation of cuboidal epithelium with delicate vascular stalks. This pattern might best be referred to as a papillary adenoma or localized hyperplasia arising within ectopic prostate. (H&E, ×250.)

tatic acid phosphatase, strong positivity can usually be demonstrated, confirming prostatic histogenesis. On occasion, the prostatic tissue shows a degree of epithelial hyperplasia (Fig. 12-8B).

Nearly all of these lesions pursue a benign course when treated by local resection, and are not thought to be pathogenetically related to carcinoma. Interestingly, there is one report of a so-called endometrioid adenocarcinoma of the prostate that was topographically related to a prostatic urethral polyp.[30] Both the neoplasm and associated prostatic ectopia showed positively for prostate-specific markers. This observation has been used as an argument against the concept of utricular or true endometrial carcinoma of the prostate, a topic that is discussed in Chapters 7 and 9.

EPITHELIAL NEOPLASMS OF THE URETHRA

Papillomas

A variety of papillomas similar to those seen in the bladder may be encountered in the urethra. Squamous cell papilloma may resemble both condyloma accuminatum and fibroepithelial polyp. It is characterized by a papillary proliferation of squamous epithelium with rather delicate fibrovascular stalks. An absence of abnormal keratinization and koilocytotic atypia distinguishes squamous papilloma from condyloma accuminatum.

Transitional cell papillomas consisting of delicate fibrovascular stalks covered by relatively normal-appearing urothelium may be rarely encountered. These tumors have delicate stalks covered by transitional epithelium with fewer than seven cell layers and showing umbrella cell differentiation. Inverted papilloma may also be seen uncommonly in the urethra, where it usually presents as a nodule to the endoscopist.[31] These lesions have a similar appearance to counterparts in the bladder. Anastomotic cords of benign transitional epithelium showing focal microcyst change are seen beneath a normal or attenuated overlying mucosa (Fig. 12-9).

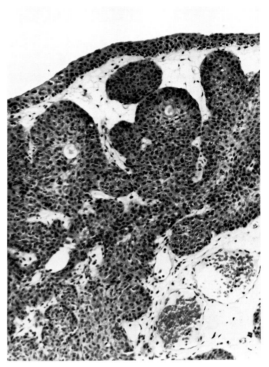

Fig. 12-9. Inverted papilloma of urethra. Note the attenuated surface urothelium with underlying anastomotic cords of benign transitional cells showing focal microcyst formation. (H&E, ×100.)

Primary Carcinoma of the Urethra

Primary carcinoma of the male urethra is an uncommon tumor, with about 600 reported cases.[32] In contrast to bladder cancer, urethral carcinoma is two to four times more prevalent in females than males. It usually affects patients in the fifth to ninth decades.

Associations include urethral stricture, venereal disease, and trauma. Cases of carcinoma developing after urethroplasty for stricture have been documented.[33] There is a strong association between urethral carcinoma and bladder cancer (see below).

Carcinoma of the male urethra usually presents clinically with bleeding, discharge, or urethral obstruction. A palpable mass or urethral fistula is commonly seen. Most urethral carcinomas originate in the bulbomembranous segment, followed in frequency by the penile and prostatic regions[34] (Fig. 12-10).

Histologically, urethral carcinomas in males are usually sqaumous cell, accounting for about 75 percent of cases (Fig. 12-11). Transitional cell carcinoma and adenocarcinoma account for about 15 and 4 percent of cases, respectively[32, 35] (Fig. 12-12). Rare examples of undifferentiated, cloacogenic, and adenosquamous carcinoma have been described.[36, 37]

The histogenetic subtype of carcinoma correlates to a certain extent with anatomic site of origin.[32, 34-35] Transitional cell carcinoma is the most frequent type noted in the bulbomembranous and penile regions. Adenocarcinoma nearly always originates in the bulbomembranous portion.[35] The exact histogenesis of urethral adenocarcinoma is particularly difficult to delineate. It may arise from multipotential surface mucosa, Cowper's glands or on rare occasions from paraurethral (Littre's) glands.[38, 39] In major resection and autopsy specimens it is useful to identify both Cowper's glands in order to rule out origin from these structures. However, Cowper's glands may be destroyed in large invasive tumors, leaving histogenesis somewhat open to speculation. At a practical level, the exact origin of urethral adenocarcinoma is not usually important. It is important, however, to rule out prostatic cancer masquerading as a urethral tumor by performing appropriate immunohistochemical studies.[35]

Urethral carcinoma may be graded using a three- or four-grade system, but this information is of less clinical importance than stage designation (Table 12-2).[40, 41] The depth of infiltration distinguishes the earlier stages of urethral carcinoma. Tumors arising in the anterior (distal) urethra tend to metastasize to inguinal lymph nodes, similar to penile carcinoma. However, inguinal lymphadenopathy in patients with urethral primaries is more likely to be caused by metastases than by reactive changes, in contrast to penile primaries.[40] Carcinoma arising in the posterior (proximal) urethra has a pattern of spread more akin to prostate cancer, with involvement of the iliac and obturator lymph nodes.

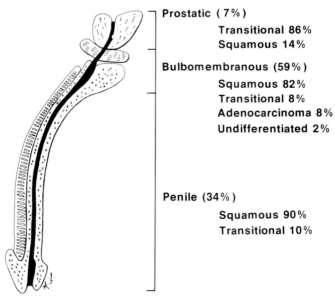

Prostatic (7 %)

Transitional 86 %
Squamous 14 %

Bulbomembranous (59 %)

Squamous 82 %
Transitional 8 %
Adenocarcinoma 8 %
Undifferentiated 2 %

Penile (34 %)

Squamous 90 %
Transitional 10 %

Fig. 12-10. Line drawing of the male urethra showing distribution of urethral carcinoma by site and histology. (Data from Johnson.[34])

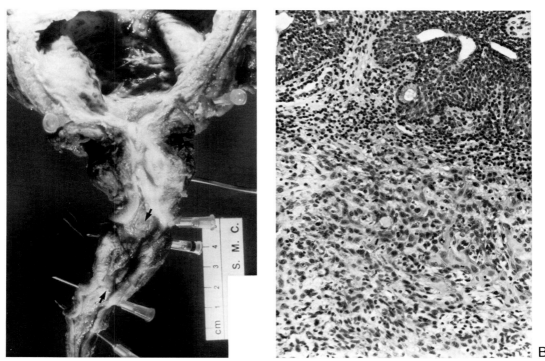

Fig. 12-11. (**A**) Gross photograph of urethrocystoprostatectomy specimen showing a noduloulcerative tumor in the bulbomembranous urethra (arrows). (**B**) Photomicrograph showing a poorly differentiated squamous cell carcinoma. Note Littre's glands at the top. (H&E, ×250.)

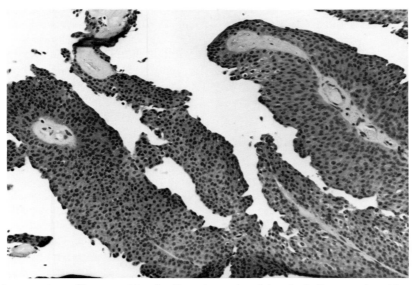

Fig. 12-12. Low-grade papillary transitional cell carcinoma involving the bulbous urethra. Note the cellular uniformity and occasional mitosis. (H&E, ×100.)

Table 12-2. Staging of Male Urethral Carcinoma

Stage Designation		Description
O		Intramural; no invasion
A		Invasion within lamina propria
B		Invasion limited to prostate gland or corpus spongiosum
C		Invasion through prostatic capsule or into corpora cavernosa, adjacent connective tissue or skin
D		Metastatic
	D1	Inguinal or pelvic lymph nodes
	D2	Distant sites

(Modified from Ray et al.,[40] with permission.)

The prognosis of urethral carcinoma is strongly related to the site of origin and stage, and is essentially unrelated to histologic subtype or grade. About 56 percent of distal urethral tumors are low stage (0,A,B), while only 14 percent of proximal tumors present as early-stage tumors.[40, 42] Overall, about two-thirds of male patients present with high-stage (C,D) tumors.[40] The overall 5-year survival rate for low-stage tumors is about 86 percent and for high-stage tumors is about 19 percent.[40]

Treatment options are protean, and may include excisional biopsy, transurethral resection, fulgarization, or urethrectomy for superficial low-grade tumors.[32, 34] Deeply invasive tumors of the distal urethra may be handled by partial or total penectomy. For tumors involving the bulbomembranous or prostatic regions, more radical surgery is often required. Total emasculation with en bloc cystoprostatectomy and pubic bone resection is sometimes recommended for bulbomembranous neoplasms, although the recurrence rate is still high and the long-term therapeutic benefit is largely unproven.[32] Radiation therapy alone has yielded poor results, and some investigators are advocating preoperative radiation followed by surgical resection.[32, 42, 43] Che-

motherapy has been applied anecdotally, yielding inconclusive results.[44]

Urethral Involvement in Bladder Cancer

Since the urethra is part of the "urothelial field," patients with bladder or upper urinary tract carcinoma are at risk of developing urethral carcinoma, usually of the transitional cell variety. Any site in the urethra may be involved, including the fossa navicularis. About 4 to 14 percent of patients who undergo radical cystoprostatectomy for bladder cancer will develop carcinoma in the urethral remnant.[32] Up to 22 percent of urethras removed at the time of cystoprostatectomy will contain foci of carcinoma in situ[45] (Fig. 12-13). The frequency of urethral involvement is related to the presence of multifocal planar carcinoma in situ, especially involving bladder neck or prostatic urethra on random biopsies. Cystoprostatectomy with en bloc total urethrectomy can be employed in the high-risk patient.[45] Alternatively, a two-stage approach may be undertaken using information derived from the surgical pathology of the initial cysto-

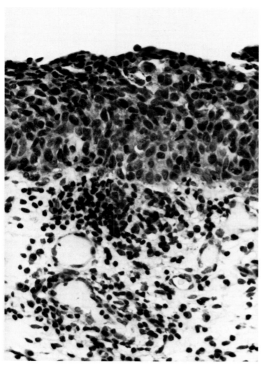

Fig. 12-13. Small cell variant of transitional carcinoma in situ involving the urethra removed with cystoprostatectomy for deeply invasive bladder carcinoma. (H&E, ×250.)

prostatectomy specimen. In the low-risk patient with a solitary lesion unrelated to the bladder neck and without accompanying carcinoma in situ, a more conservative approach may be advocated.[46] In these patients, close clinical follow-up, urethroscopy, and urethral wash cytology should be employed to monitor the urethral remnant.

MESENCHYMAL NEOPLASMS OF THE
URETHRA

Benign Connective Tissue Tumors

A variety of benign mesenchymal tumors of the urethra have been described. Hemangioma appears to be the most common mesenchymal

tumor of the male urethra.[47] Leiomyomas are the most common soft tissue tumors to affect the female urethra, but are only rarely seen in males.[48] Patients with these tumors may present with obstruction and/or bleeding. The histology is similar to counterparts in soft tissue sites.

Sarcomas

Sarcoma of the urethra is exceptionally uncommon, although leiomyosarcoma, rhabdomyosarcoma, fibrosarcoma, and unclassified sarcoma have been noted.[32, 49, 50] The histology of these tumors is similar to that seen in other sites. With large lesions, especially in the distal urethra, it is often difficult to determine whether the sarcoma arose from urethral connective tissue or penile mesenchyme, although this distinction is somewhat academic.

OTHER MALIGNANCIES OF THE URETHRA

Malignant Melanoma

Malignant melanoma of the male urethra has been well described in the literature.[51, 52] It usually occurs in the distal urethra around the fossa navicularis and external meatus, although 20 percent of reported cases were in the more proximal urethra.

Histologically, malignant melanoma of the urethra has an appearance similar to melanoma in other sites, with atypical melanocytes scattered along the epithelial-stromal junction. Intramucosal infiltration and stromal invasion by the melanin cells may be seen. The amount of melanin pigment present is variable, and amelanotic examples have been described. Histochemistry, immunocytochemistry and electron microscopy may be used to confirm a diagnosis in difficult cases. In one study using Breslow's thickness measurements, all urethral melanomas were 7 mm or thicker and had a dismal outcome.[52]

Malignant Lymphoma

Only a rare example of malignant lymphoma presenting as a urethral mass is found in the literature[53] (Fig. 12-14).

Secondary Neoplasms

The urethra is frequently involved by direct spread from carcinoma arising in the prostate gland or bladder. Rare examples of metastatic carcinoma of the urethra from distant sites such as kidney and colon have been seen.[54, 55] These patients usually present with urethral obstruction, pain, and hematuria. The diagnosis relies on clinicopathologic correlation.

SEMINAL VESICLES

SURGICAL ANATOMY AND HISTOLOGY

The seminal vesicles are paired secondary sex glands located posterior to the bladder and anterior to Denonvilliers' fascia (Fig. 12-15).

Embryologically, they arise as outpouchings from the ampulla, a dilated portion at the lower end of the mesonephric ducts.[56] The anterosuperior surface of the vesicles lies beneath the inferoposterior surface of the bladder and trigone. On occasion, the seminal vesicles may be partially situated within the capsule of the prostate gland. Seminal vesicles are variable in size and shape, usually measuring 5 to 6 cm in length and 1 to 2 cm in width. The overall size is related to patient age, functional status, and the presence of obstruction.

Histologically, the seminal vesicles consist of convoluted and capacious lumens lined by simple cuboidal to columnar epithelium and surrounded by a muscular wall that serve a contractile function. Frequently, the lining is thrown up into papillary folds, and there may be a proliferation of tubules in the underlying stroma. This feature may cause some confusion in the differential diagnosis with prostatic acinar carcinoma, especially in needle biopsy preparations that include some of these adenoid regions.[57] With age, there is often an increase in stromal fibrosis, sometimes to the extent that the epithelial architecture is markedly distorted.

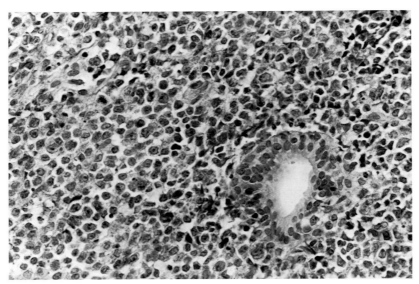

Fig. 12-14. Large cell lymphoma presenting as a urethral mass. Note the sheets of monotonous lymphoid cells around periurethral gland. (H&E, ×250.)

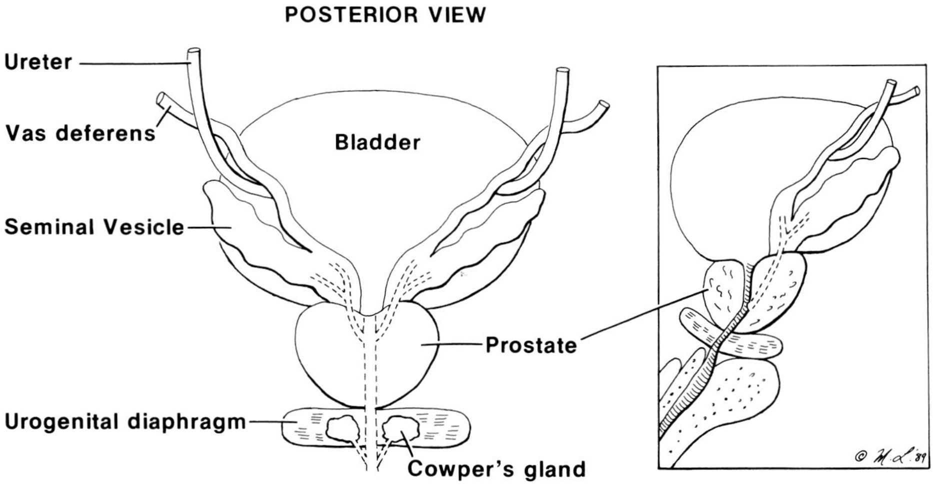

POSTERIOR VIEW

Fig. 12-15. Line drawing showing the anatomy of seminal vesicle and adjacent structures. Note location of Cowper's glands. The insert shows a parasagittal view.

AGE-ASSOCIATED EPITHELIAL ATYPIA

With advancing age, the epithelium of the seminal vesicles often shows cytologic atypia.[58, 59] Luminal cells with large irregular, hyperchromatic nuclei are seen (Fig. 12-16). Nuclear pseudoinclusions are frequently encountered. Mitoses are not seen, and the chromatin pattern is uniform and nonvesicular. Similar changes have been observed in the ejaculatory ducts and efferent ductules of the epididymides. Importantly, the cytoplasm of seminal vesicular epithelial cells frequently show lipochrome deposition. This pigment is refractile and has a yellow-brown coloration. The lipochrome deposits increase with age, and the presence of the pigment assists the surgical pathologist, especially in cases with crushed or tangentially cut seminal vesicles. The cytologic atypia, when coupled with tubular proliferation of epithelium and stromal fibrosis, can simulate infiltrating prostate cancer.[57] Atypical seminal vesicle cells have also caused cytopathologists difficulty in the interpretation of prostatic massage specimens.[60]

CONGENITAL ANOMALIES

Currently, the most common indication for seminal vesicle surgery is assessment of congenital anomalies.[61] A variety of abnormalities may be encountered because of the intimate relationship between the ureteric bud and mesonephric derivatives during embryogenesis. Of these, ureteral ectopy is probably the most common.[61] In men, ectopic ureters may terminate in the prostatic urethra, seminal vesicles, vasa deferentia, or ejaculatory ducts.[62] When ureters terminate in wolffian duct derivatives, they are often associated with ipsilateral renal dysgenesis and contralateral renal hypertrophy. Perineal and/or testicular pain may be noted, and a fluctuant cystic mass may be palpable on rectal examination. Treatment usually involves surgical exploration or unroofing of the enlarged seminal vesicle and ureterocele, with concomitant management of the renal and/or ureteral abnormality.[61]

Congenital absence of mesonephric duct-derived structures such as the vas deferens and seminal vesicles has also been described in the

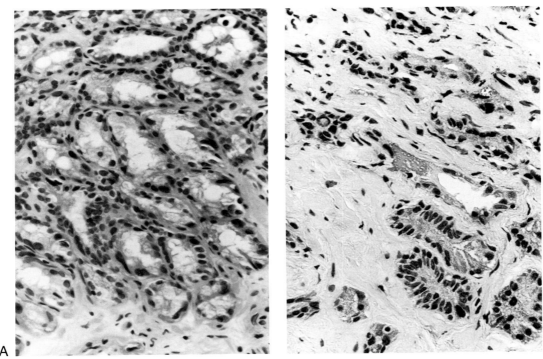

A   B

Fig. 12-16. (A) Tubular proliferation of seminal vesicle glands simulating small acinar carcinoma of prostate. (H&E, ×250.) (B) Tubular pattern of seminal vesicle glands showing cytologic atypia and stromal fibrosis. (H&E, ×250.)

setting of mucoviscidosis.[63] These disorders are rarely encountered by the general surgical pathologist, but may be occasionally seen in pediatric practice.

CYSTS OF THE SEMINAL VESICLE

Most seminal vesicle cysts are thought to arise from congenital obstruction at the level of the juncture between vesicle and ejaculatory duct.[61] The cysts are usually encountered in the third decade of life, and are nearly always solitary.[64] They may reach quite large sizes and have been termed *hydrops* by an occasional investigator.[65] Seminal vesicle cysts have been associated with renal agenesis.[66]

Cystic dilation of the seminal vesicle may also be acquired, secondary to prostatitis, leading to obstruction of the vesicle outflow tract (Fig. 12-17).

A number of other lesions enter the differen-

tial diagnosis of vesicle cysts, including cysts of wolffian and müllerian duct remnant, prostatic cysts, and diverticula of ejaculatory ducts.[61] Seminal vesicle cysts and diverticula of ejaculatory ducts may contain sperm on needle aspiration. Investigation of such cystic structures includes vasoseminal vesiculography, which affords excellent imaging detail of luminal abnormalities. Additionally, computed tomography and ultrasonography may be used in the investigation of cysts. Cysts of the seminal vesicles and related structures may be only occasionally encountered by the practicing surgical pathologist if a biopsy or cyst removal is undertaken.

VESICULITIS

Seminal vesicle surgery, usually in the form of perineal vesiculotomy, was popular in the late nineteenth and early twentieth centuries, as these organs were thought to be the source

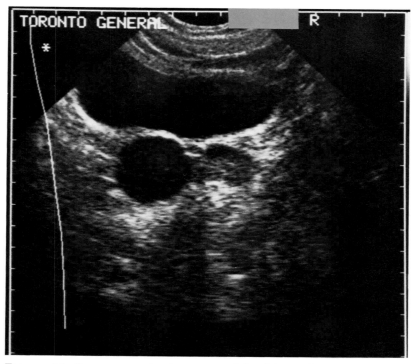

Fig. 12-17. Transurectal ultrasonogram showing a cyst of the right seminal vesicle from a 53-year-old man who presented with vague pelvic pain. (Case courtesy of Dr. Ans Toi, Department of Radiology, Toronto General Hospital, Toronto, Ontario, Canada.)

of infection leading to inflammatory rheumatism.[61] Tuberculosis of the seminal vesicles was also treated surgically until effective antibiotics were developed.[61] Today, vesiculitis may complicate epididymitis or prostatitis, but in these situations, seminal vesiculitis is rarely biopsied. On occasion, one may find inflamed seminal vesicle or ejaculatory duct tissue in transurethral resectates performed in the setting of prostatitis. Effective drugs are available to eradicate the bacteria that are the most common cause of prostatitis and vesiculitis. Tuberculosis and granulomatous fungal disease may also affect the seminal vesicles, but today these represent histologic curiosities.

LOCALIZED CALCIFICATION

Dystrophic calcification of the vas deferens and seminal vesicles may be encountered in longstanding diabetes mellitus, especially in older patients.[61] Reports of dystrophic calcification of the seminal vesicles secondary to chronic suppurative or granulomatous inflammation may be found in the older literature. Interestingly, calcification of the seminal vesicles and vas deferens has also been noted in patients with uremia.[67]

LOCALIZED AMYLOIDOSIS

Amyloid deposits are not uncommonly found in seminal vesicles removed at autopsy, radical prostatectomy, or cystoprostatectomy.[68] These deposits have been noted in about 14 percent of patients over the age of 70 years.[68] However, symptomatic localized amyloidosis of seminal vesicles is a distinctly uncommon phenomenon.[69] At the histologic level, large subepithelial nodular masses of amyloid are detected (Fig. 12-18). The diagnosis can be confirmed by ap-

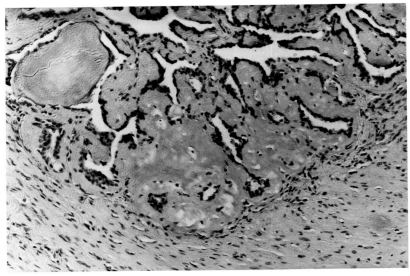

Fig. 12-18. Localized amyloidosis of seminal vesicles. Note the nodular subepithelial collections of amorphous material with distortion and irregularity of glands. (H&E, ×100.)

propriate histochemical and ultrastructural analysis.

NEOPLASMS

Secondary Neoplasms

Secondary neoplasms of the seminal vesicles are more common than primary tumors, and prostatic adenocarcinoma is the most common. Interestingly, in about 12 percent of presumed early-stage prostate cancers, involvement of the seminal vesicles is noted in radical prostatectomy specimens.[70] This pathologic upstaging is an adverse prognostic factor. Deeply invasive bladder cancer can also involve the seminal vesicles by direct extension. This is most commonly encountered in bladder lesions arising in the inferoposterior or trigonal regions. Recently, in situ spread of transitional cell carcinoma has been detected in ejaculatory ducts and seminal vesicles, although this mode is exceedingly uncommon[71] (Fig. 12-19). Direct extension of anorectal carcinoma of the glandular or undifferentiated variety may also be seen. Metastatic

involvement of the seminal vesicle from distant sources is rare.

Primary Neoplasms

Primary neoplasms of the seminal vesicles are uncommon. Rare cases of cystadenoma are found in the literature.[72, 73] An unusual epithelial/stromal tumor of the seminal vesicles with cytologic atypia has also been recently described.[74] The investigators suggested that this tumor may be a low-grade malignancy. Adenocarcinoma of the seminal vesicles may be seen, but origin at this site is often difficult to confirm, especially at an advanced stage. In a critical review of the experience at the Mayo Clinic, only 2 of 12 potential cases of seminal vesicle carcinoma were accepted.[75] The investigators also accepted 35 previously reported cases.[75, 76] In a 40-year review of the material at the Canadian Reference Centre for Cancer Pathology, only one of five cases accessioned as carcinoma of the seminal vesicle was a possible example of this tumor. The other four cases demonstrated positivity for prostatic specific markers, al-

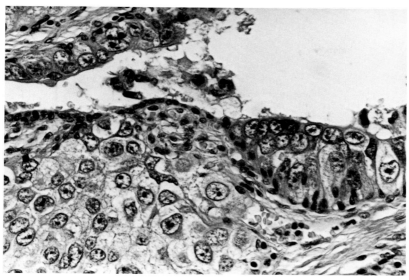

Fig. 12-19. Transitional cell carcinoma involving the seminal vesicles. Note the in situ involvement of the epithelium (middle right and upper left). An invasive component is seen in the lower left corner. (H&E, ×400.)

though the tumor epicenters appeared to be in the region of the seminal vesicle (Fig. 12-20).

Patients with adenocarcinoma of the seminal vesicle have a mean age of about 62 years, with a wide range (24 to 90 years).[75] Symptoms include those of bladder outlet obstruction and hematospermia. Seminal vesiculography, when performed, shows abnormalities. The computed

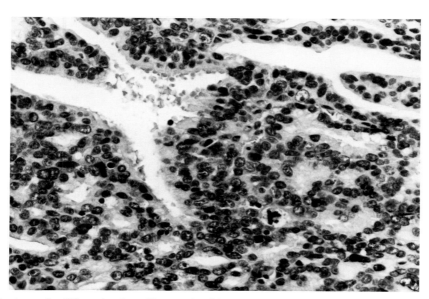

Fig. 12-20. A poorly differentiated papillary and solid neoplasm with its epicenter in the seminal vesicle. This case was coded as adenocarcinoma of the seminal vesicle, but showed focal positivity for prostate-specific antigen. (H&E, ×250.)

tomographic scan has recently proved of value in defining carcinoma of the seminal vesicle.[75] These tumors are usually papillary or anaplastic with mucin production, and show early invasion of the bladder, prostate, and rectum.

A number of criteria may be used in defining a case of probable adenocarcinoma of the seminal vesicle: (1) localization of tumor epicenter in retrovesical space superior to the prostate gland by clinical examination, imaging studies, surgical exploration, or autopsy observation; (2) absence of adjacent prostate, bladder, or anorectal cancer; (3) characteristic high-grade cytoarchitectural features, including papillary, anaplastic, and mucinous areas; (4) presence of in situ adenocarcinoma in adjacent uninvolved seminal vesicle epithelium; (5) negativity for prostate specific markers.

The prognosis for adenocarcinoma of the seminal vesicles is poor. Radical surgical treatments have been attempted with dismal results. Radiotherapy has been used, with a few long-term survivors.[75]

Occasional benign mesenchymal tumors, including fibroma, leiomyoma, and mesenchymoma, have been noted.[61, 77, 78] Sarcoma of the seminal vesicles is exceptionally rare, with examples of pleomorphic cell sarcoma, leiomyosarcoma, fibrosarcoma, and hemangiosarcoma found in the literature.[79-82] Surgical treatment has generally been employed in these cases.

ACKNOWLEDGMENTS

We thank Dr. Jane Thomas and Mrs. Anna Litvan of The Canadian Reference Centre for Cancer Pathology, Ottawa, Ontario, Canada, for providing some of the case material used to illustrate this chapter. We also thank Marcie Okunsky for her excellent secretarial assistance.

REFERENCES

1. McCallum RW: The adult male urethra. Normal anatomy, pathology and method of urethrography. Radiol Clin North Am 17:227, 1979
2. McNeal JE: The prostate and prostatic urethra: a morphologic synthesis. J Urol 107:1008, 1972
3. Duckett JW: Hypospadias. p. 1969. In Walsh PC, Gitter RF, Perlmutter AD, Stamey TA (eds): Campbell's Urology. 5th Ed. WB Saunders, Philadelphia, 1986
4. Coladny A: Urethral lesion in infants and children. p 1782. In Gillewater JY, Grayhack JT, Howards SS, Duckett JW (eds): Adult and Pediatric Urology. Year Book Medical Publishers, Chicago, 1987
5. Evan KJ, McCarthy MP, Sands JP: Adenocarcinoma of a female urethral diverticulum: a case report and review of the literature. J Urol 126:124, 1981
6. Allen R, Nelson RP: Primary urethral malignancy. Review of 22 cases. South Med J 71:549, 1978
7. Richmond SJ, Sparking PF: Genital chlamydial infections. Am J Epidemiol 103:428, 1976
8. Raghavaiah NV: Tuberculosis of the male urethra. J Urol 122:417, 1979
9. Sarma KP: On the nature of cystitis follicularis. J Urol 104:709, 1970
10. Young R: Papillary and polypoid cystitis. Am J Surg Pathol 12:542, 1988
11. Schinella R, Thurm J, Feiner H: Papillary pseudotumor of the prostatic urethra: proliferative papillary urethritis. J Urol 111:38, 1974
12. Rosenberg S, Reid R, Greenberg M, Lorincz AT: Sexually transmitted papillomaviral infection in the male. II. The urethral reservoir. Urology 32:47, 1988
13. McClure J: A case of urethral malakoplakia associated with vesical disease. J Urol 125:705, 1979
14. Sharma TC, Kagan KN, Sheils JP: Malakoplakia of the male urethra. J Urol 125:885, 1981
15. Stanton MJ, Maxted W: Malakoplakia: a study of the literature and current concepts of pathogenesis, diagnosis and treatment. J Urol 125:139, 1981
16. Ullmann AS, Fine G, Johnson AJ: Localized amyloidosis (amyloid tumor) of the urethra. J Urol 92:42, 1964
17. Stillwell TJ, Segura JM, Farrow GM: Amyloidosis of the male urethra. J Urol 141:52, 1989
18. Vijayan P, Clarke PB, Anderson CK: Leukoplakia of the male urethra. A short case report. Br J Urol 48:346, 1976
19. Bhagavan BS, Tiamson EM, Wenk RE, et al: Nephrogenic adenoma of the urinary bladder and urethra. Hum Pathol 12:907, 1982

20. Koss LG: Tumors of the urinary bladder. In Atlas of Tumor Pathology. 2nd Series, Fascicle 11, Suppl. Armed Forces Institute of Pathology, Washington DC, 1984, p. 7

21. Ingram EA, DePauw P: Adenocarcinoma of the male urethra with associated nephrogenous metaplasia. Cancer 55:160, 1985

22. Downs RA: Congenital polyps of the prostatic urethra. A review of the literature and report of 2 cases. Br J Urol 42:76, 1970

23. Mostofi FK, Price EB: Tumors and tumor-like lesions of the male urethra. p. 263. In Tumors of the Male Genital System. Atlas of Tumor Pathology, 2nd Series, Fascicle 8. Armed Forces Institute of Pathology, Washington DC, 1973

24. Butterick JD, Schnitzer B, Abell MR: Ectopic prostatic tissue in the urethra: a clinico-pathological entity and a significant cause of hematuria. J Urol 105:97, 1971

25. Stein AJ, Prioleau PG, Catalona WJ: Adenomatous polyps of the prostatic urethra: a cause of hematospermia. J Urol 124:298, 1980

26. Goldstein AMB, Bregin SD, Terry R, et al: Prostatic urethral polyps in adults: histopathologic variations and clinical manifestations. J Urol 126:129, 1981

27. Baroudy AC, O'Connell JP: Papillary adenoma of the prostatic urethra. J Urol 132:120, 1984

28. Hara S, Horie A: Prostatic caruncle: urethral papillary tumor derived from prolapse of the prostatic duct. J Urol 117:303, 1977

29. Chen JKC, Chow TC, Tsui MS: Prostatic-type polyps of the lower urinary tract: three histogenetic types? Histopathology 11:789, 1987

30. Walker AN, Mills SE, Fechner RA, et al: "Endometrial" adenocarcinoma of the prostatic urethra arising in a villous polyp: a light microscopic and immunoperoxidase study. Arch Pathol Lab Med 106:626, 1982

31. DeMeester LJ, Farrow GM, Utz TC: Inverted papilloma of the urinary bladder. Cancer 36:505, 1975

32. Hopkins SC, Grabstald H: Benign and malignant tumors of the male and female urethra. p. 1441. In Walsh PC, Gitter RF, Perlmutter AD, Stamey TA (eds): Campbell's Urology. 5th Ed. WB Saunders, Philadelphia, 1986

33. Williams G, Ashken MH: Urethral carcinoma following urethroplasty. J R Soc Med 76:370, 1980

34. Johnson DE: Cancer of the male urethra: an overview. p. 243. In Johnson DE, Boileau MA (eds):

35. Bostwick DG, Lo R, Stamey TA: Papillary adenocarcinoma of the male urethra. Case report and review of the literature. Cancer 54:2556, 1984

36. Lucman L, Vadas G: Transitional cloacogenic carcinoma of the urethra. Cancer 31:1508, 1973

37. Peterson RO: Urologic Pathology. JB Lippincott, Philadelphia, 1986, p. 437

38. Keen MR, Golden RL, Richardson JF, Melicow MM: Carcinoma of Cowper's gland treated with chemotherapy. J Urol 106:854, 1970

39. Sachs SA, Waisman J, Apfelbaum HB, et al: Urethral adenocarcinoma (possibly originating in the glands of Littre). J Urol 113:50, 1975

40. Ray B, Canto AR, Whitmore WF: Experience with primary carcinoma of the male urethra. J Urol 117:591, 1977

41. Hermanek P, Sobin LH (eds): TNM Classification of Malignant Tumors. 4th Ed. Springer-Verlag, Berlin, 1987, p. 142

42. Kaplan GW, Bulkley GJ, Grayhack JT: Carcinoma of the male urethra. J Urol 98:365, 1967

43. Bracken RB, Henry R, Ordonez N: Primary carcinoma of the male urethra. South Med J 73:1003, 1980

44. Angel JR, Kraus SD, McClung T, et al: Unusual case of urethral carcinoma. Urology 18:74, 1981

45. Schellhammer PF: Urethral carcinoma. Semin Urol 1:83, 1983

46. Raz S, McLorie G, Johnson S, Skinner DG: Management of the urethra in patients undergoing radical cystectomy for bladder cancer. J Urol 120:298, 1978

47. Roberts JW, Devine CJ Jr.: Urethral hemangioma: treatment by total excision and grafting. J Urol 129:1053, 1983

48. Lake MH, Kossow AS, Bokinsky G: Leiomyoma of the bladder and urethra. J Urol 125:742, 1981

49. Painter MR, O'Shaughnessy EJ, Larson PH, et al: Rhabdomyosarcoma of the male urethra. J Urol 99:455, 1968

50. Alabaster AM, Jordan WP Jr, Soloway MS, et al: Leiomyosarcoma of the bladder and subsequent urethral recurrence. J Urol 125:583, 1981

51. Weiss J, Elder D, Hamilton R: Melanoma of the male urethra: surgical approach and pathologic analysis. J Urol 128:392, 1982

52. Oldbring J, Mikulowski P: Malignant melanoma of the penis and male urethra. Report of nine

cases and review of the literature. Cancer 59:581, 1987

53. Chaitin BA, Manning JT, Ordonez NG: Hematologic neoplasms with initial manifestations in lower urinary tract. Urology 23:35, 1984

54. Selikowitz SM, Olsson KA: Metastatic urethral obstruction. Arch Surg 107:906, 1973

55. Abeshouse BS, Abeshouse GA: Metastatic tumors of the penis: a review of the literature and report of two cases. J Urol 86:99, 1961

56. Gray SW, Skandalkis JE: Embryology for Surgeons. WB Saunders, Philadelphia, 1972

57. Srigley JR: Small-acinar patterns in the prostate glands with emphasis on atypical adenomatous hyperplasia and small-acinar carcinoma. Semin Diagn Pathol 5:254, 1988

58. Arias-Stella J, Takano-Moron J: Atypical epithelial change in the seminal vesicles. Arch Pathol 66:761, 1958

59. Kuo T-T, Gomez LG: Monstrous epithelial cells in human epididymis and seminal vesicles. A pseudomalignant change. Am J Surg Pathol 5:483, 1981

60. Koss LG: Diagnostic Cytology and Its Histologic Bases. 3rd Ed. JB Lippincott, Philadelphia, 1979

61. Palmer JM: Surgery of the seminal vesicles. p. 2846. In Walsh PC, Gitter RF, Perlmutter AD, Stamey TA (eds): Campbell's Urology. 5th Ed. WB Saunders, Philadelphia, 1986

62. Schnitzer BJ: Ectopic ureteral opening into seminal vesicle. A report of four cases. J Urol 93:576, 1965

63. Olson JR, Weaver DK: Congenital mesonephric defects in male infants with mucoviscidosis. J Clin Pathol 22:725, 1979

64. Beeby DI: Seminal vesicle cysts associated with ipsilateral renal agenesis: a case report and review of the literature. J Urol 112:120, 1974

65. Hart JB: A case of cystic hydrops of the seminal vesicle. J Urol 86:137, 1961

66. Klein LA, Proppe KH: Case 21 - 1980. N Engl J Med 302:1246, 1980

67. Silber SJ, McDonald ED: Calcification of the seminal vesicles and vas deferens in a uremic patient. J Urol 105:542, 1971

68. Goldman H: Amyloidosis of seminal vesicles and vas deferens. Arch Pathol 75:106, 1963

69. Krane RJ, Klugo RD, Olsson CA: Seminal vesicle amyloidosis. Urology 2:70, 1973

70. Byar DE, Mostofi FK: Carcinoma of the prostate: prognostic evaluation of certain pathologic features in 208 radical prostatectomies examined by the step section technique. Cancer 30:5, 1972

71. Ro JY, Ayala AG, el-Naggar A, Wishnow KI: Seminal vesicle involvement by in situ and invasive transitional cell carcinoma of the bladder. Am J Surg Pathol 12:951, 1987

72. Damjanov I, Apic R: Cystadenoma of the seminal vesicles. J Urol 111:808, 1974

73. Lundhus E, Bundgaard N, Sorensen FB: Cystadenoma of the seminal vesicle. Scand J Urol Nephrol 18:341, 1984

74. Mazur M, et al: Cystic epithelial-stromal tumor of the seminal vesicle. Am J Surg Pathol 11:210, 1987

75. Bensen RC, Clark WR, Farrow GM: Carcinoma of the seminal vesicle. J Urol 132:483, 1984

76. Dalgaard JB, Giertsen JC: Primary carcinoma of the seminal vesicle; case and survey. Acta Pathol Microbiol Scand 39:255, 1956

77. Ordonez NG, Ayala AG, Johnston OL, Johnson DE: Retrovesical leiomyoma. Urology 27:67, 1986

78. Islam M: Benign mesenchymoma of the seminal vesicles. Urology 13:203, 1979

79. Lazarus JA: Primary malignant tumors of the retrovesical region with special reference to malignant tumors of the seminal vesicles: report of a case of retrovesical sarcoma. J Urol 55:190, 1946

80. Buck AC, Shaw RE: Primary tumors of the retrovesical region with special reference to mesenchymal tumors of the seminal vesicles. Br J Urol 41:47, 1972

81. Chiou R-K, Limas C, Lange PH: Hemangiosarcoma of the seminal vesicle: case report and literature review. J Urol 134:371, 1985

82. Schned AR, Ledbetter JS, Selkowitz SM: Primary leiomyosarcoma of the seminal vesicle. Cancer 57:2202, 1986

13

Clinical Management of Prostatic Tumors

Michael K. Brawer

Surgery remains the principal treatment for bladder outlet obstruction resulting from nodular hyperplasia, for removal of clinically localized carcinoma, and for management of many of the sequelae of advanced tumors. Consequently, the surgical pathologist plays an important role in the management of patients with these common lesions. This chapter reviews the clinical aspects of benign prostatic hyperplasia and prostatic carcinoma from a urologist's point of view, which may be helpful to the surgical pathologist.

NODULAR HYPERPLASIA (BENIGN PROSTATIC HYPERPLASIA)

The normal human prostate undergoes three important growth phases. First, during gestation, there is an early proliferation of glandular and stromal elements, followed by regression of tubules.[1] In the prepubescent boy the mean prostatic weight is approximately 1.4 g.[2] Second, after puberty, the mean weight increases to about 10.8 g.[2] Histologically, there is acinar distention and the development of tall columnar secretory epithelium. By the third decade the mean weight has risen to 18.1 g, after which there is a gradual increase. In the sixth and seventh decades, the third growth phase occurs, in which there is a steady rise in prostatic growth.[2] By the eighth decade, the mean prostatic weight is 30.9 g.[2] The development of nodular hyperplasia occurs during the second and third phases of growth, as described in Chapter 3.

Berry et al.[2] compiled data from 10 published studies on the autopsy incidence of nodular hyperplasia, and noted the virtual absence of hyperplasia prior to age 30. Above that age, there was a marked increase in incidence, so that, by the ninth decade, almost 90 percent of patients had histologic evidence of hyperplasia.

DEVELOPMENT OF NODULAR HYPERPLASIA

The development of nodular hyperplasia requires the presence of testes and a changing hormonal milieu. Following castration, dihydrotestosterone and testosterone administration will not induce the development of benign prostatic hyperplasia in dogs.[3] However, in dogs with intact testes, dihydrotestosterone will induce significant growth in benign prostatic hyperplasia.[4] In a classic report, White[5] demonstrated prostatic shrinkage and relief of bladder outlet obstruction in 87 percent of 111 men following castration.

The hormonal milieu of the aging prostate involves more than a simple drop in androgen levels. In older men, there is a decrease in levels of seminal vesicle fructose, expressed prostatic fluid acid phosphatase, and lactate dehydrogenase, all of which are under androgen control.[6] These falling sugar and enzyme levels are accompanied by falling testosterone levels.[7] By contrast, there is no change in seminal vesicle weight and prostatic fluid citric acid concentration, both of which are under the control of androgens and other hormones.[6, 8]

229

It is uncertain whether nodular hyperplasia represents a response of normal prostatic cells to an abnormal hormonal growth stimulus, a response of abnormal prostatic cells to a normal hormonal environment, or both.[9] One hypothesis is presented by McNeal in Chapter 3.

CLINICAL SIGNS AND SYMPTOMS

The clinical signs and symptoms of nodular hyperplasia result from bladder outlet obstruction and increased resistance to the flow of urine through the prostatic urethra. This resistance is a mechanical phenomenon related to compression, tortuosity, and elongation of the prostatic urethra. The amount of hyperplastic tissue does not necessarily correlate with the severity of symptoms; a patient with extensive hyperplasia may have minimal encroachment on the urethra with few obstructive symptoms, while another patient may have mild periurethral hyperplasia that causes marked narrowing of the urethral lumen and severe obstructive symptoms.

In order to maintain constant flow in the setting of increased resistance owing to nodular hyperplasia, there must be increased bladder pressure at micturition with compensatory hypertrophy of the detrusor muscle. These changes are explained by Ohm's law, which states that the pressure (E) equals flow (I) times resistance (R): (E = IR). Increased contractility results in increased detrusor pressure, thus maintaining urine flow. Detrusor hypertrophy may be associated with bladder hyperirritability, which is complicated by frequency, nocturia, and urgency. As the mass of nodular hyperplasia increases, the detrusor is unable to overcome urethral resistance, resulting in hesitancy, intermittency, dribbling, and eventual urinary retention. Ureterectasis, hydronephrosis, and renal insufficiency are late sequelae attributable to increased resistance at the level of the intramural ureter following trigonal hypertrophy. Other complications include urinary tract infections, formation of calculi, and development of bladder and urethral diverticuli.

CLINICAL EVALUATION

A careful history should be obtained from patients with suspected bladder outlet obstruction, with particular attention directed to the symptoms noted above. Palpation of the prostate should include an assessment of its configuration and size. An abnormality of consistency or symmetry suggestive of neoplasm demands further evaluation (see below). Contributory laboratory studies include chemical and microscopic urinalysis to identify proteinuria, glycosuria, crystals suggestive of urolithiasis, hematuria (nodular hyperplasia is one of the most common causes of hematuria), pyuria, and bacteriuria; urine cultures and sensitivities when indicated; complete blood count and serum chemical profile; and coagulation profile and platelet count when a bleeding diathesis is suspected.

Urodynamic evaluation in select patients may include uroflow, residual urine determination, cystometrogram, urethral resistance profile, and videocystogram. Imaging modalities may include intravenous urogram, prostatic ultrasound, renal and abdominal ultrasound, and computed tomography (CT). Cystourethroscopy appears to be the most reliable method for assessing the bladder and urethra.

TREATMENT OF NODULAR HYPERPLASIA

The presence of hyperplasia alone is not an indication for treatment. Most patients seek treatment because the symptoms of bladder outlet obstruction interfere with their lives. The severity of symptoms varies markedly between patients. One patient may not be bothered by four nightly episodes of nocturia and marked hesitancy, while another rising twice in the night to void may find his life sufficiently interrupted to desire treatment. Lytton et al.[10] calculated that a 40-year-old man has a 10 percent chance of undergoing prostatectomy for nodular hyperplasia if he lives to age 80. Birkhoff[11] noted that a 50-year-old man has a 25 percent chance of undergoing simple prostatectomy. The high frequency of hyperplasia and its tremendous impact on health care costs has increased the need for the development of alternative therapies. The controversies about indications for prostatectomy have been recently reviewed.[12]

Androgen deprivation has been shown to offer relief for symptomatic bladder outlet obstruction owing to nodular hyperplasia in 60 percent of patients. Pharmacologic castration results in shrinkage of the prostate and atrophy of the epithelial component of nodular hyperplasia.[13] A variety of drugs cause androgen deprivation, including estrogen, estrogen with androgen, progesterone, medrogestone, cyproterone acetate, flutamide (an antiandrogen), and luteinizing hormone-releasing hormone (LHRH) agonists (agents causing stimulation of the anterior pituitary with resulting down-regulation of LHRH receptors and decreased LH secretion).[14-16] The utility of these agents in treating nodular hyperplasia underscores the necessity of the testes in the development and maintenance of nodular hyperplasia in the prostate.

The other important pharmacologic agents for treating hyperplasia are adrenergic antagonists. These drugs act by blocking α-sympathetic nerve stimulation to the bladder neck, prostatic urethra, and prostatic capsule, areas that are innervated by α_1-adrenergic fibers[17] to allow for closure of the bladder neck at orgasm and subsequent antegrade ejaculation. By blocking sympathetic nerve stimulation, these agents decrease the resting tone of the innervated muscles and lower the resistance to urine flow. The α-blockers phenoxybenzamine and prazosin have been used successfully in human trials, with improvement in urinary flow and symptoms.[18-20]

Despite advances in pharmacologic management of symptomatic nodular hyperplasia, prostatectomy remains the treatment of choice. Simple prostatectomy (more appropriately called *prostatic adenectomy*) involves the removal of the obstructing "adenoma" from the transition zone and periurethral area.[21]

There are two surgical methods of simple prostatectomy. The most common method,

transurethral resection (TUR), involves insertion of a resectoscope with an electrical cutting loop on the end. Making serial cuts with the loop allows excision of "chips" measuring up to 2 cm in length. Resection is carried down to the level of the "surgical capsule," identified as a tissue plane between the compressed hyperplastic nodules and the surrounding uninvolved tissue. The second surgical method is an open prostatectomy, performed by a retropubic, suprapubic (transvesical), or perineal approach. Open prostatectomy is performed through an incision in the prostatic capsule and enucleation of the hyperplastic tissue. It is important to note that simple prostatectomy, whether transurethral or open, does not include resection of tissue from the peripheral zone of the prostate, and consequently may miss malignant tissue.

Pathologic examination of simple prostatectomy specimens varies between different institutions. Submission of eight tissue blocks from TUR specimens by the surgical pathologist will detect 89 percent of stage A1 cancers and 100 percent of stage A2 cancers, although some investigators advocate submission of all of the resected tissue in the search for carcinoma, regardless of number of tissue blocks.[22] Open prostatectomy specimens may weigh up to several hundred grams, so that selective sampling is required. The tissue should be serially sectioned and carefully examined, with histologic sampling of any yellow indurated areas. Margins are irrelevant in these specimens because there is no true barrier between the enucleated adenomas and the surrounding prostate. When carcinoma is identified in the TUR or open prostatectomy specimen, all remaining tissue should be submitted for histologic examination in order to ensure accurate staging. The number of chips involved with carcinoma or the estimated percentage of tissue involvement should be included in the pathology report.

A new approach to the surgical management of nodular hyperplasia is transurethral incision of the prostate (TUIP). In this procedure, incisions are made endoscopically to the level of the true prostatic capsule. The rationale is that the prostatic capsule contributes to increased dynamic tone by binding the expanding adenoma, resulting in centrally directed compression of the urethra and increased resistance to flow. Capsular incisions made by TUIP result in a decrease in dynamic tone, with resulting decreased resistance and increased flow, similar to adrenergic antagonists. Hart[23] reported improved flow in 87 of 89 patients undergoing TUIP, with significant symptomatic relief. No tissue is removed for pathologic examination with TUIP.

PROSTATIC CARCINOMA

The clinical management of prostatic carcinoma requires familiarity with the epidemiology, etiology, and natural history, as well as an understanding of clinical evaluation and treatment. New approaches to the evaluation and management of carcinoma in the last decade include the use of prostate-specific antigen (PSA), transrectal prostatic ultrasonography, and nerve-sparing (potency-maintaining) radical prostatectomy. Other aspects of prostatic carcinoma, including premalignant lesions, incidental carcinoma, grading, radiation injury, and unusual tumors of the prostate, are discussed in other chapters.

EPIDEMIOLOGY

Prostatic carcinoma is the second most common visceral cancer in men in the United States, with 90,000 new cases annually.[11, 24, 25] Mortality recently eclipsed colorectal carcinoma as the second most common cause of male cancer deaths, with 26,000 deaths annually.[24, 25]

The autopsy incidence of prostatic carcinoma significantly exceeds the clinical incidence. Thorough serial step-sectioning of prostates obtained at postmortem examination revealed carcinoma in more than 30 percent of men over age 50.[26, 27] Franks[27] showed a steady increase in incidence with advancing age, noting that 100 percent of men in the tenth decade had

carcinoma of the prostate. The significant difference between clinically manifest carcinoma and incidental carcinoma was poignantly illustrated by Stamey[28]; he calculated that for every man dying of carcinoma of the prostate, 380 had tumors. The marked variability in the clinical significance of different tumors poses a multitude of problems concerning biologic potential, prognosis, and treatment in individual cases.

PROGNOSTIC CLUES

Other than stage, tumor grade is probably the most useful prognostic clue. Grossman[29] demonstrated a strong correlation between histologic grade and the presence or absence of pelvic lymph node metastases. Twenty-two percent of patients with grade 1 carcinoma had lymph node metastases, compared with 54 percent with grade 2, and 77 percent with grade 3. Similarly, Paulson et al.,[30] using the Gleason score, demonstrated pelvic lymph node metastases in 14 percent of scores 2 to 5, 32 percent of score 6, 50 percent of score 7, 75 percent of score 8, and 100 percent of scores 9 and 10. Other aspects of histologic grading are discussed in other chapters.

Recently, tumor volume has been shown to correlate strongly with capsular penetration, seminal vesicle invasion, and lymph node metastases. In a series of 68 radical prostatectomy specimens in which the tumor volume was quantitated, Stamey et al.[31] noted that only 6 of 34 prostates (18 percent) with tumor volumes less than 3 cc had evidence of capsular penetration, compared with 27 of 34 (79 percent) with tumor volume greater than 3 cc. Similarly, these investigators noted seminal vesicle invasion in only 1 of 34 patients with small-volume tumors, but in 15 of 34 patients (44 percent) with large-volume tumors. All six patients with pelvic lymph node metastases at the time of exploration had tumor volumes greater than 4 cc.

Other proposed clues of tumor aggressiveness include morphometric assessment of nuclear roundness, nucleolar size, DNA content, and ploidy and oncogene expression.[32-38] Despite positive correlation with malignant potential, none of these methods has advanced to the point of influencing clinical decisions for individual patients.

ETIOLOGY

The etiology of prostatic carcinoma remains enigmatic. Similar to nodular hyperplasia, carcinoma requires the presence of an intact hypothalamic-pituitary-gonadal axis in an aging man. Zumoff et al.[39] showed that patients with carcinoma have decreased testosterone and increased estrogen levels when compared to normal controls. An inherited predisposition has been suggested by study of relatives of patients with carcinoma of the prostate.[40] Race also seems to be a significant factor. Black men develop carcinoma earlier, present with higher-stage tumors, and have a higher mortality than whites;[41] however, one report suggests these findings may be a reflection of socioeconomic differences.[42] Jackson et al.[43] compared prostatic carcinoma in Nigerian and American blacks, and found a significantly increased (six-fold) incidence of clinically manifest carcinoma in the Americans, but an equal incidence at autopsy. National differences are also evident for prostate cancer. Scandinavia has the highest incidence, the United States is twelfth in incidence, and nations in the Orient have the lowest incidence.[24] Akazaki and Stemmerman[44] showed that the autopsy incidence of Japanese living in Japan was equal to those migrating to Hawaii, but the clinical incidence was twice as high in the latter group. A diet high in saturated fat may correlate, and it has been shown that patients with prostatic carcinoma have increased cadmium and decreased zinc concentrations in their prostates.[45] Occupational exposure to cadmium and other heavy metals, including workers in the rubber, textile, shipbuilding, janitorial, farming, painting, and printing industries, seems to contribute to a slightly higher risk of prostate cancer.[46] A history of venereal disease exposure shows a positive correlation with prostate carcinoma.[40, 47] Viral infections[48-50] and the presence of oncogenes have also been shown to correlate.[51]

NATURAL HISTORY

The natural history of carcinoma of the prostate is quite variable. The majority of men die with, and not of, this neoplasm. Whitmore[52] has stated that these tumors may progress in a stage-skipping fashion, with, for example, stage A (incidental) tumors metastasizing widely (stage D) without first being clinically palpable (stage B). Conversely, Stamey et al.[31] demonstrated a linear correlation of tumor volume and stage, tumor grade, capsular penetration, seminal vesicle invasion, and metastases. These seemingly contradictory views may be explained by a tumor's ability to grow centrally rather than eccentrically toward the rectal surface, thus remaining clinically undetectable while achieving significant volume and therefore greater biologic potential.

DIAGNOSIS

The majority of patients with prostatic carcinoma present with an abnormal rectal examination. Approximately 50 percent of patients with prostatic induration are found to have cancer.[53] Another 20 percent of cases are diagnosed following histologic examination of simple prostatectomy specimens performed for presumed benign disease.[54]

The clinical impression of the urologist is very important in the evaluation of prostatic nodules. Catalona[55] showed that carcinoma was not found in biopsies of palpably normal glands, compared with a frequency of 45 percent positive biopsies in prostates with marked induration. Needle biopsy is commonly used for evaluation of palpable prostatic nodules, but transrectal fine-needle aspiration is gaining in popularity. Fine-needle aspiration cytology is limited by the small sample obtained, the expertise needed for interpretation, and the inability to assign tumor grade in malignant specimens.

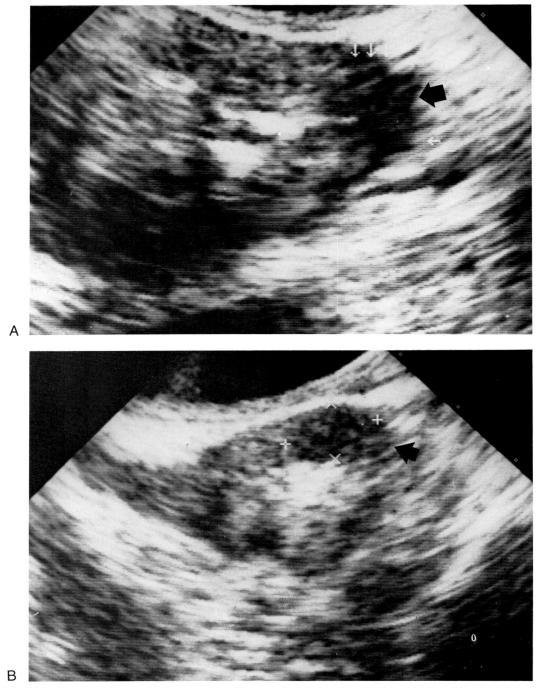

Fig. 13-1. Transrectal prostatic ultrasonogram. Hypoechoic peripheral zone lesion, which, on biopsy, revealed a Gleason 3+3 carcinoma (black arrow). (**A**) Axial. (**B**) Left parasagittal.

False-negative biopsies attributable to limited sampling are not infrequent. In a compilation of seven series, false-negative needle biopsies were confirmed in 105 of 682 patients (15 percent).[56-62] Transrectal aspiration has a false-negative rate of between 2 and 29 percent.[63, 64]

Transrectal ultrasonography (TRUS) has been used to guide the biopsy needle in an effort to improve the accuracy of prostatic biopsy, and is believed by most investigators to provide the best available method for imaging of the prostate. The majority of carcinomas of the prostate are hypoechoic and arise in the peripheral zone[65-69] (Fig. 13-1). TRUS allows precise localization of the biopsy needle within the lesion of interest. The transrectal ultrasound probe in combination with a spring-loaded biopsy (Bard Biopsy) instrument provides an excellent 15-mm-long 18- or 20-gauge core specimen.

It is important to note that a number of histologic entities give rise to hypoechoic lesions indistinguishable from carcinoma (Table 13-1). In our experience, 35 percent of TRUS-guided biopsies of peripheral zone hypoechoic lesions reveal carcinoma. Recently we reported a series of 22 patients who had undergone 1 to 3 digitally guided needle biopsies of indurated glands that were benign. Repeat biopsy under TRUS revealed carcinoma in 11 (50 percent). Interestingly, of six patients with prostatic intraepithelial neoplasia in digitally guided specimens, five had carcinoma on the TRUS biopsy.[70]

STAGING

Once the diagnosis of carcinoma is made, accurate staging is critical to allow rational treatment decisions. In the United States, the most commonly employed clinical staging system is the Jewett modification of the Whitmore system (Fig. 13-2).[71] Almost 41 percent of patients present with extraprostatic or disseminated tumors,[72, 73] accounting, in part, for the high mortality of prostatic carcinoma.

Following a careful history and physical examination, the patient should undergo appropriate staging studies, which may include determi-

Table 13-1. Differential Diagnosis of Peripheral Zone Hypoechoic Lesions

Adenocarcinoma
Prostatic intraepithelial neoplasia
Benign hyperplasia
Acute inflammation
Chronic inflammation
Granulomatous inflammation
Fibrosis
Skeletal muscle
Cystic atrophy
Normal

nation of serum prostatic acid phosphatase (PAP) and PSA, radioisotope bone scan, chest and skeletal radiography, TRUS, CT, magnetic resonance imaging, and bipedal lymphangiography. CT is commonly employed for pelvic lymph node assessment, although it has a false-negative rate of up to 80 percent.[74] Because of this lack of sensitivity of imaging pelvic lymph nodes, most clinicians perform lymph node dissection prior to radical extirpative surgery.

There is considerable controversy about how extensive the pelvic lymph node dissection

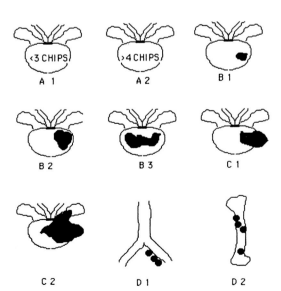

Fig. 13-2. Modified Whitmore-Jewett clinical staging system for prostatic carcinoma. Many classify hormonally resistant metastatic carcinoma as D3.

should be. The usual complete lymph node dissection includes the lymph node-bearing tissue within the following boundaries: the genitofemoral nerve laterally, the bifurcation of iliac artery cranially, the circumflex iliac vein caudally, and the obturator nerve medially. There is a widely held belief that lymph node dissection is of no therapeutic value in prostatic carcinoma. Hence, many surgeons perform a limited dissection, examining only those lymph nodes medial to the external iliac vein and lateral to the obturator nerve.[75] Pelvic lymph node dissection is usually undertaken immediately prior to radical prostatectomy, with frozen-section evaluation of the lymph nodes for metastases. Intraoperative clinical assessment of lymph node status is problematic without histologic confirmation. In a recent report, 33 of 40 pelvic lymph node dissections that were believed intraoperatively to be grossly normal were found to contain carcinoma.[76] However, even intraoperative frozen sections may be inconclusive, with up to 19 percent of cases shown to be falsely negative.[77]

The management of patients with prostatic carcinoma has been significantly advanced by the identification of a new tissue-specific marker: PSA.[78] This 34-kD glycoprotein is found exclusively in the cytoplasm of prostatic epithelium, and is present in the serum of men with prostatic tissue. Antibodies directed against PSA allow immunohistochemical identification of the prostate as the site of origin for some metastatic carcinomas of unknown origin, and also provide for accurate measurement of serum PSA levels. Multiple studies have demonstrated increased diagnostic sensitivity of serum PSA when compared to PAP in all stages of prostatic carcinoma.[79-83] However, there is overlap of PSA levels within different stages, so it is less useful in predicting pathologic stage[80-84] (Fig. 13-3).

One of the most important uses of serum PSA determination is in the follow-up of patients after definitive therapy. After successful surgical ablation of carcinoma, persistent or rising serum PSA levels indicate advanced pathologic stage and recurrent neoplasm.[82, 83]

Little data exist concerning serum PSA levels following radiation therapy. Hudson et al.[84] demonstrated that serum PSA fell to undetectable levels in 3 of 18 patients following definitive external beam radiation therapy.[84] PSA also appears to be a good predictor of response to endocrine therapy in disseminated tumors.[79, 84]

TREATMENT

Considerable controversy exists regarding appropriate treatment for each stage of prostatic carcinoma. This results in part from the discrepancy between pathologic findings and clinical manifestations, as discussed above. Because most patients with prostate cancer are over 60 years of age, an assessment of intercurrent disease is critical. Treatment decisions must balance the patient's health with the potential for morbidity and mortality attributable to different regimens.

Most urologic oncologists believe that patients with an expected survival of 10 years or more should receive treatment for clinically localized prostatic carcinoma. If the tumor has metastasized by the time of diagnosis, there are two options: early hormonal manipulation or withholding treatment until the patient becomes symptomatic.

Treatment of clinically localized prostatic carcinoma includes radical prostatectomy or radiation therapy. Radical prostatectomy was introduced in 1866 as treatment for localized carcinoma.[85] There are two surgical approaches to radical prostatectomy: the perineal approach and the retropubic approach, both of which involve removal of the prostate and attached seminal vesicles. Pelvic lymphadenectomy is usually performed in conjunction with or preceding radical prostatectomy. Details of the operative approach are beyond the scope of this chapter. Of importance in tissue sampling are the surgical margins of excision, including the urethral margin distal to the apex of the prostate; the prostatic investment of Denonvilliers' fascia posteriorly; the periprostatic adipose tissue, including the superficial branches of the dorsal vein anteriorly;

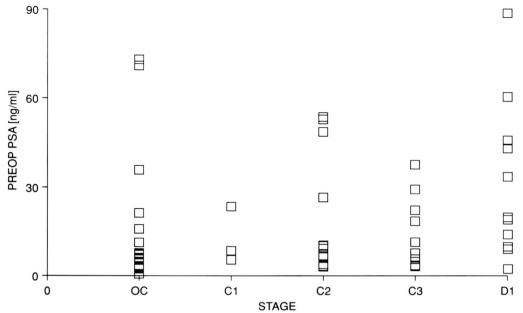

Fig. 13-3. Preoperative serum PSA (Hybritech Tandem, San Diego, CA) and pathologic stage in radical prostatectomy patients. *OC*, organ confined; *C1*, capsular invasion; *C2*, capsular penetration; *C3*, seminal vesicle involvement; *D1*, pelvic lymph node metastases.

and the bladder neck superiorly. The seminal vesicles remain attached to the prostate, together with the ejaculatory ducts and the distal vas deferens.

Recently, Walsh et al.[86] introduced the nerve-sparing radical retropubic prostatectomy. By identifying the nerve plexuses that innervate the corpora cavernosa and allow for penile erection, these investigators modified the radical retropubic prostatectomy to avoid injury to these plexuses. They report maintenance of potency in approximately 70 percent of patients.[87]

The pelvic nerve plexus follows a course outside the capsule of the prostate in the lateral pelvic fascia. In a review of a 100 men undergoing nerve-sparing radical retropubic prostatectomy, Eggleston and Walsh[87] noted that, of 7 patients with positive surgical margins, all had extensive extraprostatic tumor, and none had surgical margins positive only at the site of the nerve-sparing modification of the conventional radical prostatectomy. Thus, it was believed that this operation did not compromise the com-

pleteness of surgical excision of neoplasm. It would seem that, as suggested earlier, the critical determinant in pathologic stage is the volume of carcinoma and not the specific operative technique.

The method of processing the radical prostatectomy specimen varies among surgical pathologists. Our protocol involves weighing and measuring the prostate, coating the external surface with India ink, and fixing it in 10 percent neutral buffered formalin for at least 24 hours. After fixation, the distal (apical) and proximal (bladder neck) margins are excised circumferentially and submitted for histologic examination. The prostate is then serially step-sectioned at 3-mm intervals perpendicular to the rectal surface. Large sections are bisected in the midsagittal plane and the right side section identified by a small wedge cut from the medial surface. Smaller sections are placed whole in the cassettes and processed routinely. Representative sections of the seminal vesicles are submitted separately.

Histologically, the tumor is graded using the Gleason system, and the tumor volume is estimated (percentage of prostate involved by tumor). All surgical margins are carefully evaluated for the presence of carcinoma, including the extent and depth of capsular penetration and invasion. The seminal vesicles are also examined for the presence of neoplasm. The importance of careful examination of the margins and capsule cannot be overemphasized; the distinction between capsular penetration and capsular invasion is critical to stratify patients for potential adjunctive therapy (radiation therapy or hormonal manipulation).

Radiation therapy is also useful in the treatment of localized prostatic carcinoma. Radiation may be delivered by external beam or by interstitial injections, the latter employing radioactive gold, iodine, or iridium. Historically, interstitial radiation has been administered by retropubic exposure of the prostate, usually following pelvic lymph node dissection. Recently, percutaneous placement of interstitial radiation has been performed by perineal exposure, aided by TRUS imaging of the prostate.

There is considerable debate concerning the efficacy of surgery vs. radiation in the treatment of prostatic carcinoma. One prospective randomized trial compared radical prostatectomy and external beam radiation therapy, and showed a statistically significant advantage of surgery in halting tumor progression.[88] The adequacy of this study has been questioned, and other reports suggest equivalent disease-free survival for radiation therapy and surgical therapy. Further studies of this issue are needed.

Androgen ablation therapy has remained the standard for treatment of metastatic prostatic carcinoma since the classic report of Huggins and Hodges[89] in 1941. Various forms of androgen ablation exist, including surgical excision of androgen sources (orchidectomy), inhibition of luteinizing hormone-releasing factor (estrogens, progesterones, cyproterone acetate, LHRH agonists), inhibition of adrogen synthesis (aminoglutethimide, spironolactone, cyproterone acetate), and the recently introduced antiandrogen therapy (cyproterone acetate, flutamide,

medrogestone). The advantages and side effects of each of these therapies is beyond the scope of this chapter.

After failure of hormonal therapy, which occurs in virtually all patients, mean survival is less than 1 year.[90] Despite multiple nonhormonal chemotherapeutic trials, no significant survival benefit has been reported to date for single-agent or combination protocols.

It is clear that the surgical pathologist plays a critical role in the management of patients with benign prostatic hyperplasia and prostatic carcinoma. Further advances in the care of men with these ubiquitous lesions will require close collaboration between clinicians and pathologists.

REFERENCES

1. Zondek LH, Zondek T: Congenital malformation of the male accessory sex glands in the fetus and neonate. p. 17. In Spring-Mills E, Hafez ESE (eds): Male Accessory Sex Glands. Elsevier North-Holland Biomedical Press, New York, 1980

2. Berry SJ, Coffey DS, Walsh PC et al: The development of human benign prostatic hyperplasia with age. J Urol 132:474, 1984

3. Walsh PC, Wilson JD: The induction of prostatic hypertrophy in the dog with androstanediol. J Clin Invest 57:1093, 1976

4. Gloyna RE, Siiteri PK, Wilson JD: Dihydrotestosterone in prostatic hypertrophy. II. The formation and content of dihydrotestosterone in the hypertrophic canine prostate and the effect of dihydrotestosterone on prostate growth in the dog. J Clin Invest 49:1746, 1970

5. White JW: The results of double castration in hypertrophy of the prostate. Surgery 22:1, 1895

6. Stearns EL, MacDonnell JA, Kaufman BJ, et al: Declining testicular function with age: hormonal and clinical correlates. Am J Med 57:761, 1974

7. Vermeulen A, Rubens R, Verdonck L: Testosterone secretions and metabolism in male senescence. J Clin Endocrinol 34:730, 1972

8. Grayhack JT, Lebowitz JM: Effect of prolactin on citric acid of internal lobe of prostate of Sprague-Dawley rat. Invest Urol 5:87, 1967

9. Grayhack JT: Directions for future research. In Hinman F (ed): Benign Prostatic Hypertrophy. Springer-Verlag, New York, 1983

10. Lytton B, Emery JM, Harvard BW: The incidence of benign prostatic obstruction. Trans Am Genitourinary Surg 59:65, 1968

11. Birkhoff JD: Natural history of benign prostatic hypertrophy. In Hinman F (ed): Benign Prostatic Hypertrophy. Springer-Verlag, New York, 1983

12. Graverson PH, Gasser TC, Wasson JH, et al: Controversies about indications for transurethral resection of the prostate. J Urol 141:475, 1989

13. Wendel E, Brannen GE, Putong PB, et al: The effect of orchiectomy and estrogens on benign prostatic hyperplasia. J Urol 108:116, 1972

14. Auclair C, et al: LHRH analogs as potential therapy for benign prostatic hyperplasia and hormone dependent cancers. Arch Androl 7:237, 1981

15. Sandow J, Beier B: LHRH agonists: mechanism of action and effect on target tissues. Prog Clin Biol Res 185A:121, 1985

16. Peters CA, Walsh PC: The effect of nafarelin acetate, a luteinizing-hormone-releasing hormone agonist, on benign prostatic hyperplasia. N Engl J Med 317:599, 1987

17. Caine M, Raz S, Zeigler M: Adrenergic and cholinergic receptors in the human prostate, prostatic capsule, and bladder neck. Br J Urol 47:193, 1975

18. Gerstenberg T, Blaabjerg J, Nielsen ML, et al: Phenoxybenzamine reduces bladder outlet obstruction in benign prostatic hyperplasia: a urodynamic investigation. J Urol 18:29, 1980

19. Caine M, Perlberg S, Shapiro A: Phynoxybenzamine for benign prostatic obstruction: review of 200 cases. Urology 17:542, 1981

20. Hedlund H, Angersson KE, Ek A: Effects of prazosin in patients with benign prostatic obstruction. J Urol 130:275, 1983

21. McNeal JE: The zonal anatomy of the prostate. Prostate 2:35, 1981

22. Rohr LR: Incidental adenocarcinoma in transurethral resections of the prostate. Am J Surg Pathol 11(1):53, 1987

23. Hart RD Jr: Transurethral incision of the prostate. J Am Osteopath Assoc 83:267, 1982

24. Silverberg E: Statistical and epidemiologic data on urologic cancer. Cancer 60 (Suppl):692, 1987

25. Silverberg E, Lubera JA: Cancer Statistics, 1988. Ca 38:5, 1988

26. Holund B: Latent prostatic cancer in a consecutive autopsy series. Scand J Urol Nephrol 14:29, 1980

27. Franks LM: Latent carcinoma of the prostate. J Pathol Bacteriol 68:603, 1954

28. Stamey TA: Cancer of the prostate. Monogr Urol 4:65, 1983

29. Grossman IC, Carpiniello VC, Greenberg SH, et al: Staging pelvic lymphadenectomy for carcinoma of the prostate: review of 91 cases. J Urol 124:632, 1980

30. Paulson CF, Piserchia PV, Gardner W: Predictors of lymphatic spread in prostatic adenocarcinoma: Uro-Oncology Research Group Study. J Urol 123:697, 1980

31. Stamey TA, McNeal JE, Freiha FS, Redwine E: Morphometric and clinical studies on 68 consecutive radical prostatectomies. J Urol 139:1235, 1988

32. Diamond DA, Berry SJ, Jewett HJ, et al: A new method to assess metastatic potential of human prostate cancer: relative nuclear roundness. J Urol 128:729, 1982

33. Epstein JI, Berry SJ, Eggleston JC: Nuclear roundness factor: a predictor of progression in untreated stage A2 prostate cancer. Cancer 54:1666, 1984

34. Benson MC, Walsh PC: The application of flow cytometry to the assessment of tumor cell heterogeneity in the grading of human prostatic cancer: preliminary results. J Urol 135:1194, 1986

35. Tannenbaum M, Tannenbaum S, DeSanetis PN, et al: Prognostic significance of nucleolar surface area in prostate cancer. Urology 19:546, 1982

36. Zetterberg A, Esposti PL: Cytophotometric DNA-analysis of aspirated cells from prostatic carcinoma. Acta Cytol 20:46, 1976

37. Tavares AS, Costa J, Costa MJ: Correlation between ploidy and prognosis in prostatic carcinoma. J Urol 109:676, 1973

38. Yokota J, Tsunetsugu-Yokota Y, Battifora H, et al: Alterations of *myc*, *myb*, and *ras*[Ha] proto-oncogenes in cancers are frequent and show clinical correlation. Science 231:261, 1986

39. Zumoff B, Levin J, Strain GW, et al: Abnormal levels of plasma hormones in men with prostate cancer: evidence toward a ''two-disease'' theory. Prostate 3:579, 1982

40. Schuman LM, Mandel J, Blackard C, et al: Epidemiologic study of prostatic cancer: preliminary report. Cancer Treat Rep 61:181, 1977

41. Ries LG, Pollack ES, Young JL Jr: Cancer patient survival: Surveillance, epidemiology and

end result program, 1973-1979. J Natl Cancer Inst 70:693, 1983

42. Blair A, Fraumeni JF Jr: Geographic patterns of prostate cancer in the United States. J Natl Cancer Inst 61:1379, 1978

43. Jackson MA, Ahluwalia BS, Herson J, et al: Characterization of prostatic carcinoma among blacks: a continuation report. Cancer Treat Rep 61:167, 1977

44. Akazaki K, Stemmermann GN: Comparative study of latent carcinoma of the prostate among Japanese in Japan and Hawaii. J Natl Cancer Inst 50:1137, 1973

45. Kipling MD, Waterhouse JAH: Cadmium and prostatic carcinoma. Lancet 1:730, 1967

46. Winkelstein W Jr, Ernster Vl: Epidemiology and etiology. p.1. In Murphy GP (ed): Prostatic Cancer. PSG Publishing, Littleton, MA, 1979

47. Steele R, Lees REM, Kraus AS, et al: Sexual factors in the epidemiology of cancer of the prostate. J Chronic Dis 24:29, 1971

48. Baker LH, Mebust WK, Chin Tdy, et al: The relationship of herpes virus to carcinoma of the prostate. J Urol 125:370, 1981

49. Lang DJ, Kummer JF, Hartley DP: Cytomegalovirus in semen: Persistence and demonstration in extracellular fluids. N Engl J Med 291:121, 1974

50. Farnsworth WE: Human prostatic reverse transcriptase and RNA-virus. Urol Res 1:106, 1973

51. Viola MV, Fromowitz F, Oravez S, et al: Expression of *ras* oncogene p21 in prostate cancer. N Engl J Med 314:133, 1986

52. Whitmore WF: The natural history of prostatic cancer. Cancer 31:1104, 1973

53. Jewett HJ: Significance of the palpable prostatic nodule. JAMA 160:838, 1956

54. Denton SE, Choy SH, Valk WL: Occult prostatic carcinoma diagnosed by the step section technique of the surgical specimen. J Urol 93:296, 1965

55. Catalona, WJ: Yield from routine prostatic needle biopsy in patients more than 50 years old referred for urologic evaluation: a preliminary report. J Urol 124:844, 1980

56. Fortunoff S: Needle biopsy of the prostate: a review of 346 biopsies. J Urol 87:159, 1962

57. Sika JV, Lindquist HD: Relationship of needle biopsy diagnosis of prostate to clinical signs of prostatic cancer: an evaluation of 300 cases. J Urol 89:737, 1963

58. Hoskins JH, Mellinger GT: Needle biopsy of the prostate. Family Physician 11:48, 1966

59. Bertelsen S: Transrectal needle biopsy of the prostate. Acta Chir Scand (Suppl) 357:225, 1966

60. Zincke H, Campbell JT, Utz DC, et al: Confidence in the negative transrectal needle biopsy. Surg Gynecol Obstet 136:78, 1973

61. Ostroff EG, Almario J, Kramer H: Transrectal needle method for biopsy of the prostate: review of 90 cases. Am J Surg 41:659, 1975

62. Bissada NK, Roundtree GA, Sulieman JS: Factors affecting accuracy and morbidity in transrectal biopsy of the prostate. Surg Gynecol Obstet 145:869, 1977

63. Chodak GW, Steinberg GD, Bibbo M, et al: The role of transrectal aspiration biopsy in the diagnosis of prostatic cancer. J Urol 135:299, 1986

64. Ljung BM, Cherrie R, Kaufman JJ: Fine needle aspiration biopsy of the prostate gland: a study of 103 cases with histological followup. J Urol 135:955, 1986

65. McNeal JE: Origin and development of carcinoma in the prostate. Cancer 23:27, 1969

66. Lee F, Gray JM, McLeary RD, et al: Transrectal ultrasound in the diagnosis of prostate cancer: location, echogenicity, histopathology, and staging. Prostate 7:117, 1985

67. Lee F, Littrup PJ, McLeary RD, et al: Needle aspiration and core biopsy of prostate cancer: comparative evaluation with biplanar transrectal US guidance. Radiology 163:515, 1987

68. Egender G, Furtschegger A, Schachtner W, et al: Transrectal ultrasonography in diagnosis and staging of prostatic cancer. World J Urol 4:163, 1986

69. Cooner WH, Mosley BR, Rutherford CL Jr, et al: Clinical application of transrectal ultrasonography and prostate specific antigen in the search for prostate cancer. J Urol 139:758, 1988

70. Brawer MK, Nagle RB: Transrectal ultrasound guided prostate needle biopsy following negative digitally guided biopsy: AUA Abstract. J Urol 141:182A, 1989

71. Jewett HJ: The present status of radical prostatectomy for stages A and B prostatic cancer. Urol Clin North Am 2:105, 1975

72. Donohue RE, Mani JH, Whitesel JA, et al: Pelvic lymph node dissection: guide to patient management in clinically locally confined adenocarcinoma of prostate. Urology 20:559, 1982

73. Murphy GP, Natarajan N, Pontes JE, et al: The national survey of prostate cancer in the United States by the American College of Surgeons. J Urol 127:928, 1982

74. Benson KH, Watson RA, Spring DB, et al: The value of computerized tomography in evaluation of pelvic lymph nodes. J Urol 126:63, 1981

75. Paulson DF, Piserchia PV, Gardner W: Predictors of lymphatic spread in prostatic adenocarcinoma: Uro-Oncology Research Group Study. J Urol 123:697, 1980

76. Epstein JI, Oesterling JE, Eggleston JC, Walsh PL: Frozen section detection of lymph node metastases in prostatic carcinoma: accuracy in grossly uninvolved pelvic lymphadenectomy specimens. J Urol 136:1234, 1986

77. Catalona WH, Stein AJ: Accuracy of frozen section detection of lymph node metastases in prostatic carcinoma. J Urol 127:460, 1982

78. Wang MC, Valenzuela LA, Murphy GP, Chu TM: Purification of a human prostate specific antigen. Invest Urol 17:159, 1979

79. Ercole CJ, Lange PH, Mathisen M, et al: Prostatic specific antigen and prostatic acid phosphatase in the monitoring and staging of patients with prostatic cancer. J Urol 138:1181, 1987

80. Lange PH, Ercole CJ, Lightner DJ, et al: The value of serum PSA determinations before and after radical prostatectomy. J Urol 141:873, 1989

81. Killian CS, Yang N, Emrich LJ, et al: Investigators of the National Prostatic Cancer Project (45) Prognostic importance of prostate-specific antigen for monitoring patients with stages B_2 to D_1 prostate cancer. Cancer Res 45:886, 1981

82. Oesterling JE, Chan DW, Epstein JI, et al: Prostate specific antigen in the preoperative and postoperative evaluation of localized prostatic cancer treated with radical prostatectomy. J Urol 139:766, 1988

83. Stamey TA, Yang N, Hay AR, et al: Prostate-specific antigen as a serum marker for adenocarcinoma of the prostate. N Engl J Med 317:909, 1987

84. Hudson MA, Bahnson RB, Catalona WJ: Clinical use of prostate specific antigen in patients with prostate cancer. J Urol 142:1011, 1989

85. Kuchier H: Uber Prostatavergrosserungen. Deutsch Klin 18:458, 1866

86. Walsh PC, Donker PJ: Impotence following radical prostatectomy: insight into etiology and prevention. J Urol 128:492, 1982

87. Eggleston JC, Walsh PC: Radical prostatectomy with preservation of sexual function: pathological findings in the first 100 cases. J Urol 134:1146, 1985

88. Paulson DF, Lin GH, Hinshaw W, et al: The uro-oncology research group: Radical surgery versus radiotherapy for adenocarcinoma of the prostate. J Urol 128:502, 1982

89. Huggins C, Hodges CV: Studies on prostatic cancer: I. The effect of castration, of estrogen and of androgen injection on serum phosphatases in metastatic carcinoma of the prostate. Cancer Res 1:293, 1941

90. Catalona, WJ: Prostate Cancer. Grune & Stratton, Orlando, FL, 1984, p.172

Index

Page numbers followed by f denote figures; those followed by t denote tables.